Healthcare Analytics and Advanced Computational Intelligence

This book aims to apply state-of-the-art advanced computational intelligence frameworks in healthcare. It presents recent and real-life applications of computationally intelligent healthcare. It also discusses problems and solutions to remote healthcare and emergency healthcare services. *Healthcare Analytics and Advanced Computational Intelligence* highlights modern ambient intelligence-enabled healthcare models along with advanced topics like quantum computing in healthcare and cryptomedical systems.

Healthcare Analytics and Advanced Computational Intelligence examines designing the latest medical systems and models that will allow the societal acceptance of ambiance computing in healthcare, medical imaging, health analytics, machine intelligence, sensory computing, medical data analytics, disease detection, telemedicine, and their applications. It includes diverse case studies dealing with various clinical-based applications. These intelligent models are primarily structured to deal with complex real-world issues in clinical data analytics by means of state-of-the-art techniques with general implementation, domain-specific solutions, or hybrid methods which integrate computational intelligence with conventional statistical methods.

The book is written for researchers and academicians in diverse areas. Engineers from technical disciplines such as computer engineering are likely to purchase the book. Various sub-streams such as machine learning, big data analytics, healthcare analytics, and computational intelligence will find the book significant for their curriculum.

Artificial Intelligence for Sustainable Engineering and Management

Sachi Nandan Mohanty, College of Eng., Pune
Deepak Gupta, Maharaja Agrasen Institute of Technology, Delhi

Artificial intelligence is shaping the future of humanity across nearly every industry. It is already the main driver of emerging technologies like big data, robotics and IoT, and it will continue to act as a technological innovator for the foreseeable future. Artificial intelligence is the simulation of human intelligence processes by machines, especially computer systems. Specific applications of AI include expert systems, natural language processing, speech recognition, and machine vision. The future of business intelligence combined with AI will see the analysis of huge quantities of contextual data in real time. So, the tool will quickly capture customer needs and priorities and do what is needed.

Green Metaverse for Greener Economies
Edited by Sukanta Kumar Baral, Richa Goel, Tilottama Singh, and Rakesh Kumar

Healthcare Analytics and Advanced Computational Intelligence
Edited by Sushruta Mishra, Meshal Alharbi, Hrudaya Kumar Tripathy, Biswajit Sahoo, and Ahmed Alkhayyat

https://www.routledge.com/AI-for-Sustainable-Engineering-and-Management-series/book-series/AISEM

Healthcare Analytics and Advanced Computational Intelligence

Edited by
Sushruta Mishra, Meshal Alharbi,
Hrudaya Kumar Tripathy, Biswajit Sahoo,
and Ahmed Alkhayyat

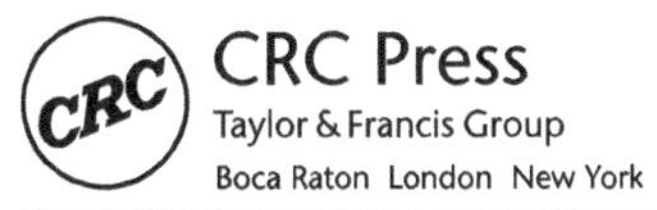

CRC Press is an imprint of the
Taylor & Francis Group, an informa business

Cover image: © Shutterstock Images

First edition published 2025
by CRC Press
2385 NW Executive Center Drive, Suite 320, Boca Raton FL 33431

and by CRC Press
4 Park Square, Milton Park, Abingdon, Oxon, OX14 4RN

CRC Press is an imprint of Taylor & Francis Group, LLC

Library of Congress Cataloging-in-Publication Data
Names: Mishra, Sushruta, editor.
Title: Healthcare analytics and advanced computational intelligence / edited by Sushruta Mishra [and four others].
Description: First edition. | Boca Raton : CRC Press, 2024. | Series: Artificial intelligence for sustainable engineering and management | Includes bibliographical references and index. |
Identifiers: LCCN 2023058992 (print) | LCCN 2023058993 (ebook) |
ISBN 9781032601908 (hbk) | ISBN 9781032624884 (pbk) | ISBN 9781032624891 (ebk)
Subjects: LCSH: Medical informatics. | Computational intelligence. |
Artificial intelligence--Medical applications.
Classification: LCC R858 .H368 2024 (print) | LCC R858 (ebook) | DDC 610.285--dc23/eng/20240319
LC record available at https://lccn.loc.gov/2023058992
LC ebook record available at https://lccn.loc.gov/2023058993

ISBN: 978-1-032-60190-8 (hbk)
ISBN: 978-1-032-62488-4 (pbk)
ISBN: 978-1-032-62489-1 (ebk)

DOI: 10.1201/9781032624891

Typeset in Times
by KnowledgeWorks Global Ltd

Contents

Preface

Computational Intelligence spans over diverse intelligence-based approaches, which primarily involve computationally intelligent models along with hybrid predictive models to address real-world problems which normal traditional methods fail to achieve due to problem complexities, presence of uncertainties, and also the stochastic domain of processes. Recently, computational intelligent approaches have displayed promising results in healthcare sector thereby enhancing the significance of healthcare research. The aim of this edited book is to present recent works where computational intelligence algorithms are specifically designed to solve complex real-world problems in healthcare data analytics.

The first chapter provides a generic viewpoint on human and system interaction in modern healthcare. The second chapter dives into the detailed aspects of cognitive computing-based healthcare using ambient intelligence. Third chapter discusses the role of machine learning models in remote medicine. Fourth chapter deals with the application of the Internet of Medical Things inter-connected clinical services. An analytical study is presented in the fifth chapter in context to the usage of cryptographic techniques in sustainable healthcare. Sixth chapter attempts to integrate quantum computing concept in medical domain utilizing machine learning models. Seventh chapter highlights the role of sign language recognition and recommendation using predictive analytics. Eighth chapter addresses the emergency healthcare scenario using Intelligent Ambulance Services Management. Ninth chapter gives an insight on precision drug delivery using advanced computational models. Tenth chapter highlights the significance of modern intelligent techniques in brain tumor assessment. Eleventh chapter presents an analysis on cardiac disease risks pattern recognition using advanced predictive analytics. Twelfth chapter summarizes the design and deployment of medical chatbots that can be used to simulate user interactions. The final chapter studies the relevance of vehicular networks in smart healthcare.

About the Editors

Sushruta Mishra is working as an Assistant Professor in the School of Computer Engineering, KIIT University, Bhubaneswar, Odisha, India. He pursued his MTech from IIIT, Bhubaneswar, Odisha, India, and has completed his PhD in Computer Science from KIIT University, India. Dr Mishra has more than 11 years of teaching experience in various educational institutions. He has handled many subjects such as Computer Networks, Data Mining, the Internet of Things, Software Engineering, and Machine Learning, among others, during his academic experience. He has a research experience of around ten years, and his research interest includes Image Processing, Machine Learning, the Internet of Things, and Cognitive Computing. He has published more than 150 research articles in reputed indexed international journals, edited books, and conferences.

Meshal Alharbi is an Assistant Professor of Artificial Intelligence in the Department of Computer Science at Prince Sattam Bin Abdulaziz University in the Kingdom of Saudi Arabia. He received PhD degree in Computer Science from Durham University, UK, in 2020, and an MSc degree in Computer Science from Wayne State University, USA, in 2014. He has ten years of experience in teaching/research/industry. His research interests lie in Artificial Intelligence Applications and Algorithms, Agent-Based Modelling and Simulation Applications, Disaster/Emergency Management and Resilience, Optimization Applications, and Machine Learning.

Hrudaya Kumar Tripathy is working as an Associate Professor in the School of Computer Engineering, KIIT University, Bhubaneswar, Odisha, India. Dr Tripathy is from Odisha and is an Indian by birth. He has received his PhD degree in Computer Science from Berhampur University, Berhampur, Odisha, India, in Computer Science in 2010. He completed his post-doctoral research at Utara Universiti, Malaysia, in 2016. He has an academic experience of around 20 years. He has handled various subjects like Software Engineering, Machine Learning, Business Intelligence, etc. His research interests include Neural Networks, Pattern Recognition, Software Engineering, Machine Learning, and Big Data. He has published several research papers in various journals and conferences. He has sound knowledge in the domain of autism spectrum disorder (ASD) analysis. He was involved in aggregating data records from many regional autistic centers. He has participated in few seminars and talks in autistic centers and NGOs related to the risks and disorders associated with autism. He has published three research papers in Scopus indexed publications. He also successfully led a project on behavioral analysis of autistic students at KIIT University.

Biswajit Sahoo is Director General and Professor at the School of Computer Engineering, Kalinga Institute of Industrial Technology, Deemed to be University, Bhubaneswar, Odisha, India. Graduated from NIT, Durgapur, West Bengal, with a Bachelor of Engineering in Electronics & Communication Engineering, he earned a Master of Engineering in Computer Science & Engineering from IIEST Sibpur, West Bengal. Having successfully completed his doctorate, Dr Sahoo holds PhD degree from the Utkal University, Bhubaneswar, Odisha. With a three-year of industrial experience as a Chip Level Maintenance Engineer at Bells Control, Calcutta, he has expert knowledge of telecom equipment and computers. Moreover, Dr Sahoo has 25 years of experience in teaching both UG and PG courses at different colleges and universities in Odisha. The research work of Dr Sahoo has been published in more than 30 national and international journals and conferences in repute. His research interests include Algorithms, Bioinformatics, and Parallel Computing.

Ahmed Alkhayyat received BSc degree in Electrical Engineering from Al Kufa University, Najaf, Iraq, in 2007, MSc degree from the Dehradun Institute of Technology, Dehradun, India, in 2010, and the PhD degree from Çankaya University, Ankara, Turkey, in 2015. He is currently the Dean of International Relationship and the Manager for the world ranking with The Islamic University, Najaf. His research interests include the IoT in Healthcare Systems, Software-Defined Networking (SDN), Network Coding, Cognitive Radio, Efficient-Energy Routing Algorithms and Efficient-Energy Media Access Control (MAC) Protocol in Cooperative Wireless Networks, Wireless Body Area Networks, and Cross-Layer Designing for Self-Organized Networks. He contributed to organizing several IEEE conferences, workshops, and special sessions. To serve the community, he acted as a reviewer for several journals and conferences.

Contributors

Angelia Melani Adrian
Department of Informatics Engineering
De La Salle Catholic University
Kota Manado, Indonesia

Oindrila Ajha
School of Computer Engineering
Kalinga Institute of Industrial Technology
Bhubaneswar, Odisha, India

Anshuman Behera
School of Computer Engineering
Kalinga Institute of Industrial Technology
Bhubaneswar, Odisha, India

Aradhana Behura
Department of Computer Science
National Institute of Technology
Rourkela, Odisha, India

Aadarsh Choudhary
Xformics Canada Inc,
Richmond Hill, ON, Canada

Souryadipta Das
School of Computer Engineering
Kalinga Institute of Industrial Technology
Bhubaneswar, Odisha, India

Tarek Gaber
School of Science, Engineering, and Environment
University of Salford
Manchester, UK

Sayan Garai
School of Computer Engineering
Kalinga Institute of Industrial Technology
Bhubaneswar, Odisha, India

Debolina Ghosh
Department of Computer Science and Engineering
Manipal University
Jaipur, Rajasthan, India

Uday Bhanu Ghosh
Itron Inc.
Bangalore, Karnataka, India

Shayan Irfan
School of Computer Engineering
Kalinga Institute of Industrial Technology
Bhubaneswar, Odisha, India

Kratika Kansal
School of Computer Engineering
Kalinga Institute of Industrial Technology
Bhubaneswar, Odisha, India

Prachi Kashyap
School of Computer Engineering
Kalinga Institute of Industrial Technology
Bhubaneswar, Odisha, India

Kashish Kaur
School of Computer Engineering
Kalinga Institute of Industrial Technology
Bhubaneswar, Odisha, India

Abhishek Kesharwani
R&D Engineer Samsung Research Institute
Noida, India

Rukaiya Khan
Department of Computer Science
C.V. Raman Global University
Bhubaneswar, Odisha, India

Tanmay Khatri
University of Melbourne
Melbourne, Australia

Priyanka Malakar
Narula Institute of Technology
Kolkata, West Bengal, India

Anjana Mishra
Department of Computer Science
C.V. Raman Global University
Bhubaneswar, Odisha, India

Pratyush Mishra
School of Computer Engineering
Kalinga Institute of Industrial Technology
Bhubaneswar, Odisha, India

Aryan Mohanty
Department of Computer Engineering
Zs Associates
Bangalore, Karnataka, India

Saswat Mohanty
School of Computer Engineering
Kalinga Institute of Industrial Technology
Bhubaneswar, Odisha, India

Francis Palma
Faculty of Computer Science
University of New Brunswick
Fredericton, NB, Canada

Ananya Pareek
School of Computer Engineering
Kalinga Institute of Industrial Technology
Bhubaneswar, Odisha, India

Raseswari Sarangi
School of Computer Engineering
Kalinga Institute of Industrial Technology
Bhubaneswar, Odisha, India

Samikshya Sarangi
School of Computer Engineering
Kalinga Institute of Industrial Technology
Bhubaneswar, Odisha, India

Khaled Shaalan
Faculty of Engineering & IT
The British University
Dubai, UAE

Jagannath Singh
School of Computer Engineering
Kalinga Institute of Industrial Technology
Bhubaneswar, Odisha, India

Jay Prakash Singh
Department of Computer Science and Engineering
Manipal University
Jaipur, Rajasthan, India

Rishika Singh
School of Computer Engineering
Kalinga Institute of Industrial Technology
Bhubaneswar, Odisha, India

Saakshi Smriti
School of Computer Engineering
Kalinga Institute of Industrial Technology
Bhubaneswar, Odisha, India

Shubham Suman
Department of Information Technology
University of Luxembourg
Luxembourg

Tridiv Swain
PricewaterhouseCoopers LLP,
Kolkata, West Bengal, India

Tapaswini Tripathy
Department of Computer Science
C.V. Raman Global University
Bhubaneswar, Odisha, India

Aditi Yadav
School of Computer Engineering
Kalinga Institute of Industrial Technology
Bhubaneswar, Odisha, India

1 Human-Computer Interaction and Healthcare

A Deep Insight

Aryan Mohanty

1.1 INTRODUCTION

Our everyday lives have become more intertwined with computer technology. They have transformed and will continue to transform the way we conduct business. Every aspect of our daily lives, from work and school to our communities and the greater society we are a part of, is affected by this. When it comes to computers, interfacing has always been an issue. When it comes to interacting with technology, humans have gone a long way. In the previous several decades, new technologies and systems have been produced on a daily basis, and research in this sector has progressed at a fast rate. There has been a steady rise in the quality and breadth of research relating to human-computer interaction (HCI) during the last several decades. There have been several studies instead of developing conventional interfaces that have concentrated on subjects such as multi-modality vs. uni-modality, intelligent adaptive interfaces against command/action based interfaces, and last but not least, active vs. passive interfaces instead.

The delivery, administration, and accessibility of medical services have all changed as a result of technology's incorporation into the medical sector [1]. Technologies have the ability to completely transform healthcare systems, from electronic health records and telemedicine to wearable technologies and applications for mobile health. The efficacy of these advances in technology, however, strongly depends on the discipline of HCI, which aims to make sure that communication between medical staff, patients, and computer systems is smooth, effective, and user-centered. Exploring human behavior, cognition, and patterns of interaction using technology is a key component of the interdisciplinary area of HCI. Practitioners and researchers attempt to improve the usability, effectiveness, and overall user experience of technology in a variety of fields, particularly healthcare, by implementing HCI concepts, techniques, and user-focused design methods. In the context of medical care, HCI is crucial in solving the particular difficulties and demands of this intricate and important field [2].

HCI has become a vital field at the nexus of technology and healthcare, offering ground-breaking approaches to improve patient care, healthcare delivery, and user experience in general. In order to develop efficient and patient-centered healthcare systems,

DOI: 10.1201/9781032624891-1

HCI covers a multidisciplinary approach that combines ideas from psychology, design, computer science, and medicine. The goal of this research study is to offer a thorough understanding of the essential themes, issues, and developments in the nexus of HCI and healthcare. In order to provide user-friendly interfaces, streamlined processes, and better results, HCI in healthcare focuses on understanding the intricate interactions between healthcare personnel, patients, and computer systems. HCI facilitates the creation of technologies that are in line with the particular requirements and tastes of many stakeholders in the healthcare ecosystem by applying user-centered design concepts.

This chapter aims to provide a deep insight into the intersection of HCI and healthcare, exploring the importance and advancements in this domain. By delving into the research and practical applications of HCI in healthcare, we can gain a comprehensive understanding of how HCI principles are transforming the healthcare landscape and improving patient care particularly in clinical workflow optimization.

1.2 DEFINITION AND TERMINOLOGY

HCI focuses on the study of interactive computer systems for human use and the fundamental phenomena underlying them. To design user-friendly interfaces and seamless experiences, it focuses on comprehending how users interact with computer systems. Designing user-friendly, effective, and efficient interfaces requires taking into account various aspects of user demands, objectives, and cognitive processes. Figure 1.1 shows the key elements of an HCI.

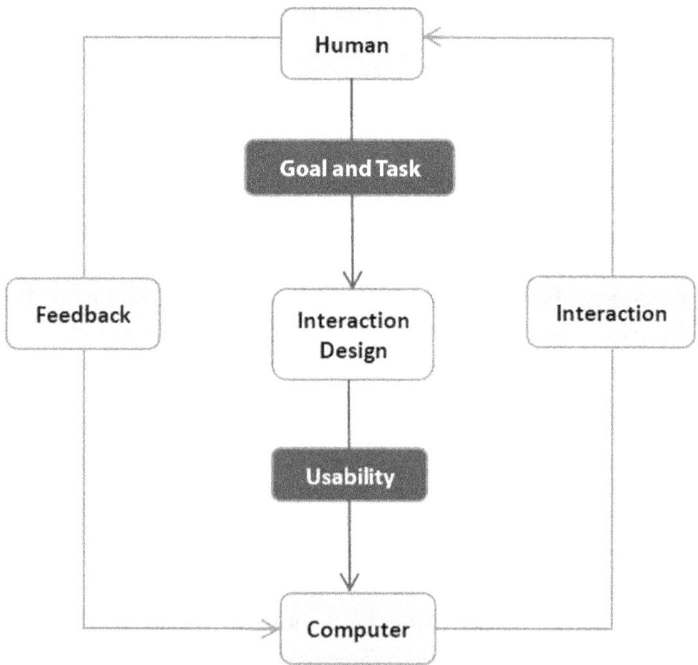

FIGURE 1.1 Key elements of human-computer interaction (HCI).

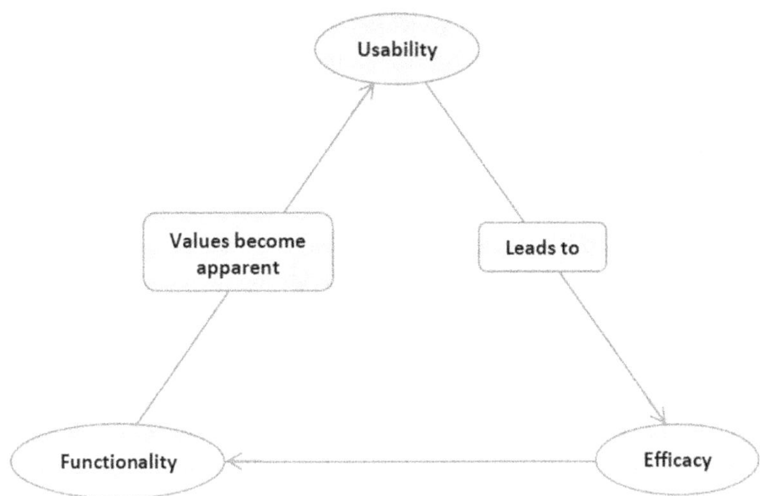

FIGURE 1.2 Relationship between functionality, usability, and efficacy.

When computers or, more generally, machines, began to be developed, the notion of "human-computer interaction," additionally known as "man-machine interaction" or "interfacing," naturally came to light. This is because most modern technology is meaningless unless humans properly use it. The two most essential criteria in HCI design—functionality and usability—are presented in this straightforward argument [3]. A system's functionality is characterized by the activities or services that are offered to users. Although a feature's worth is only apparent when the user is able to put it to good use. Usability refers to the extent to which a system with a specific feature can be used constructively and adequately to attain specified aims for specific individuals. When the system's functionality and usability are correctly balanced, the system's true efficacy is achieved [4], which is shown in Figure 1.2.

1.3 HISTORY OF HCI

Electronic Numerical Integrator and Calculator (ENIAC), the first general-purpose electronic computer created in 1946, paved the way for HCI. At 10 feet tall and 1000 square feet in area, it drew in all the kinetic energy of a small town. When graphical user interface (GUI) and the Internet came into existence, the significance of HCI was made more explicit. Further HCI research has been an enormous success, affecting computers dramatically [5].

Many of the interface toolkits and builders that are used in current software were first developed in academic institutions, which is another excellent example. Hypertext technology in browsers makes it possible to go worldwide with a single mouse click, a feat made possible through HCI research. More than anything else, user interface (UI) advances have spurred this exponential growth. Universities and a few corporate research labs are also working to develop new UIs for computers in the near future.

The beginnings of HCI may be found in the early days of computing when academics first started looking at how to make computers more user-friendly and logical.

a. ***Early Developments (1940–1960):*** Early computer systems were big and mainly utilized by scientists and mathematicians in the 1940s [6]. These systems primarily interacted with users using punch cards and switches, which needed particular training. Researchers started delving into the idea of GUIs in the 1950s. NLS (oN-Line System), a system created by Douglas Engelbart in the 1960s, offered technologies including Windows, hypertext, and the mouse.
b. ***The Rise of the GUI (1970–1980):*** During this time, the Xerox Palo Alto Research Centre (PARC) was crucial to the advancement of HCI [7]. The Alto computer, which had a UI that was graphical and a mouse, was created by researchers at PARC, including Alan Kay. The first commercial computer with a GUI, the Xerox Star, was released by Xerox in the late 1970s. Although the Star did not achieve success in the marketplace, it had an impact on later GUI designs.
c. ***WIMP Paradigm (1980–1990):*** During this time, the WIMP paradigm (Windows, Icons, Menus, Pointer system) gained popularity. The Microsoft Windows and Apple Macintosh operating systems made it more widely used. In 1984, Apple unveiled the Macintosh, a computer with a mouse-friendly GUI. It introduced ideas such as the desktop metaphor and the usage of icons to represent files [8]. The 1990 introduction of Microsoft Windows 3.0 contributed to the growing popularity of GUIs for IBM-compatible PCs.
d. ***Web and Mobile Interfaces (1990–2000):*** The World Wide Web's introduction in the early 1990s presented new potential and problems for HCI. Web-based UIs needed to be made to work with a variety of gadgets used by users. In the late 2000s, as mobile devices proliferated, HCI grew to encompass touch-based interactions, tiny displays, and many other factors [9]. Mobile HCI has been greatly influenced by companies like Apple with the iPhone and Google with Android.
e. ***Ubiquitous Computing and Beyond (2000–Present):*** The 21st century saw the rise of computing that is everywhere, in which technology is smoothly incorporated into daily life. As a result, creating interfaces for various devices and situations presented additional hurdles. Innovative interaction methods including voice command, augmented reality, virtual reality, and wearable technology have all been studied in HCI research. Usability testing and user-centered design are now fundamental components of the HCI process, ensuring that technology is created with users' requirements and preferences in mind.

As technology advances and new paradigms for HCI develop, the history of HCI is a never-ending journey. The goal of researchers and designers alike is to develop UIs that are simple to use, inclusive of all demographics, and easily accessible.

1.4 GOALS OF HCI

Increasing the usability and responsiveness of computers to user needs is one of the fundamental objectives of HCI. HCI is concerned with the following topics [10, 11].

- ***Usability:*** A system's usability is determined by how simple it is for users to understand, operate, and remember it. A useful system is one that users can remember how to operate even after a significant amount of time has passed.
- ***Effectiveness:*** A system's effectiveness is determined by how successfully it accomplishes its objectives. An efficient system aids users in completing activities swiftly and effortlessly.
- ***Safety:*** The likelihood that a system may hurt users is measured in terms of safety. A safe system is one that is intended to eliminate or significantly reduce user mistakes and harm.
- ***User-Centered Design:*** HCI encourages a user-centered design philosophy that entails comprehending users' needs, objectives, and preferences. HCI seeks to build systems that satisfy the needs of users and fit with their mental models by incorporating users in all stages of the design process.
- ***Efficiency and Productivity:*** HCI aims to increase users' productivity and efficiency by creating interfaces that simplify activities, lighten cognitive burdens, and assist users in successfully completing their objectives. This entails taking into account elements like information organization, navigation, and interaction methods.
- ***Safety and Reliability:*** HCI attempts to create systems that are error-free and safe to use. To guarantee that users can engage with technologies securely and dependably, it entails taking into account elements like mistake prevention and error recovery systems and giving users direct input.
- *Flexibility and Adaptability:* HCI researches how to design interfaces that can change to accommodate various people, environments, and devices. HCI aims to create adaptable systems that can take into account user preferences, varied interaction styles, and various settings.
- ***Ethical Considerations:*** HCI covers ethical issues relating to the development and application of technology. It entails taking into account the privacy, security, and ethical ramifications of gathering and using user data in addition to dealing with concerns about bias, openness, and fairness in computational systems.

It's an ongoing purpose of HCI to develop systems that bridge the gap between users' mental models of what they want to accomplish and computers' understanding of their work.

1.5 IMPORTANCE OF HCI

Every day, we utilize a wide range of technology, including our cell phones, TV remotes, air conditioner remotes, keyboards, and other items like ATMs, the Internet, or mobile apps [12]. As a general rule, we take our time to grasp the design, and we don't spend our time distinguishing between good and terrible design. Interaction is the term used to describe the relationship that exists between a user and a device or software. When it comes to producing interactive goods, interaction design focuses on helping people in both their personal and professional lives. Every company wants to get in on the action design industry.

Users are drawn to software by its UI, which is one of its most essential features. An interface is a piece of software that allows users to interact with a computer system [13]. Interaction and interface are both parts of HCI. HCI presents the idea of improving the user experience (UX) of computers and software. In order to achieve a particular purpose, a device's services must be designed in such a way that the user, device, and the benefits the device provides have a positive connection. HCI is a need in aviation because we need to be able to effectively communicate the functioning of aircraft software and hardware to pilots. When designing ATMs, train tickets, hot drinks, banking software, management software, airplanes, and cars, HCI is an essential factor. Not only is it critical for your product's end customers, but it's also a significant priority for the software development industry. Computer-based systems should be improved in terms of safety and usefulness as well as effectiveness, efficiency, usability, and attractiveness [14].

No one will want to use a software product that is frustrating to use, has poor functionality, or has a terrible UI, and sales will suffer as a consequence. Organizations may miss essential features or have an unattractive UI because non-technical individuals use computers.

1.6 IMPORTANCE OF HCI IN HEALTHCARE

The field of medicine and health relies on precise and rigorous human-computer interface (HCI) design, especially when it comes to medical monitoring equipment. These devices require accurate expression, simple operation, and timely responsiveness due to their monitoring and reference functions. Therefore, the design of Human Machine Interface (HMI) in medical monitoring equipment interfaces holds significant importance. HCI plays a vital role in ensuring effective interaction between humans and these devices, improving usability and overall user experience [15].

HCI is of utmost importance in the healthcare sector, greatly influencing the development and use of healthcare technology. The user experience is at the forefront of healthcare technology development thanks to HCI, which places a strong emphasis on comprehending human behavior, cognitive processes, and interaction patterns with technology. Healthcare technology can be improved to address the particular requirements, preferences, and difficulties of healthcare professionals, patients, and other stakeholders by incorporating HCI principles, methodologies, and user-centered design approaches.

There are several medical gadget models from various national brands accessible in both marketplaces and hospitals. These devices have various operational strategies despite providing comparable services. Since the learning curve is steep as a result, mistake rates are greater. Due to the direct connection between high-end medical devices and user safety, careful HCI design must be given top priority during their development. To improve usability, this entails carefully evaluating user behavior and implementing suitable materials, colors, and touch elements. The objective is to lessen medical staff's tolerance for mistakes and minimize errors [16].

Usability is a crucial component of HCI in the medical field [17]. Healthcare workers work in hectic, high-stress settings where accuracy and efficiency are crucial. Designing intuitive and user-friendly interfaces that simplify operations, lighten cognitive load, and reduce mistakes is made possible by HCI principles. Utilizable healthcare technology guarantees that healthcare workers can complete their responsibilities quickly, access patient data, and make wise judgments, thereby improving patient outcomes and care. Along with improving usability, HCI encourages patient ownership and involvement. HCI promotes active involvement, collaborative decision-making, and self-management of health issues by incorporating patients in their own healthcare journey. The development of platforms that enable patients to access their medical information, monitor their advancement, and participate in individualized treatment plans is made possible by user-centered design concepts. Additionally, HCI enables the development of technologies that support telemedicine, virtual consultations, and remote surveillance, hence enhancing autonomy for patients and increasing access to medical care [18].

A further key factor is how HCI affects clinical decision support. Clinical decision-support platforms may provide healthcare practitioners with fast, accurate, and context-aware information to enhance patient safety, diagnosis, and treatment planning by implementing HCI principles. Healthcare practitioners may easily incorporate decision support technologies into their clinical processes because of designed effectively interfaces, which help them make choices based on evidence and minimize diagnostic mistakes [19].

1.6.1 HCI for Optimized Clinical Workflows

Today, the management of people's health and welfare is greatly influenced by digital technology, both in terms of how healthcare is delivered and how individuals perceive it. Digital technology may address a wide range of health and wellness concerns, and both the number of users and their individual differences are substantial [20]. Numerous researches in the field of HCI have discussed user requirements for specific contexts, the usability, user experience, and safety of certain health technology, as well as cutting-edge interactive digital treatments in healthcare. To date, HCI has had a very small but discernible influence on medical procedures, the experiences of medical personnel, and patient outcomes.

Healthcare systems and the methods in which individuals interact with their health and well-being are undergoing rapid transformation on a global scale. These changes are happening on a number of levels. Individually, innovative engagement tools are creating fresh opportunities for contact between healthcare providers and patients on the perceptual, cognitive, and emotional levels.

At this time, fresh large-scale research is made possible by the dramatically rising volume of heterogeneous biological data, necessitating specialized and customized computational solutions. The most recent machine learning (ML) approaches have recently demonstrated exceptional performance and made a significant contribution to clinical research, eventually seeking to advance precision medicine and enhance healthcare processes. These desirable advantages, from diagnosis to therapy, are, nevertheless, accompanied by fresh, pressing problems. In fact, this information excess may be too much for physicians' analytical skills to handle while making everyday decisions. The requirement to properly integrate imperfectly organized, uncertain, and sometimes contradicting information from numerous sources always complicates decision-making for healthcare practitioners.

Healthcare is a crucial industry with high-risk, time-sensitive jobs that are characterized by unusual quirks such as inherent intra-subject and inter-subject variability, institutional harmonization, and legal concerns [21]. The idea that experts cannot fail is crucial in these highly specialized and dynamic work situations, especially in the clinical setting when experts with varied educational backgrounds and degrees of experience collaborate. For instance, providing safe, timely, and effective treatments in critical and emergency care demands a well-structured collaborative plan [22]. The ultimate objective in real-world settings is to employ user-centered Clinical Decision Support Systems (CDSSs) and sophisticated artificial intelligence (AI) approaches to bridge the gap between healthcare information processes and AI technologies [23]. Therefore, by specifically taking into consideration efficient and safe interaction paradigms, the correct combination of AI software and human intelligence skills will enable the delivery of care that is more effective than what these two "intelligence types" can achieve independently.

The translation into clinical situations may be compromised by the sophisticated computational tools' complexity and lack of usability. Additionally, because they may make the use of current AI-based technologies in clinical practice more difficult, interpretability and explainability problems must be taken into account [24]. The design of software geared toward medical decision-making must take into account HCI [25, 26]. To successfully communicate, medical practitioners frequently rely on digital technologies like CDSSs, Electronic Health Records (EHRs), and imaging systems. These solutions solve the issues with insufficient data gathering during in-person clinic visits [27] by enabling the integration and analysis of data from numerous sources, including EHRs, wearable technology, and virtual consultations. Additionally, patient participation in shared decision-making procedures supports a patient-centered approach to healthcare [28].

However, adopting poorly designed UIs in these systems may frustrate doctors who have trouble using electronic technologies. Usability testing is essential to resolving this problem in order to verify interface designs with an emphasis on a "physician-centered" approach. Data management and content presentation are effortlessly incorporated into CDSSs when AI and Cognitive Informatics (CI) are used [29]. It's notable that CI finds use in a variety of contexts, but it notably helps telemedicine teams communicate while analyzing data and making decisions.

A seamless integration of AI with HCI is necessary to guarantee accurate and secure conclusions. In order to support doctors in their everyday work effectively, CDSSs prioritize interactive solutions that make use of their specialized knowledge and evidence-based reasoning. Efforts are being undertaken to improve the different elements stated in this study, with the goal of optimizing clinical workflows.

1.7 VISIONS FOR THE FUTURE

Digital health has been portrayed as having an ideal future in which advancements would always be favorable. Healthcare and medicine are reportedly being transformed by "big data [30]." This vision is predicated on the idea that people will freely contribute their data, which includes genetic details, medical issues, and other biomarkers. Sharing this information is being done for the larger good as well as for personal gain. The vision also predicts that the understanding of health and care would advance far faster by fusing this personal data with socioeconomic, environmental, and other pertinent data. The delivery of healthcare is anticipated to undergo a fundamental change as a result of the integration of various data sources, while prices are kept in line with benefits. The vision places a strong emphasis on the use of creative, engaging, and understandable AI algorithms in order to accomplish this. In order to analyze the combined data, facilitate decision-making, and eventually enable the transformation of care delivery, these cutting-edge algorithms will play a critical role.

Future HCI experts (including academics) will have a crucial role in making sure that user experience, usability, and safety concerns are addressed and that HCI is acknowledged as a crucial process that must be included from the start of any digital health development process.

For instance, HCI will be crucial in making sure that future AI systems are "explainable" [31].

It is becoming more and clearer that HCI techniques must be expanded in order to develop sophisticated adaptive systems. Although there is a sizable body of literature on the design of work systems and the difficulties involved, little focus has been placed on the intricate details of designing interfaces, task structures, and other elements of digital technologies that will be included in these complex adaptive systems. When several users are involved in diverse roles and there is system interoperability, this is very important. Further study and investigation into developing efficient interfaces and structures that can seamlessly integrate with these complex adaptive systems are urgently needed to close this gap, ensuring effective user collaboration and smooth communication with other interconnected systems [32].

Learning to collaborate with technology developers and healthcare professionals is a crucial first step in HCI. Another is to focus on concerns that span the full pathway from user demands to broad deployment, taking into account both more regional difficulties that fall within the "comfort zone" of HCI as well as therapeutic results, scalability, and sustainability [33–35]. Experts analyze the life cycles of development from HCI and health systems research to highlight similarities and differences, but what is required is a development method that combines the best of both worlds [36, 37].

In conclusion, the study of HCI is crucial to realizing the promise of health technology in the future. Due to the fundamentally multidisciplinary character of this project, HCI experts must work with other important stakeholders, such as technologists, healthcare workers, patients, and several other relevant parties. The requirements and aspirations of the whole healthcare ecosystem are met by HCI initiatives thanks to this collaborative approach. Furthermore, it is critical to take into account additional processes that are sometimes disregarded in HCI research but are necessary for attaining significant advancements in healthcare. To accept and widely disseminate HCI-driven advances in healthcare, these processes involve recognizing technical potential, early adopters, and thorough planning. For HCI innovations to really enhance patient care and overall healthcare outcomes, these stages must be addressed.

Therefore, research efforts should encompass broader aspects such as interdisciplinary collaboration, stakeholder engagement, technology exploration, and strategic planning for the effective adoption and dissemination of HCI-driven solutions in the healthcare domain. This will maximize the beneficial effects of HCI in healthcare. Researchers in the field of HCI can significantly progress healthcare technology and eventually improve the well-being of patients and healthcare personnel by adopting this holistic approach.

1.8 CONCLUSION

Designing systems that include HCI is an essential aspect of the process. The quality of a system is directly related to how its users perceive and interact with it. There has been a huge focus on improving the design of HCI. Researchers are concentrating their efforts to create forms of interaction that are more intuitive and natural-feeling while still being multimodal, intelligent, and flexible. Additionally, we also summarized the latest advances in passive HCI in healthcare and discussed their potential applications in areas of HCI intending to inform the HCI community about the benefits and vision of passive HCI systems in healthcare.

The complexity of healthcare systems makes it necessary to create fresh approaches for creating and implementing interactive health technologies that successfully address the many demands and values of users. With an emphasis on comprehending the impact and effectiveness of HCI-driven robots functioning in closed-loop interaction with humans, future research efforts should prioritize increasing the synergy between healthcare and HCI domains. Researchers may develop novel strategies that optimize the design and implementation of interactive health technologies, ensuring that they are in line with the complex healthcare environment and satisfy the many user requirements by merging experiences from both fields. To assess their efficacy and improve their design, HCI-driven robots must be thoroughly investigated in closed-loop interactions. This will improve the experiences and results of all involved parties in healthcare.

REFERENCES

1. Singh, A., Newhouse, N., Gibbs, J., Blandford, A. E., Chen, Y., Briggs, P., & Bardram, J. E. (2017, May). HCI and Health: Learning from Interdisciplinary Interactions. In Proceedings of the 2017 CHI Conference Extended Abstracts on Human Factors in Computing Systems (pp. 1322–1325). Denver, CO.
2. Stephanidis, C., Salvendy, G., Antona, M., Chen, J. Y., Dong, J., Duffy, V. G., & Zhou, J. (2019). Seven HCI grand challenges. International Journal of Human–Computer Interaction, 35(14), 1229–1269.
3. Karray, F., Alemzadeh, M., Abou Saleh, J., & Arab, M. N. (2008). Human-computer interaction: Overview on state of the art. International Journal on Smart Sensing and Intelligent Systems, 1(1), 137.
4. Hewett, T. T., Baecker, R., Card, S., Carey, T., Gasen, J., Mantei, M., & Verplank, W. (1992). *ACM SIGCHI Curricula for Human-Computer Interaction.* ACM, New York, NY.

5. Sahoo, P. K., Mishra, S., Panigrahi, R., Bhoi, A. K., & Barsocchi, P. (2022). An improvised deep-learning-based Mask R-CNN model for laryngeal cancer detection using CT images. Sensors, 22(22), 8834.
6. Ceruzzi, P. E. (2003). *A History of Modern Computing*. MIT Press, Cambridge, MA.
7. Reinschluessel, A. V., & Zagermann, J. (2023). Exploring hybrid user interfaces for surgery planning. IEEE International Symposium on Mixed and Augmented Reality Adjunct (ISMAR-Adjunct), 208–210.
8. Arcadi, G., Dutra, M., Ghosh, P., Lindner, M., Mambrini, Y., Pierre, M., & Queiroz, F. S. (2018). The waning of the WIMP? A review of models, searches, and constraints. The European Physical Journal C, 78, 1–57.
9. Lee, B., Isenberg, P., Riche, N. H., & Carpendale, S. (2012). Beyond mouse and keyboard: Expanding design considerations for information visualization interactions. IEEE Transactions on Visualization and Computer Graphics, 18(12), 2689–2698.
10. Gupta, S., Bagga, S., & Sharma, D. K. (2020). Hand Gesture Recognition for Human Computer Interaction and Its Applications in Virtual Reality. In Advanced Computational Intelligence Techniques for Virtual Reality in Healthcare (pp. 85–105). Springer, Cham.
11. Issa, T., & Isaias, P. (2022). Usability and Human–Computer Interaction (HCI). In Sustainable Design: HCI, Usability and Environmental Concerns (pp. 23–40). Springer, London.
12. Mohapatra, S. K., Mishra, S., Tripathy, H. K., & Alkhayyat, A. (2022). A sustainable data-driven energy consumption assessment model for building infrastructures in resource constraint environment. Sustainable Energy Technologies and Assessments, 53, 102697.
13. Rogers, Y., Sharp, H., & Preece, J. (2023). Interaction Design: beyond Human-Computer Interaction. John Wiley & Sons, Hoboken, NJ.
14. Blandford, A. (2019). HCI for health and wellbeing: Challenges and opportunities. International Journal of Human-Computer Studies, 131, 41–51.
15. Alrizq, M., Solangi, S. A., Alghamdi, A., Nizamani, M. A., Memon, M. A., & Hamdi, M. (2022). An architecture supporting intelligent mobile healthcare using human-computer interaction HCI principles. Computer Systems Science and Engineering, 40(2), 557–569.
16. Issa, T., & Isaias, P. (2015). Sustainable Design: HCI. Usability and Environmental Concerns (Human Computer Interaction). Springer, Berlin.
17. Bitkina, O. V., Kim, H. K., & Park, J. (2020). Usability and user experience of medical devices: An overview of the current state, analysis methodologies, and future challenges. International Journal of Industrial Ergonomics, 76, 102932.
18. Bharti, U., Bajaj, D., Batra, H., Lalit, S., Lalit, S., & Gangwani, A. (2020, June). Medbot: Conversational artificial intelligence powered chatbot for delivering tele-health after COVID-19. In 2020 5th International Conference on Communication and Electronics Systems (ICCES) (pp. 870–875). IEEE, Coimbatore, India.
19. Sutton, R. T., Pincock, D., Baumgart, D. C., Sadowski, D. C., Fedorak, R. N., & Kroeker, K. I. (2020). An overview of clinical decision support systems: Benefits, risks, and strategies for success. NPJ Digital Medicine, 3(1), 17.
20. Mishra, S., Thakkar, H. K., Singh, P., & Sharma, G. (2022). A decisive metaheuristic attribute selector enabled combined unsupervised-supervised model for chronic disease risk assessment. Computational Intelligence and Neuroscience, 2022, 8749353.
21. Dutta, P., & Mishra, S. (2022). A comprehensive review analysis of Alzheimer's disorder using machine learning approach. Augmented Intelligence in Healthcare: A Pragmatic and Integrated Analysis, 1, 63–76.
22. Sivani, T., & Mishra, S. (2022). Wearable Devices: Evolution and Usage in Remote Patient Monitoring System. In Connected e-Health (pp. 311–332). Springer, Cham.

23. Nemeth, C., Nunnally, M., O'Connor, M., Klock, P. A., & Cook, R. (2005). Getting to the point: Developing IT for the sharp end of healthcare. Journal of Biomedical Informatics, 38(1), 18–25.
24. Patel, V. L., Zhang, J., Yoskowitz, N. A., Green, R., & Sayan, O. R. (2008). Translational cognition for decision support in critical care environments: A review. Journal of Biomedical Informatics, 41(3), 413–431.
25. Franklin, A., Liu, Y., Li, Z., Nguyen, V., Johnson, T. R., Robinson, D., & Zhang, J. (2011). Opportunistic decision making and complexity in emergency care. Journal of Biomedical Informatics, 44(3), 469–476.
26. Miotto, R., Wang, F., Wang, S., Jiang, X., & Dudley, J. T. (2018). Deep learning for healthcare: Review, opportunities and challenges. Briefings in Bioinformatics, 19(6), 1236–1246.
27. Mez, J., Daneshvar, D. H., Kiernan, P. T., Abdolmohammadi, B., Alvarez, V. E., Huber, B. R., & McKee, A. C. (2017). Clinicopathological evaluation of chronic traumatic encephalopathy in players of American football. JAMA, 318(4), 360–370.
28. Chakraborty, S., Sahoo, K. S., Mishra, S., & Islam, S. M. (2022, April). AI Driven Cough Voice-Based COVID Detection Framework Using Spectrographic Imaging: An Improved Technology. In 2022 IEEE 7th International Conference for Convergence in Technology (I2CT) (pp. 1–7). IEEE, Mumbai, India.
29. Suman, S., Mishra, S., Sahoo, K. S., & Nayyar, A. (2022). Vision navigator: A smart and intelligent obstacle recognition model for visually impaired users. Mobile Information Systems, 2022, 9715891.
30. Tripathy, H. K., Mishra, S., Suman, S., Nayyar, A., & Sahoo, K. S. (2022). Smart COVID-shield: An IoT driven reliable and automated prototype model for COVID-19 symptoms tracking. Computing, 104, 1–22.
31. Raghuwanshi, S., Singh, M., Rath, S., & Mishra, S. (2022). Prominent Cancer Risk Detection Using Ensemble Learning. In Cognitive Informatics and Soft Computing (pp. 677–689). Springer, Singapore.
32. Patel, V. L., Kannampallil, T. G., & Kaufman, D. R. (Eds.). (2015). *Cognitive Informatics for Biomedicine: Human Computer Interaction in Healthcare.* Springer, Berlin.
33. Raghupathi, W., & Raghupathi, V. (2014). Big data analytics in healthcare: Promise and potential. Health Information Science and Systems, 2(1), 1–10.
34. Goebel, R., Chander, A., Holzinger, K., Lecue, F., Akata, Z., Stumpf, S., & Holzinger, A. (2018). Explainable AI: The New 42? In International Cross-Domain Conference for Machine Learning and Knowledge Extraction (pp. 295–303). Springer, Cham.
35. Greenhalgh, T., Wherton, J., Papoutsi, C., Lynch, J., Hughes, G., Hinder, S., & Shaw, S. (2017). Beyond adoption: A new framework for theorizing and evaluating nonadoption, abandonment, and challenges to the scale-up, spread, and sustainability of health and care technologies. Journal of Medical Internet Research, 19(11), e8775.
36. Mohanty, A., & Mishra, S. (2022). A Comprehensive Study of Explainable Artificial Intelligence in Healthcare. In Augmented Intelligence in Healthcare: A Pragmatic and Integrated Analysis (pp. 475–502). Springer, Singapore.
37. Patnaik, M., & Mishra, S. (2022). Indoor Positioning System Assisted Big Data Analytics in Smart Healthcare. In Connected e-Health (pp. 393–415). Springer, Cham.

2 Deep Dive into Cognitive Assisted Ambient Intelligent System for Quality Healthcare

Uday Bhanu Ghosh, Abhishek Kesharwani, and Tanmay Khatri

2.1 INTRODUCTION

Ambient Intelligence (AmI) is a multi-disciplinary research field that explores critically acclaimed ways for formulating symbiotic relationships between people and technological advancements. It aims to facilitate interaction with both people and the environment around them, making it more natural and seamless [1]. Advanced services that AmI systems typically distribute allow devices to reach a common ground where they can work and share information together in order to support people in their everyday activities. For example, lights and HVAC can be controlled by these systems, hence proving their ability to meet the day-to-day requirements and needs of the people using them. By communicating with each other on a ubiquitous basis, these devices can provide the necessary support for those who rely on them. AmI systems are nowadays forecast as a type of distributed services architecture which can empower various services that are networked together to achieve a common goal [1], where each service is devised through the application of artificial intelligence methods and computer networking technologies [2–4]. Using Internet of Things (IoT), we have access to detailed information about our environment, emphasizing more on the capabilities of AmI. AmI aims at providing highly sophisticated as well as intelligent solutions obtained among various varied application areas by studying the context of the user. The field of Artificial Intelligence is rapidly evolving, with new techniques and hardware being developed all the time. AmI research focuses on both the fundamental aspects of data capture and fusion, as well as AI-based methods for processing large amounts of information more accurately [5]. As a result, in some cases, hardware-adapted systems can be developed and situations that were not possible to handle in other contexts can be addressed.

AI has long been working to find ways to incorporate the physical world into its interface design, develop smart environments, make situational awareness a priority, allow for context-specific environmental programming, and perfect the experience as a whole. Despite these advances, AI still faces a number of challenges [6]. In Figure 2.1, we try to define AmI subdomains.

DOI: 10.1201/9781032624891-2

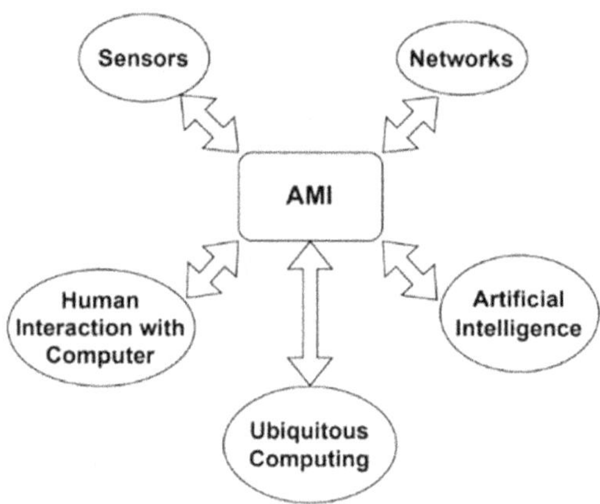

FIGURE 2.1 Scope of AmI.

Over the next decade, finding answers to how AmI can be used to solve real-life problems will be more important than embedding AmI into people's lives. Throughout our world, the human mind is surrounded by intellectual spontaneous interfaces that connect people to all kinds of objects and surroundings that respond indistinguishably and sometimes invisibly to the presence of different individuals. AmI will introduce multiple new requirements for the growth of the Information Society since it affects the people living in our society often more invisibly. In addition to changing the type, content, and functionality of the developing products and services, AmI will create multiple new requirements for the growth of the Information Society. There is a common belief that AMI can contribute significantly to education. Classrooms are impacted by information technologies in a variety of ways. Students can benefit from them by gaining access to information, creating a stimulating learning environment, participating in active learning, and improving their enthusiasm. In the AmI areas, many research efforts are focused on smart homes or cooperative backgrounds, but few procedures address the need for smart homes and an intelligent environment to care for people as a companion, to teach them, and to monitor their health. Pervasive computing is an evolving multi-disciplinary area that affects protocols, infrastructure, systems, devices, etc. Among people, AmI helps people by suggesting new ways of communicating, tailoring it to the needs of each person as well as the environment in which they live [7]. Through ubiquitous computing elements that communicate abundantly among themselves, AmI strives to adapt the technology to the needs of the people. Our ordinary environment will gradually become more intelligent and responsive over time thanks to emerging technologies. It is possible that in the near future, people will be surrounded by more and more intelligent articles through which the environment will capture and identify certain individuals and objectively return them in an untraceable manner. We are all connected through AmI, which implies intelligence about us. Society exists in a digital and persuasive environment which is adaptive, penetrating, aware, and cautious of its presence. Software methods that are spread, non-intrusive, and intelligent are being analyzed in this new area. The digital background helps people in their day-to-day lives and provides them with a comfortable standard of living.

2.2 BACKGROUND STUDY

The European Commission in 2001 coined the term AmI, when the Information Society Technology Advisory Group (ISTAG) of the European Community announced the AmI challenge [8], later updated in 2003 [9]. In recent years, many similar projects and research programs have been conducted worldwide, despite the term's origin in Europe. Over the past few years, several collections of papers have been published and special issues [10–14] have also been published, as well as several specialized workshops and conferences. As described by Gaggioli [15], AmI is an attempt at a subjective digital environment which is both intelligent and responsive to people's presence. It is embedded in our everyday lives, augmenting our experience of the world. Eventually, the system will recognize and express emotion as a result of learning from the behavior of users and being sensitive to context. The term embedded refers to small, possibly miniature devices blending into people's lives and surroundings as they go about their daily lives. Furthermore, Aarts [16] identifies five technology features that are closely related: embedded, contextually aware, personalized, adaptive, and anticipatory.

An area of computer science known as ambient computing deals with developing intelligent systems that can operate in an unstructured environment. By combining natural language processing, ontology-related work, and computer perception, AmI system that combines the naturalness of natural language processing with the smartness of artificial intelligence by combining Natural Language Processing (NLP), ontology-related work, and computer perception techniques such as situation detection and speech recognition. They point out that NLP and AmI can be mutually beneficial in a roadmap article by Gurevych and Muhlhauser [17]. Unstructured information can be transformed into structured knowledge using natural language processing and speech interfaces. The AmI approach can provide contextual information that can be used to resolve ambiguities in natural language.

A Multi-agent Architecture for Mobile Sensing Systems, written by Francisco [18], A new method for mobile sensing systems proposed for planning in large cities is based on the use of intelligent agents and multi-agent systems. In this system, expert learning agents are implemented in each domain where data collection takes place, and these agents are able to carry out machine learning tasks. The advantage of this system is that it is scalable and can handle a large amount of data effectively.

The purpose and objective of various studies was to predict and analyze the failures of composite resin restorations applied to teaching dental students. The study was conducted by students enrolled in dental studies at the Complutense University situated in Madrid. The results obtained showed that a huge number of the failures were due to incorrect placement of the restoration, improper curing, and inadequate occlusion adjustment [19], which examines the reasons and types of failure of posterior composite resin restorations. A large number of dental students took part in studies which were focused on improving both their cognitive knowledge and skills so that posterior teeth restorations would be more successful. In this study, resin restorations placed by students were predicted to fail more likely than non-resin restorations.

This paper explains how artificial intelligence can be used to generate profiles of individuals for information recovery and analysis. The system described herein uses a neural network to learn from a database of facts about people and then generate new profiles based on that information. This system could be used to help locate missing persons, or to investigate crime scenes [20]. It presents a system that can retrieve personal information from the Internet using several input criteria. Despite having the same name, the system can distinguish between the data of different individuals. For the study important information was gathered about the people living in Spain which was further compiled from various other sources in order to draw a huge database. When it comes to web crawling and scraping, this study identified the most useful and reliable tools. Additionally, different AI methodologies were also involved that have been put under test to determine which are the most accurate results and perform best with face recognition and topic modeling [21]. AmI envisions a future where technological advances result in increased intelligence in our everyday surroundings, making our lives easier and more convenient. This concept was first proposed in 2001 and has since been influential in shaping research and development efforts in the field. There are four possible scenarios commissioned by the Advisory Group on Information Society Technologies. Information and communications technology (ICT) research discussions were structured using the results acquired from the above-mentioned scenarios.

According to Aarts and Diederiks [22], Philips' ExperienceLab has been researching ambient lifestyles for the past 25 years, and has now published a guide on how to create them. This book explores how to design and implement an ambient lifestyle, from concept to experience. This book contains a wealth of research from Philips Research Laboratories, ranging from topics such as artificial intelligence to sustainable living. No matter your interests, you'll be sure to find something fascinating within its pages. In the report, they describe a number of killer applications, with the Ambient Intelligent Light television coming out on top. Incubator projects have resulted in startups like amBX, Serious Toys, and Lumalive as a result of several concepts. ExperienceLab concepts, however, rarely led to business activity, since it was difficult to determine what added value they would have for people and what business model to apply for their market entry.

2.3 METHODOLOGY AND FRAMEWORKS OF VARIOUS AMI APPLICATIONS

This section discusses some relevant models in the context of AmI applications.

2.3.1 AmI for Home Applications

A large portion of AmI's vision is directed toward the home environment. When we are aware of and proactive about your context, we can support everyday living with AmI at home [23]. The person can use the bathroom mirror to see a reflection of themselves and be reminded to take their medication. The car stereo can play the same music as during breakfast so that the person can feel like they are in the same space and time as when they ate breakfast. It is not uncommon for ideas and functionalities to be distant visions, such as self-monitoring and self-painting walls, lighting, and furniture that recognizes moods and emotions. However, with the rapid advancements in technology, many of these ideas are becoming reality. For example, there are now self-monitoring appliances available on the market that can communicate with each other to provide a seamless experience for the user. Additionally, there are also lighting fixtures and furniture that can be controlled by voice or smartphone to change colors or adjust according to the user's needs; some have already developed prototypes, such as dormitories that learn the preferences of their single residents about the level of lighting and heating, and the open or closed windows. Commercially available AmI-based devices include temperature-sensitive heaters, motion-activated lighting, and light-activated blinds. Pervasive technology is used in homes that provide residents with AmI services under a variety of names. A smart home is described in many ways, including as a warehouse, an intelligent home, an integrated environment, and an interactive, dynamic, responsive environment. Technology that is designed for the home has traditionally been motivated by the goal of reducing the amount of work required to maintain a household, as well as improving the quality of life for those who live there. In the past several years, AmI has been motivated to develop at home for this reason. Technological advances, expectations, and the trend toward blurring the lines between work, rest, and entertainment are also contributing factors. Figure 2.2 highlights the cognitive regions space.

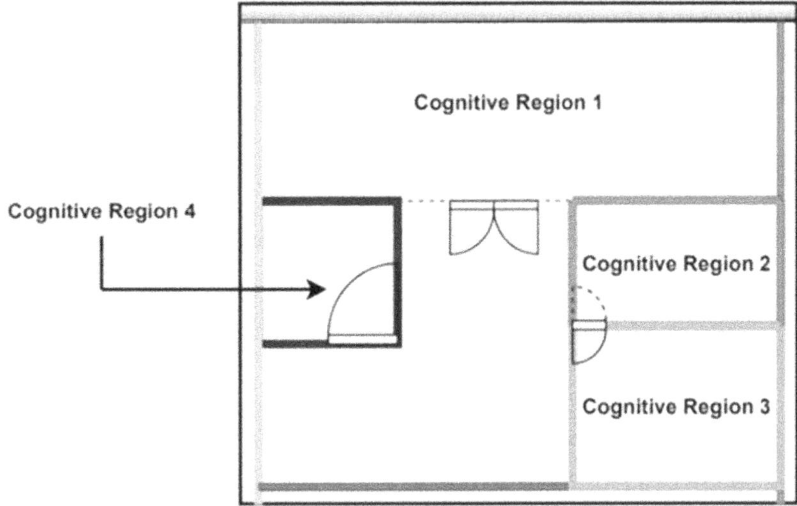

FIGURE 2.2 A sample of cognitive regions.

2.3.2 AmI for Remote Care of Elderly Assistance

As life expectancy increases due to improvements in healthcare and quality of life, there is a growing need for support of independent living for the elderly. AmI is one technological solution that can help meet this need. According to the United Nations, the elderly constituted 12–17% of the European population in 2002. The elderly now make up a significant portion of the population, 15% of the UK population, up from 11% in 1951 and 5% in 1911. Over 60s have now outnumbered under-16s in the United Kingdom. The elderly population is expected to continue to grow, according to several studies. By 2020, 1 in 6 of the US population will be over 65 years of age, the fastest-growing age group in the country [24]. Health care and maintaining quality of life face such challenges as a result of demographic changes. Resources are increasingly being shifted away from institutionalized care toward home-based care and preventative care. The benefits of home automation supported by AmI can be much greater than those of institutional care for the elderly. By providing a preventative approach, it is hoped that caregivers and institutional services will be reduced, leading to additional cost-effectiveness advantages. As a result, the main objective of AmI research has been to support independent living for elderly people, especially those who might be experiencing the early stages of cognitive or physical impairment and may prefer to live in their own homes but may need to be monitored for their safety and well-being in order to do so. This chapter explores a wide range of activities related to the use of technology to improve the efficiency of paper production. This includes everything from more efficient systems and equipment, to studies of user attitudes toward paper production. Figure 2.3 denotes the generic prosperity representation.

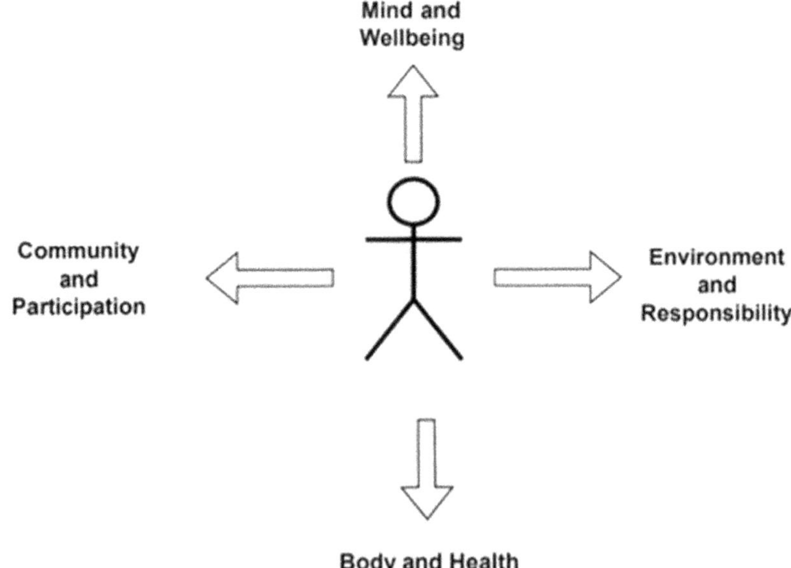

FIGURE 2.3 Synergistic prosperity pictorial representation.

2.3.3 AmI in Quality Healthcare

The quality of medical examination and treatment has improved significantly with the implementation of electronic medical applications. Doctors can now view X-rays and pathology slides remotely and assist or perform surgery via the robot remotely. This technological advancement has had a significant impact on the medical field and will continue to do so in the future [25]. PEM is a wearable personal electrocardiogram monitor that helps detect events and cardiology and improve decision making by sending messages to care providers in the event of an anomaly.

Three different alarm levels are reserved: primary, indicating a serious event requiring urgent assistance; weak, indicating that the user must make an appointment with his or her doctor; and Tips, show the tip on the Patient Relationship Management (PRM) screen. Figure 2.4 depicts the traditional ambient intelligent system process. AmI technology has the potential to enable continuous monitoring of patients in their homes, which could lead to earlier detection of health problems or cognitive decline. This type of monitoring is not possible in a clinical setting, and it has the potential to significantly improve patient care [26–28].

2.3.4 AmI for Business Recommendation System

Responsive environments are those that react to a customer's presence based on the customer's identity and profile. In these environments, devices are controlled by software agents that enable consistent experiences. This survey looks at different aspects

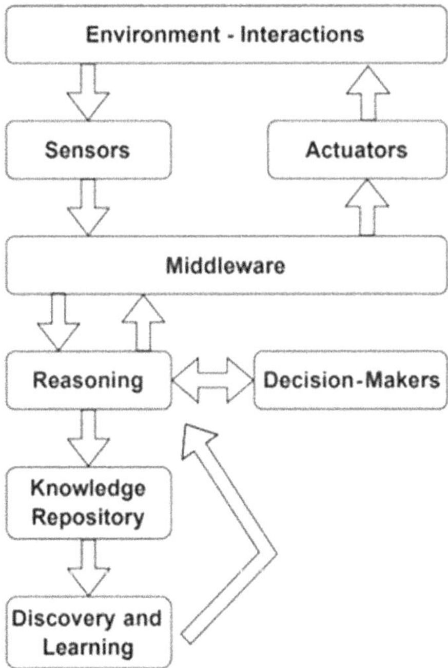

FIGURE 2.4 AmI response flow chart.

of stores and businesses from this angle. A proposed framework that allows stores and shoppers to interact with each other in a context-dependent manner. This will bring e-commerce and AmI closer together, making commerce more popular. A c is a type of artificial intelligence used to predict what a user might want to buy or see. They are commonly used on sites like Amazon and Netflix. In open, connected environments, recommendation systems can be used to adapt known user profiles in one domain for use in another. Shops as Responsive Environments acknowledges that software agents can be used to create responsive environments, defined as environments that can adapt to the needs and preferences of individuals.

The book provides an overview of how to design and implement such systems, with an emphasis on how they can be used to create personalized shopping experiences [29, 30]. An environment that reacts to the events occurring in it is described as a reactive medium. In a reactive environment, the software agent provides the reactive behavior, and the physical world is a combination of the physical agent and the software agent. A common architecture is described, but this article focuses on applying that architecture to an AmI-enhanced library. There are sensors throughout the bookstore and between the shelves. A Bluetooth-enabled store mobile phone, PDA, or loyalty card can be used to detect and identify customers. In-store customer profiles include information such as what they've purchased in the past and their preferences, and stores can link customers' identities to their profiles. By using all this information, we hope to maximize sales by providing customers with a pleasant shopping experience and encouraging them to purchase. This can be achieved through various devices in the store, such as music players and LCD monitors. When choosing music to play on music players, the customers closest to them should consider their preferences, and on the LCD screen, books or other items they may be interested in will be displayed. Likewise, store windows should have bright lights highlighting items that locals might find interesting. It's also important to adjust the display when multiple customers are nearby so that all tastes can be catered for.

2.3.5 AmI in Information Management with AI Approach

We've seen how AI, databases, and agent technology can be used for time- and event-driven reasoning, temporal reasoning, abduction, case-based reasoning, learning, and fuzzy logic. We now need to investigate how these technologies can be used to make AmI applications context-aware, enable distributed planning and self-organization, and create embodiment systems.

The Context-Aware Data Management paper presented by Feng [31] and Li [32]. For too long, database systems have been focused on content-based access, which is all about efficiency. But now, we need artificial intelligence applications that require a more individualized, context-aware approach to data management. This new approach is all about usefulness, rather than just efficiency. Context-aware data management systems should be capable of handling queries like: "Get the Document I edited for publication last week after discussion with the Journal editor," or "Find nearby restaurants based on my order history from food delivery apps." Different users will have different answers to such questions, and the same user will have different answers at different times. Context is defined by the authors as the situation in which the user attempts to access the database. Context can be categorized into two types: user-centered and environment-centric. There are several subcategories within each [29]. A user-centric context may include information about the user's interests, habits, and background. It may also include physiological data from body sensors or emotional data from multimodal sensors, as well as information about the user's features. Physical environment, time, location, temperature, etc., can be considered environment-centric contexts. A user's location and activity can be used to determine the surrounding environment, whether it be a social or computational environment, such as a traffic jam or surrounding people from service providers.

2.3.6 AMI FOR COGNITIVE TELEREHABILITATION

In previous publications [33, 34], this system has been described as an extension. A few relevant social features were included in the first one [33] in order to increase motivation and reduce isolation. This multi-user therapy proposal can be designed to create a more entertaining environment. As part of the second paper [35], both the therapist and the patient were presented in the same physical location during the physical-cognitive rehabilitation process. Through the linking of cognitive activities with physical exercises, our system combines cognitive rehabilitation with physical rehabilitation. In order to monitor this activity, a Kinect is used to track the patient's physical movements. Although physical and cognitive activities may be arduous, patients are more likely to find enjoyment in these activities if they are combined. This, in turn, will help motivate patients in their rehabilitation [35]. The objective of this company is to take advantage of economies of scale by integrating operations that are typically separate. Figure 2.5 represents a diagrammatic representation of

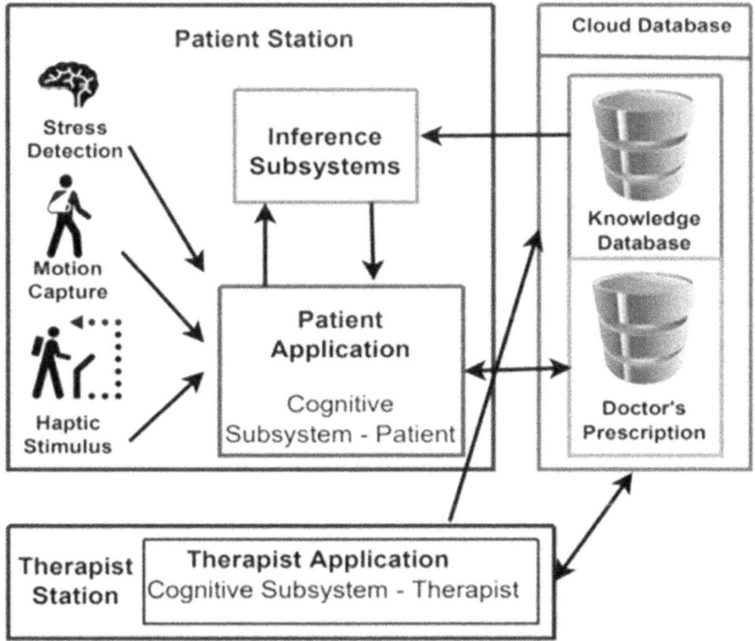

FIGURE 2.5 Cognitive telerehabilitation based on AMI architecture.

the above discussion, pointing out the overall flow of AMI-based cognitive system for telerehabilitation.

2.4 USE CASES OF AMI

2.4.1 Patient Application System

Thanks to the work of Jaquero, this paper emphasized a developed patient interface that makes it easy for patients to access their medical information and get the care they need [36]. Do not try to include too much information in the interface, as this can be overwhelming and lead to users ignoring important details. Stick to the basics and only include information that is absolutely necessary. By reducing the user's interface elements as much as possible, we hope to reduce the cognitive load presented to users by processing these elements. Considering that the system is used by patients with cognitive deficits in this specific case, this is relevant.

An explanation text is displayed at the beginning of the rehabilitation exercise to explain providing instructions for the exercise to the patient. To complete the exercise successfully, the user should be able to understand the text. During the creation of the exercise, the therapist writes the text and sets the length of the display. During the rehabilitation exercise execution, the user is guided by this text. Below is a summary of the patient's current "Score." If the patient selects valid objects, the score will increase; Werbach and Hunter's gamification strategy encourages users to score higher by providing negative feedback for incorrect object selection [37]. A central part of the interface displays the exercise itself. On this interface, the therapist places objects, the patient interacts (by default his/her left and right hands), and the picture from the camera is shown. The therapist can display additional information beyond the user-interface objects to help the patient with their exercises. This allows for a more customized experience that caters to exactly what the patient needs in order to carry out their exercises.

2.4.2 AmI-Enabled Smart Homes

Smart homes are equipped with a variety of sensors and actuators that can monitor activities, movements, and potentially hazardous situations such as fire or smoke. Homes also often include computing devices linked to the aforementioned sensors and actuators to provide greater control over things like windows, cooking appliances, and more. Radio Frequency Identification (RFID) sensors can be used to detect the presence of an object or a person. For example, the sensor could be used to detect if a weight is on a chair or if someone wearing an ID card walks through a door in another room. Depending on the sensor information, additional processing may be needed to produce useful data, such as location [38] or the task the resident is trying to perform [39, 40]. Smart homes can be programmed to respond in some way to prevent disasters [41, 42]. The device can also be used to learn how occupants behave [43]. People living alone with cognitive impairment often use the concept of Smart Home as a support system. People living in such homes enjoy a better quality of life, are more independent, and can stay in their homes longer, reducing the costs of institutionalization. Most homes have alarm systems as standard equipment. The

Smart Home concept is much more than that, including systems that track residents' activities, compare them to their records, act if needed, and provide support and advice on security, health, medical, and entertainment aspects. For example, in the event of an emergency, fire, unconsciousness, or fall, people have panic buttons in their homes or around their necks. The user may not trigger the alarm enough time [44]. To alleviate this problem, we are moving toward alarms that have the ability to trigger automatically, such as those that respond to vital signs like blood pressure or pulse. In Smart Home, lights are turned on to anticipate the needs of the resident or even to remind him that he should move in a certain direction. We have many systems that automatically turn on lights when motion is detected, but Smart Homes can do more than just detect motion. In a home setting, AmI services will include the following. Automate many daily tasks and reduce the burden of home management. For example, automatically controlling appliances and other objects can reduce the amount of labor associated with housework and maintenance. For example, by controlling lights and blinds, you can improve utility efficiency. In addition, safety and security can be enhanced by preventing accidents, instantly recognizing and reporting accidents, tracking individuals, and providing sophisticated access control [30]. Access control and alarms can be included in safety/security, as well as automated security safeguards for appliances such as the iron and the oven. Health and biomedical monitoring may also be included. Self-monitoring buildings and alerting each other when rebuilding and repairs are needed can also be included. By providing entertainment and increasing comfort, you can improve your quality of life, helping older people and people with disabilities live independently. Next, we will discuss it in detail, as it is an important application in itself.

2.4.3 Emotion Aware AmI Multiagent Framework

This paper focuses on a multi-agent system consisting of cognitive agents capable of realizing adaptive AmI environments. This environment can recognize the user's presence and, more importantly, their emotional state. Architecturally, the proposed method divides the habitat into several cognitive regions. Services are sent by agents to specific locations in the environment, such as rooms, floors, or buildings. For example, an HVAC service might deliver time-based emotional services, while a lighting service might deliver a music service. This is achieved by cognitive regions that combine environmental features with the user's emotional state and temporal knowledge [45–47], agents in the framework of we provide actions that change over time and are therefore able to provide distinct services according to the same sentiments and environmental conditions. When service delivery is affected by temporal factors such as season or time of day, this option is particularly useful. The smart lighting agent can decide to activate different luminaries in winter and summer, or the music agent can play different styles of music at different volumes in the morning and at night. These decisions are based on a new type of fuzzy perception engine that can directly deal with the emotional and temporal problems common in immersive computer environments. The tool is a combination of Russell's two-dimensional emotion model and Timed Automata-based fuzzy cognitive map, allowing agents to infer the best service collection from emotional analysis, Human contact, environmental characteristics, and the concept of time. Thanks to this way of thinking, cognitive agents can manage and understand a group of cognitive systems that work together to cover a certain area in time, as well as the relationship between these systems.

2.4.4 Music Agent Usability Case Study

The user's interactions with the test bed begin in a realistic environment that has been designed to provide services and collections. Figure 2.6 represents TAFCM demo architecture. The user chooses a vote from the real range [1, 2] (the higher, the better) to express their satisfaction level for three usability aspects.

The design aspect of responsiveness measures the effect of a system's behavior on the user's emotional state and environmental characteristics. This is directly related to the design of the system, especially the modeling of TAFCM (Timed Autonomous Machine-Based Fuzzy Cognitive Mapping).

This metric measures how quickly the system responds to user requests, relative to how fast the correct response will occur according to the underlying automaton. A low value indicates that the response system closely resembles the controller, while a high value indicates a significant mismatch between the two values.

The usefulness of the system lies in its ability to improve quality of life.

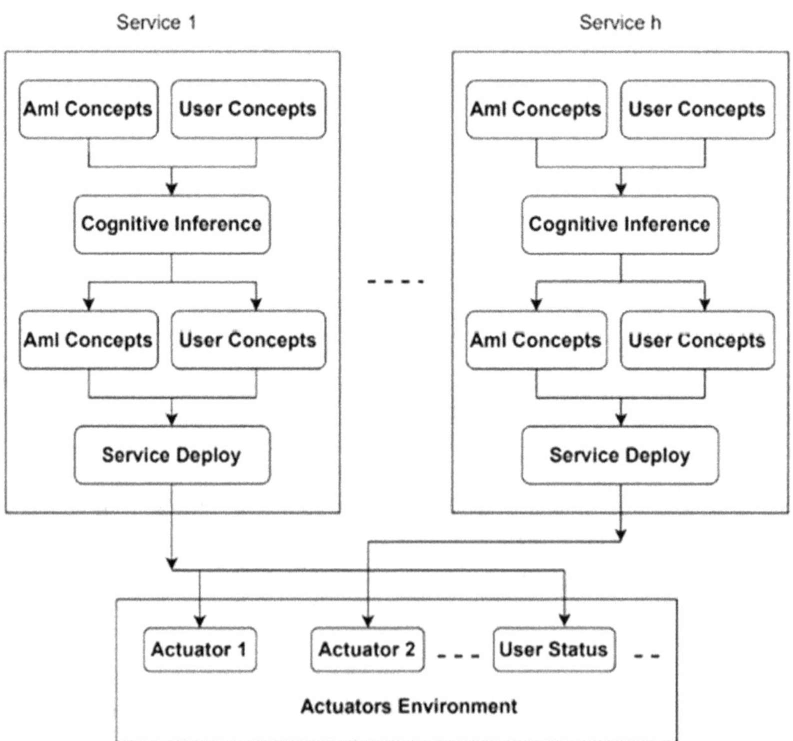

FIGURE 2.6 Depiction of timed automata based FCMs for AMI-based architecture.

TABLE 2.1
Tabular Representation of Usability Test

Test	Correctness			Practicality			Effectiveness		
	Min	Avg	Max	Min	Avg	Max	Min	Avg	Max
Morning	6	7.2	8.2	5.3	7.8	7.2	7.1	7.8	9.2
Afternoon	3	9	9.3	4.2	8.2	8.1	8.3	8.1	9.4
Evening	4	6.5	8.7	4.1	5.9	7.9	7.4	8.6	9.2
Night	7	7.2	7.9	5.6	7.6	6.9	6.7	7.9	9.3

The results in Table 2.1 show that the proposed method mostly meets the needs of users in all aspects. Minimum, maximum, and average scores demonstrate this fact. The main objective of usability testing is to observe and analyze the decision-making process of actors over a period of time, to assess the dynamics involved. To do this, 50 users were invited to participate in a test bench, which simulates a cognitive life support environment.

2.4.5 LivingLab Home Initiative

The LivingLab Home initiative aims to create interactive environments for older adults and explore the social impact of these technologies. The three-story, 5040-square-foot home serves as an in-house laboratory for interdisciplinary research and evaluation. Some of the program's goals include designing interactive environments for older adults and exploring the social impact of these technologies.

Less Invasive Surfactant Administration (LISA) system is designed to help people live independently by providing support and prompting when needed [18, 19]. The system uses agents that each monitor a different aspect of user behavior, such as drug use or mobility. Officers then coordinate their responses to provide needed assistance.

This project addresses high-level inference skills from three main aspects: machine learning, target recognition, and feedback generation. Machine learning is used to learn residents' regular activity schedules and generate correlation models between sensor readings and specific activities. Target detection is used to infer residents' goals from observed actions, based on a system called PHATT (Probabilistic Hostile Agent Task Tracker) [35]. PHATT uses a library of simple hierarchical task network maps. Response generation selects system response based on detected target.

Feedback generation is done in three steps. Figure 2.7 shows a task network. The first step is when individual domain agents generate a context-free response. These responses are based solely on their own domain information and are sent to the central response dispatching agent. The second step is where the central response coordinator prioritizes responses and aggregates them. The third step is when the Central Response Coordination Agent decides which response to send to a device, such as a phone.

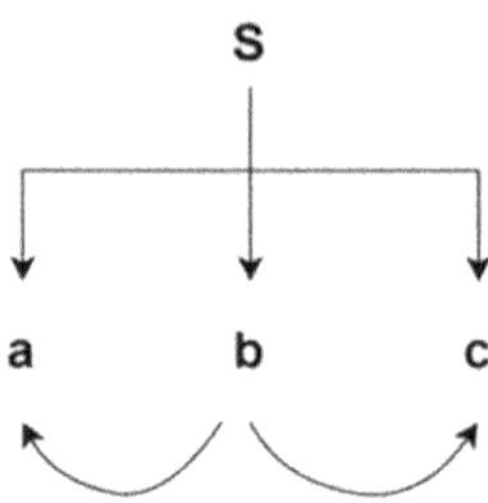

FIGURE 2.7 Representation of hierarchical task network.

2.5 CONCLUSION

A selection of AmI applications were examined in this study, including smart home, elderly care, healthcare, and business and commerce. For this reason, we comprehensively analyze trends, requirements, and challenges as well as technical developments and implemented demonstrators. Furthermore, in the context of AmI, we discuss various AI and data management technologies, including event-condition-action rules, production rules, learning, fuzzy logic, scheduling, plan detection, temporal reasoning, and reasoning based on cases. The survey also placed an emphasis on how current technologies are being used and what enhancements are deemed necessary. Agents have also been considered in various other ways, including as abstraction tools to model devices and their interactions.

We then consider the role of affective computing and human emotions in environmental intelligence. We consider different approaches to emotion detection and classification, including self-reports, physiological metrics, seat and hand pressure sensors, and speech act features. We also looked at studies correlating some of these different techniques and examining people's preferences in evaluating their emotions according to the two main models of human emotions: the basic emotions and the dimensional emotion models. People can be influenced by the ways in which how computer systems interact with humans. Using AmI technologies as a focus, we examine their social and ethical implications and challenges.

AmI technology has the potential to revolutionize the way we interact with our environment. By using simple data and reasoning mechanisms, AmI can provide a wealth of information and functionality. However, realizing the full potential of AmI requires advances in knowledge representation and reasoning, as well as AI and agent-oriented technologies. AmI technology has evolved significantly with new developments in computing power and data processing. This has led to a more sophisticated understanding of the world around us and our interaction with it. The introduction of AmI into our everyday lives has the potential to revolutionize the way we interact with technology.

This document explores how AmI's ethical principles can be applied to support teaching and learning and childcare. The authors argue that the personalized interaction that AmI systems enable can have a profound impact on user experience.

To test this claim, two alternative scenarios are proposed: a configuration in which Smart Space provides only consistent textual/graphical feedback and a configuration in which it provides personalized multimodal communications to the user. The effectiveness of each approach is evaluated by collecting and comparing user responses.

REFERENCES

1. Aarts, E., and Roovers, R. 2004. Embedded system design issues in ambient intelligence. T. Basten, M. Geilen, and H. Groot, Eds., Ambient Intelligence: Impact on Embedded System Design, Springer, New York, NY, 11–29.
2. Lyytinen, K., and Yoo, Y. 2002. Issues and challenges in ubiquitous computing. Commun. ACM, 45, 12, 63–65.
3. Fenza, G., Senatore, S., and Loia, V. 2008. A hybrid approach to semantic web services matchmaking. Int. J. Approx. Reason., 48, 3, 808–828.
4. Gaeta, M., Capuano, N., Gaeta, A., Orciuoli, F., Pappacena, L., and Ritrovato, P. 2004. "A service oriented virtual organisation for e-Learning," in Learning Grid of Excellence Working Group.
5. Carneiro, D., Pimenta, A., Gonçalves, S., Neves, J., and Novais, P. 2016. Monitoring and improving performance in human–computer interaction. Concurr. Comput. Pract. Exp., 28, 1291–1309. https://doi.org/10.1002/cpe.3635
6. Aarts, E., and Grotenhuis, F. 2011. Ambient intelligence 2.0: Towards synergetic prosperity. J. Ambient Intell. Smart Environ., 3, 3–11.
7. Ramkumar, M. O., Sarah Catharin, S., and Nivetha, D. Preceding of International Conference on Systems Computation Automation and Networking 2019: Survey of Cognitive Assisted Living Ambient System Using Ambient Intelligence as a Companion.
8. Ducatel, K., Bogdanowicz, M., Scapolo, F., Leijten, J., and Burgelman, J.-C. 2001. Scenarios for Ambient Intelligence in 2010. IST Advisory Group Final Report, European Commission (EC), Brussels.
9. Ducatel, K., Bogdanowicz, M., Scapolo, F., Leijten, J., and Burgelman, J.-C. 2003. Ambient Intelligence: From Vision to Reality. IST Advisory Group Draft Report, European Commission.
10. Werner, W., Rabaey, J. M., and Aarts, E. H. L. 2005. Ambient Intelligence. Springer, Berlin.
11. Cai, Y., and Abascal, J. 2006. Ambient Intelligence for Everyday Life, vol. 3864, Springer, Berlin.
12. Augusto, J. C., and Nugent, C. D. 2006. Smart homes can be smarter. J. C. Augusto and C. D. Nugent, Eds., Designing Smart Homes: The Role of Artificial Intelligence, Eds., Lecture Notes in Artificial Intelligence, vol. 4008, Springer, Berlin, 1–15.
13. Augusto, J. C., and Nugent, C. D. 2006. Designing Smart Homes the Role of Artificial Intelligence, Lecture Notes in Artificial Intelligence, vol. 4008, Springer, Berlin.
14. Aarts, E. H., Aarts, E. H. L., and Encarnação, J. L. 2009. True Visions: The Emergence of Ambient Intelligence, Springer, Berlin.
15. Gaggioli, A. 2005. Optimal experience in ambient intelligence. G. Riva, F. Vatalaro, F. Davide and M. Alcaniz, Eds., Ambient Intelligence, IOS Press, Amsterdam, 35–43.
16. Aarts, E. 2004. Ambient intelligence: A multimedia perspective. IEEE Intell. Syst, 19, 1, 12–19.
17. Gurevych, I., and Muhlhauser, M. 2007. Natural language processing for ambient intelligence. Special Issue of KI-Zeitschrift Ambient Intelligence und Künstliche Intelligenz, 10–16.

18. Laport, F., Serrano, E., and Bajo, J. 2019. A multi-agent architecture for mobile sensing systems. J. Ambient Intell. Human Comput. https://doi.org/10.1007/s12652-019-01608-4
19. Aliaga, I. J., De Paz, J. F., Vera, V., García, A. E., and Bajo, J. 2020. Prediction and failure analysis of composite resin restorations in the posterior sector applied in teaching dental students. J. Ambient Intell. Human Comput. https://doi.org/10.1007/s12652-020-01804-7
20. Chamoso, P., Bartolomé, Á, García-Retuerta, D., Prieto, J., and De La Prieta, F. 2020. Profile generation system using artificial intelligence for information recovery and analysis. J. Ambient Intell. Human Comput. https://doi.org/10.1007/s12652-020-01942-y
21. Ducatel, K., Bogdanowicz, M., Scapolo, F., Leijten, J., and Burgelman, J. C. 2001, Scenarios for Ambient Intelligence in 2010: Final Report, ISTAG, Cameroon.
22. Aarts, E. H. L., and Diederiks, E., Eds. 2006. Ambient Lifestyle: From Concept to Experience, BIS Publishers, Amsterdam.
23. Encarnacao, J. L., and Kirste, T. 2005. Ambient intelligence: Towards smart appliance ensembles. M. Hemmje et al., Eds., Lecture Notes in Computer Science, vol. 3379, Sprinter, Berlin, 261–270.
24. Corchado, J. M., Bajo, J., and Abraham, A. 2008. GerAmi: Improving healthcare delivery in geriatric residences. J. IEEE Intell. Syst. (Special Issue on Ambient Intelligence), 3, 2, 19–25.
25. Riva, G. 2003. Ambient intelligence in health care. Cyber Psych. Behav., 6, 3, 295–300.
26. Fifer, S. K., and Thomas, N. 2002. A second and more promising round of e-health enterprises. Manag. Care Interface, 15, 52–56.
27. Haux, R. 2006. Individualization, globalisation and health—About sustainable information technologies and the aim of medical informatics. Int. J. Med. Informatics, 75, 795–808.
28. Rumetshofer, H., Puhretmair, F., and Wob, W. 2003. Individual information presentation based on cognitive styles for tourism information systems. A. J. Frew, M. Hitz, and P. O'Connor, Eds., Proceedings of the International Conference on Information and Communication Technologies in Tourism, Springer Verlag, Berlin, 440–449.
29. Da Silva, F. S. C., and Vasconcelos, W. W. 2007. Managing responsive environments with software agents. J. Appl. Artif. Intell., 21, 4, 469–488.
30. Da Silva, F. S. C., and Vasconcelos, W. W. 2005. Agent-based management of responsive environments. In Proceedings of Advances in Artificial Intelligence, 9th Congress of the Italian Association for Artificial Intelligence, Springer, Milan, Italy, 224–236.
31. Feng, L., Apers, P. M. G., and Jonker, W. 2004. Towards context-aware data management for ambient intelligence. In Proceedings of the 15th International Conference on Database and Expert Systems Applications (DEXA). Lecture Notes in Computer Science, vol. 3180, Springer, Zaragoza, Spain, 422–431.
32. LI, Y., Feng, L., and Zhou, L. 2008. Context-aware database querying: Recent progress and challenges. D. Stojanovic, Ed., Context-Aware Mobile and Ubiquitous Computing for Enhanced Usability: Adaptive Technologies and Applications, IGI, Hershey, PA, 147–170.
33. Oliver, M., Molina, J. P., Fernández-Caballero, A., and González, P. 2017. Collaborative computer-assisted cognitive rehabilitation system. Adv. Distrib. Comput. Artificial Intell. J., 6, 57–74.
34. Oliver, M., González, P., Montero, F., Molina, J. P., and Fernández-Caballero, A. 2016. Smart computer-assisted cognitive rehabilitation for the ageing population. Advances in Intelligent Systems and Computing, Springer International Publishing, New York, vol. 476, pp. 197–205.
35. Franco-Martin, M. A., et al. 2011. Usability of cognitive (Gradior) and physical training with mild dementia, mild cognitive impairment and healthy elderly people: Long lasting memories, preliminary findings. Eur. J. Neurol., 18, 80.

36. López-Jaquero, V., Montero, F., and Teruel, M. A. 2017. Influence awareness: Considering motivation in computer assisted rehabilitation. J. Ambient Intell. Humaniz. Comput. 10, 2185–2197
37. Werbach, K., and Hunter, D. 2012. For the Win: How Game Thinking Can Revolutionize Your Business, Wharton, Philadelphia.
38. Favela, J., Rodriguez, M., Preciado, A., and Gonzalez, V. M. 2004. Integrating context-aware public displays into a mobile hospital information system. IEEE Trans. Inf. Technol. Biomed, 8, 3, 279–286.
39. Geib, C. W., and Goldman, R. P. 2001. Probabilistic plan recognition for hostile agents. In Proceedings of the 14th International Florida Artificial Intelligence Research Society Conference. AAAI Press, Key West, FL, 580–584.
40. Geib, C. W. 2002. Problems with intent recognition elder care. In Proceedings of the AAAI Workshop on Automation as Caregiver, Edmonton, AB.
41. Augusto, J. C., Nugent, C. D., Martin, S., and Olphert, C. 2005. Towards personalization of services and an integrated service model for smart homes applied to elderly care. S. Giroux and H. Pigot, Eds., Proceedings of the International Conference on Smart Homes and Health Telematics, IOS Press, Montreal, From Smart Homes to Smart Care, 151–158.
42. Augusto, J. C., Liu, J., Mccullagh, P., Wang, H., and Yang, J.-B. 2008. Management of uncertainty and spatio temporal aspects for monitoring and diagnosis in a smart home. Inter. J. Computat. Intell. Syst., 1, 4, 361–378.
43. Hagras, H., Callaghan, V., Colley, M., Clarke, G., Pounds-Cornish, A., and Duman, H. 2004. Creating an ambient-intelligence environment using embedded agents. IEEE Intell. Syst., 12–20. DOI:10.1109/MIS.2004.61
44. Abascal, J., Bonail, B., Marco, A., Casas, R., and Sevillano, J. L. 2008. AmbienNet: An intelligent environment to support people with disabilities and elderly people. In Proceedings of the 10th International ACM SIGACCESS Conference on Computers and Accessibility (ASSETS), 293–294.
45. Aarts, E. H. L., and Eggen, B., Eds. 2002. Ambient Intelligence in HomeLab. Neroc.
46. Kientz, J. A., Patel, S. N., Jones, B., Price, E., Mynatt, E. D., and Abowd, G. D. 2008. The Georgia tech aware home. CHI '08: CHI '08 Extended Abstracts on Human Factors in Computing Systems, ACM, New York, 3675–3680.
47. Rutishauser, U., Joller, J., and Douglas, R. 2005. Control and learning of ambience by an intelligent building. IEEE Trans. Systems, Man and Cybernetics, Part A: Systems and Humans, 35, 1, 121–132.
48. Plocher, T., and Kiff, L. M. 2003. Mobility monitoring with the Independent LifeStyle Assistant (I.L.S.A.). In Proceedings of the International Conference on Aging, Disability and Independence (ICADI), University of Florida, St. Petersburg, FL, 170–171.
49. Guralnik, V., and Haigh, K. Z. 2002. Learning models of human behaviour with sequential patterns. In Proceedings of the AAAI Workshop on Automation as Caregiver, AAAI Press, Edmonton, AB.

3 Emergence of Telemedicine Applications Using Machine Learning

Anshuman Behera, Pratyush Mishra, Saswat Mohanty, Raseswari Sarangi, and Tarek Gaber

3.1 INTRODUCTION

Machine learning is important because it helps with the development of new products and gives business insight into patterns in customer practices and business operations. From the paper by Shen et al. [1, 2], many of the top businesses operating today, including Facebook, Google, and Uber, are starting to heavily rely on machine learning. Machine learning today substantially sets many firms apart from their rivals [3]. As a distinct medical field, telemedicine has yet to gain recognition. The integration of telemedicine into healthcare facilities is part of a larger investment in technology and care delivery models. Regardless of the delivery method, cost recovery fees remain consistent. This implies that the programming and invoicing of remote services are identical. Greater opportunities have been created for the development of the global health industry, especially telemedicine, as a result of the ongoing development of technologies that allow the expansion of Internet connections and the growth of data processing capacity. This chapter will discuss the important, from the paper by Pacis et al. [4] current and possible future application of various artificial intelligence concepts to telemedicine goals. These objectives, patient monitoring, health information technology, intelligent computer diagnostics, simulation and training systems, and information analysis and collaboration, will be used to classify each concept and application that is discussed. By automating hospital logistics, time management, medical needs provision, and operational efficiency can all be improved. Telemedicine is the use of interactive digital communication to transfer medical information so that doctors can collaborate remotely while conducting consultations, medical examinations, and procedures.

3.2 MOTIVATION AND SCOPE

Telemedicine has made it unnecessary to attend a doctor's office or clinic, a kids' park, go for a stroll, or wait in a waiting room while you're unwell. You may visit your doctor while relaxing on your couch or bed. Virtual visits are typically

 DOI: 10.1201/9781032624891-3

simpler to fit into a busy schedule [5]. Your schedule may not require you to take time off or schedule child care if you choose telemedicine. Better evaluation: Specialist doctors, such as allergists, can conduct remote assessments and counseling for mental health through telemedicine, allowing them to better understand the specific factors causing allergies in patients' homes. Telemedicine also makes it simple to have access to mental health assessments and counseling services. Some methods that enable new patients to book an appointment with a nearby general practice (GP) can save time.

In India, 68% of the population lives in rural areas where healthcare services are minimal and telemedicine can bridge the gap by overcoming barriers to distance through the joint efforts of government and private healthcare institutions [6, 7]. The future of the world is becoming more connected as technology and internet connectivity develop. The substantial change applies equally to healthcare. Future emergency care and specialized medicine fields like diagnostic technology and mental health will be better understood thanks to extensive research and technological advancements. By integrating AR, VR, 3D printing, robots, and AI, customers can personalize healthcare delivery with greater value. The integration of telemedicine and technology will revolutionize healthcare, providing a modern solution for a better patient experience. Telemedicine encompasses diverse communication avenues, including voice, audio, text, and digital data exchange.

The main highlights of the work are as follows:

- Store and forward, remote monitoring, and in-person interaction are all part of telemedicine. Each contributes positively to healthcare as a whole and, when used correctly, may actually help patients and healthcare professionals.
- Store-and-forward telemedicine does away with the need for a face-to-face examination by the doctor. Patient information, such as medical photographs, can instead be given to the professional as needed after being collected from the patient. If it is set up and handled properly, telemedicine may help doctors save time and give patients better treatment.
- A variety of technical instruments are used in self-monitoring and self-testing to remotely monitor a patient's clinical symptoms and general health. In the treatment of chronic ailments, it is often used. The benefits of remote monitoring include lower costs, more frequent monitoring, and improved patient satisfaction.
- Interactive services can provide those who require medical care with timely guidance. Numerous methods, including the phone, the internet, and house visits, can be used to do this. The taking of the history and consultation with the current symptoms may be followed by an assessment comparable to what is usually done during face-to-face appointments.

3.3 APPLICATION FEASIBILITY

Various potential applications of telemedicine are discussed in this section. Figure 3.1 illustrates some of these vital applications.

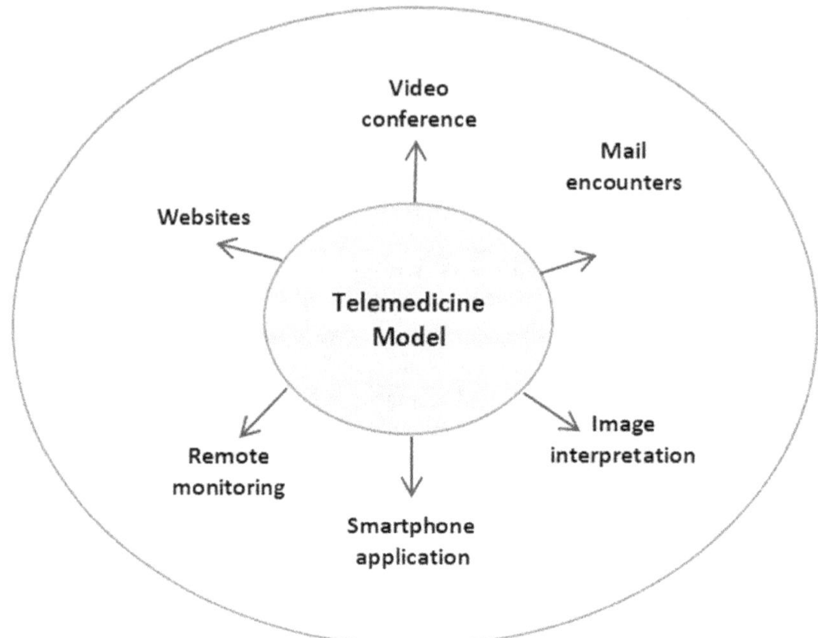

FIGURE 3.1 Telemedicine applications using machine learning.

3.3.1 Video Conference

Patients no longer have to wait as long to contact doctors and other healthcare professionals, thanks to medical video conferencing, which reduces the time lost in the initial stages of treatment. From the paper by Mishra et al. [8], this ensures appropriate medical care in the shortest amount of time, which is very helpful in the treatment of critical illnesses. Based on this procedure, the relevant authorities will review the situation right away and take the necessary corrective action.

This facility will allow professionals to design corrective measures without wasting time traveling to the scene to begin the required measures in cases of disasters brought on by natural calamities or as a result of infamous and criminal acts of mankind. In these circumstances, every minute counts, and the use of this contemporary technology enables providers to gain crucial time that will ultimately save thousands of lives.

There may be a great distance between you and the best medical professional. Patients may not be able to physically travel in these situations to seek a consultation with a doctor or other provider of medical and health services [9, 10]. The patient and healthcare provider can consult using telemedicine video conferencing technology. This facility will allow specialists to design corrections without wasting time traveling to the site to start the necessary measures in cases of disasters brought on by natural calamities or as a result of infamous and criminal acts of mankind. One minute counts in these situations, and the use of this cutting-edge technology enables medical professionals to gain crucial time that will ultimately save thousands of lives. From the paper by Sahoo et al. [11], there may be a great distance between you and the best medical professional. In these situations, it might not be viable for patients to physically travel to seek a consultation with a doctor or provider of medical and health services. The patient and healthcare provider can consult via video conference using telemedicine technology. This tends to increase the number of cases that professionals can handle, which is good for patients. Doctors can now use this methodology instead of the traditional method of sitting down at a table with their colleagues, which decelerates the process and inadvertently increases the cost of healthcare for patients.

3.3.2 Remote Monitoring

Patients are treated remotely through a process called remote patient monitoring (RPM), which is a subset of telehealth. Patients use wearable devices that serve as read-out for medical staff, translating real-time results. The patient can still be monitored whether they're at work, home, and school or on the road. RPM, which enables remote treatment for patients, has several advantages for both patients and healthcare facilities. This method of treatment is advantageous for both parties because it enables them to receive care in the convenience of their homes while using fewer resources and at a lower cost. With improvements in internet connectivity, digital marketing, and healthcare technology, humans make technological progress every day. From the paper by Sahoo et al. [11] the use of RPM is expanding daily. Not only is telemedicine economical, but it also helps both parties. For patients receiving remote treatment, there are sophisticated systems in place that aim to offer comfort, quality, and improved services. The fundamental objective of telemedicine equipment standardization and proliferation is to improve the experience for patients and medical professionals. From the paper by Qadir et al. [12], those who will use the gadgets need to understand how they work. The data that will be examined by these tools must be straightforward and understandable. Most significantly, a mobile device management system should be able to assist in giving end customers whenever they want rapid technical support. Setting up notifications for any unusual behavior and remotely accessing or monitoring device performance are examples of troubleshooting chores. For better analysis, RPM keeps track of the patient's weight, vital signs, blood pressure, blood sugar, blood oxygen level, and other factors. These measurements are baseline information that is gathered through RPM and examined by professionals at the hospitals. People are increasingly at ease remaining in and working from home, as was shown during the epidemic. Because it enables you as a healthcare provider to expand your facilities, RPM is a technology that is worthwhile investing in. Every day, technology advances, and those who don't change with the times risk damaging their own businesses.

3.3.3 Image Interpretation

A constant issue in the healthcare industry is image quality when providing telehealth services. Health professionals now show more interest in the provision of Telediagnosis services than in previous years. From the paper by Haleem et al. [13]

telediagnosis may involve face-to-face communication with patients or interprofessional cooperation. To accomplish this, high-quality medical pictures, graphics, and videos must be transmitted in real-time. Medical professionals employ a variety of digital platforms to connect with patients, leveraging social media and messaging channels alongside structured telemedicine consultations for guidance. These virtual consultations can either be a first encounter or a continuation of a prior interaction between a patient and healthcare professional. In the face of rising data needs, the importance of a sturdy broadband network foundation becomes ever more vital. The perceptions of medical professionals in India and Pakistan with regard to the problems with the caliber of medical images, graphics, and videos used to diagnose and treat patients are discussed in this paper. Numerous medical images are produced daily to aid in the diagnosis and treatment of disease applications. From the perspective of telemedicine, analysis and storage of medical data are crucial tasks and data transport is also required. In the analysis, storage, and transmission of medical data, preprocessing, segmentation, and compression methods are becoming more and more crucial. Before continuing with processing, a suitable filtering technique is needed since noise taints medical images. Although efficient lossy compression algorithms are also available for medical photos, they are stored in a lossless manner. It's crucial to compress medical photos for the database to be used effectively. From the paper by Dutta et al. [14] depending on whether the image is grayscale or RGB, the primary goal of image compression is to decrease the number of bits used to describe the image while maintaining the image quality and pixel intensity level to the greatest extent possible. Less or no quality detail loss is preferred when compressing significant portions because medical photos also contain diagnostic information about a disease. Planning treatment could become challenging or lead to incorrect diagnosis otherwise.

3.3.4 Mail Encounters

During the past decade, email has been utilized in various healthcare settings for diverse diseases. By linking the environment via the Internet or computer, we can significantly enhance human connections. The Internet can strengthen the doctor-patient bond. A collaborative relationship between doctor and patient, built on trust, moral obligation, and patient well-being, is what this type of relationship entails. The foundation of exceptional healthcare lies in the harmonious relationship between medical staff. Telemedicine provides patients with greater access to doctors, fostering new ways of connecting them [15]. Several studies highlight the diverse uses of email in doctor-patient communication, including enhancing the bond between healthcare professionals and patients, boosting interactions between physicians and patients, facilitating correspondence among individuals at home with medical institutions, simplifying things for everyone involved, motivating healthcare workers, and automating tasks to streamline workflows while ensuring seamless connections during critical situations. These objectives include fostering improved communication within hospitals by saving healthcare personnel's valuable time searching for patients or following up on their whereabouts, therefore promoting uninterrupted care delivery while minimizing potential errors due to oversight in documentation management practices involving sensitive patient data protection under strict confidentiality protocols embedded into software applications tailored exclusively towards supporting these functions across disparate domains without compromising security standards established through rigorous audits conducted periodically throughout each hospital network integration process—all resulting in increased efficiency gains over extended periods rather than just short bursts.

3.3.5 Websites

Patients in rural areas who previously had difficulty visiting a doctor can now do so virtually. On different systems through an interface, knowledge transfer occurs efficiently, benefiting doctor–patient relationships. By streamlining these procedures via digital channels, telemedicine tools help shorten the time between medical need and assistance. Both applications feature user profiles. Information such as names, photos, age, etc., can all go into creating comprehensive patient profiles, which are accessible through this platform. Before receiving the call, the medical consultant will be better able to assess and comprehend the patient thanks to this. One of the key components of a telemedicine online application is medical reporting. This covers the doctor's credentials, expertise, and patient testimonials. In telemedicine web applications, having a platform where patients and physicians may interact is crucial [16]. This feature enables the patient and doctor to communicate with each other via an interactive medium, such as a video call. One of the essential components of a telemedicine online platform is physician evaluations. The addition of this functionality will aid people in selecting the best physician for their needs. A feature that assists the doctor in scheduling an appointment during his free time is appointment management so that patients are aware of the availability of everything. It's crucial to incorporate many payment mechanisms into a web application for telemedicine. Users will benefit from this functionality while making a payment. The online application for telemedicine has made healthcare services conveniently and swiftly accessible. Telemedicine apps on the web help patients avoid multiple hospital visits for related concerns. Once the delay has been eliminated, medical care procedures are conducted sooner. By leveraging app functionality based on ease of access, doctors check up on patients across diverse digital platforms. Under this system, patients will regularly interact with medical professionals before updating progress through our application. Thus, personalized service delivery is achieved alongside efficient time management. Utilizing these platforms allows individuals to avoid hospitals altogether. This change allows them to save on travel fees [17, 18]. Doing this will reduce travel costs for medical professionals. By transitioning away from traditional modes of documentation, doctors could alleviate some of their dependence on physical materials. From improved learning to more thorough assessments, the expansion of healthcare apps has significantly impacted how patients receive treatment. Via various approaches, doctors closely observe patients' states. During routine consultations, patients will share updates via the app after receiving medical advice. As a consequence, highly individualized services are provided while simultaneously saving time. There's a chance that those living in isolated areas won't have access to some clinics. However, by bringing physicians and clinics online, web-based telemedicine program have found a solution to this issue. With the help of this software, people in faraway locations may easily contact medical consultants.

3.3.6 Mobile Applications

From the paper by Shen et al. [1] the trend of mobile healthcare applications, which are referred to as mobile telehealth applications, is tied closely to telehealth. The doctor and patient can communicate using their favorite mobile or desktop digital device with the use of a telehealth program. The world is heavily digitized, and the rise of mobile healthcare applications has begun to alter the landscape of the healthcare sector. A subset of telehealth called telemedicine makes use of a variety of contemporary technology to provide medical care remotely using software and communication tools. As a result, the market for mobile applications for telemedicine is expanding more quickly. From the paper by Zhang et al. [19], in a short amount of time, telehealth mobile applications provide patients with a number of advantages, including accessibility to medical services, prompt medical attention and digital preservation of medical data, a centralized patient management and monitoring system, and efficient time management of medical professionals. From the paper by Tripathy et al. [20], due to the utilization of technologies like artificial intelligence, big data, blockchain, and IoT in the development of mobile healthcare apps, demand for these services is rising. Using data-capable mobile devices with cellular or Wi-Fi access, a mobile app facilitates consultations between healthcare practitioners and patients from any place, even while on the road. From the paper by Zhang et al. [19] mobile apps are a type of cloud computing in which locally installed client software interacts with servers to provide services via networks. Cloud systems are software based, and client apps are made to access software on servers that handle communications using microphone and camera features that have been integrated into or added to local computing equipment. They differ greatly from conventional, stand-alone hardware video conferencing systems because they are more scalable and flexible. Enhanced processor abilities enable smooth video chats via apps, eliminating reliance on external devices. These devices feature integrated cameras, contributing to the trend of camera-equipped mobile computers such as tablets, smartphones, and more.

3.4 DISCUSSION AND ANALYSIS

Thanks to this arrangement, nurses may stay connected with trained doctors even if patients develop concerns about shifting conditions. By using telemedicine applications, nurse admit rates decline substantially due to reduced need for hospitalizations. Recognition of how telemedicine reduces hospital visits abounds. From the paper by Pacis et al. [4]. More readily available Adding to the first point, research demonstrates that telehealth services are most advantageous in situations where care would otherwise be unavailable or severely constrained due to a lack of care resources. As telemedicine becomes more and more popular, healthcare professionals are able to stay in touch with and reach out to their patients, providing a stable and dependable communication option.

3.5 FUTURE CHALLENGES

For clubs and organizations, collecting online payments from customers may be challenging. Medicare and other commercial and public health insurance programs formerly had restrictions on the number of telehealth sessions they would cover. From the paper by Sivani et al. [21] the majority of these Medicare limits were, however, eased by the government during the COVID-19 pandemic. In turn, this presents a chance for insurance companies. It is now simpler for healthcare institutions to accept payments or reimbursements, thanks to the removal of this limitation. When it comes to health information, both patients and providers have serious privacy concerns. From the paper by Alwashmi et al. [22] even on the patient's end, you must make sure that all communication endpoints are secure and encrypted. Data privacy is an issue due of the possibility of cyberattacks on both sides. Depending on the telehealth services you provide, you can deal with enormous volumes of data every day, including patient records, videos, and medical imaging scans. Large-scale management of sensitive patient data is extremely difficult and calls for specialized knowledge and expertise. Keeping such data secure may be a difficult task, especially in light of how crucial it is. From the paper by Pace et al. [23] it might be difficult to convert your practice to digital. Patients who lack digital literacy frequently quit applications too soon. So that patients may use the application from any location, you must provide solutions that are easily accessible, adaptable, and simple to use. In the end, if your solution is unusable or overly complex, you risk losing clients.

3.6 CONCLUSION

The current era is marked by the rapid expansion of computer intelligence, a transformative technology that will surpass existing capabilities and revolutionize both manual tasks and current technologies. By shedding light on the significance of this technology's deployment in medicine, this article offers valuable insights. The technology's user-friendly nature has led to its broad application in multiple domains. Within a telemedicine app, adding more patient beds is just one of the options while figuring out how to carry out a procedure that will impact many lives. Diversified telemedicine offers boundless growth potential. From the paper by Pacis et al. [4] even though telemedicine has been able to keep up with advances in artificial intelligence, there are still problems that need to be fixed. Since carrying out this study will be its main contribution, it is imperative to start looking at methods to make this technology affordable so that it may be used in rural regions and underserved medical settings.

REFERENCES

1. Shen, Y. T., Chen, L., Yue, W. W., & Xu, H. X. (2021). Digital technology-based telemedicine for the COVID-19 pandemic. Frontiers in Medicine, 8, 646506.
2. Bhaskar, S., Bradley, S., Sakhamuri, S., Moguilner, S., Chattu, V. K., Pandya, S., & Banach, M. (2020). Designing futuristic telemedicine using artificial intelligence and robotics in the COVID-19 era. Frontiers in Public Health, 708, 556789.

3. Suman, S., Mishra, S., Sahoo, K. S., & Nayyar, A. (2022). Vision navigator: A smart and intelligent obstacle recognition model for visually impaired users. Mobile Information Systems, 2022, 1–15.
4. Pacis, D. M. M., Subido, E. D. Jr, & Bugtai, N. T. (2018, February). "Trends in Telemedicine Utilizing Artificial Intelligence," AIP Conference Proceedings (Vol. 1933, No. 1, p. 040009). AIP Publishing LLC.
5. Raghuwanshi, S., Singh, M., Rath, S., & Mishra, S. (2022). Prominent Cancer Risk Detection Using Ensemble Learning. In Cognitive Informatics and Soft Computing: Proceeding of CISC 2021 (pp. 677–689). Springer Nature Singapore, Singapore.
6. Patnaik, M., & Mishra, S. (2022). Indoor Positioning System Assisted Big Data Analytics in Smart Healthcare. In Connected e-Health: Integrated IoT and Cloud Computing (pp. 393–415). Springer International Publishing, Cham.
7. Sridhar, K. V. (2008, September). "Implementation of Prioritised ROI Coding for Medical Image Archiving Using JPEG2000," 2008 International Conference on Signals and Electronic Systems (pp. 239–242). IEEE.
8. Mishra, S., Thakkar, H. K., Singh, P., & Sharma, G. (2022). A decisive metaheuristic attribute selector enabled combined unsupervised-supervised model for chronic disease risk assessment. Computational Intelligence and Neuroscience, 2022, 1–7.
9. Alanzi, T. (2021). A review of mobile applications available in the App and Google Play Stores used during the COVID-19 outbreak. Journal of Multidisciplinary Healthcare, 14, 45–57.
10. Abouzid, M., El-Sherif, D. M., Eltewacy, N. K., Dahman, N. B. H., Okasha, S. A., Ghozy, S., & Islam, S. M. S. (2021). Influence of COVID-19 on lifestyle behaviors in the Middle East and North Africa region: A survey of 5896 individuals. Journal of Translational Medicine, 19(1), 1–11.
11. Sahoo, P. K., Mishra, S., Panigrahi, R., Bhoi, A. K., & Barsocchi, P. (2022). An improvised deep-learning-based mask R-CNN model for laryngeal cancer detection using CT images. Sensors, 22(22), 8834.
12. Qadir, J., Mujeeb-U-Rahman, M., Rehmani, M. H., Pathan, A. S. K., Imran, M., Hussain, A., & Luo, A. (2017). IEEE access special section editorial: Health informatics for the developing world. IEEE Access, 5, 27818–27823.
13. Haleem, A., & Javaid, M. (2020). Medical 4.0 and its role in healthcare during COVID-19 pandemic: A review. Journal of Industrial Integration and Management, 5(04), 531–545.
14. Dutta, P., & Mishra, S. (2022). A comprehensive review analysis of Alzheimer's disorder using machine learning approach. Augmented Intelligence in Healthcare: A Pragmatic and Integrated Analysis, 1, 63–76.
15. Filkins, B. L., Kim, J. Y., Roberts, B., Armstrong, W., Miller, M. A., Hultner, M. L., & Steinhubl, S. R. (2016). Privacy and security in the era of digital health: What should translational researchers know and do about it? American Journal of Translational Research, 8(3), 1560.
16. Manogaran, G., Thota, C., Lopez, D., & Sundarasekar, R. (2017). Big Data Security Intelligence for Healthcare Industry 4.0. Cybersecurity for Industry 4.0: Analysis for Design and Manufacturing (pp. 103–126), Springer, Berlin.
17. Hathaliya, J., Sharma, P., Tanwar, S., & Gupta, R. (2019, December). "Blockchain-Based Remote Patient Monitoring in Healthcare 4.0," *2019 IEEE 9th International Conference on Advanced Computing (IACC)* (pp. 87–91). IEEE, Tiruchirappalli, India.
18. Yan, H., Xu, L. D., Bi, Z., Pang, Z., Zhang, J., & Chen, Y. (2015). An emerging technology—wearable wireless sensor networks with applications in human health condition monitoring. Journal of Management Analytics, 2(2), 121–137.
19. Zhang, K., Liu, W. L., Locatis, C., & Ackerman, M. (2016). Mobile videoconferencing apps for telemedicine. Telemedicine and e-Health, 22(1), 56–62.

20. Tripathy, H. K., Mishra, S., Suman, S., Nayyar, A., & Sahoo, K. S. (2022). Smart COVID-shield: An IoT driven reliable and automated prototype model for COVID-19 symptoms tracking. Computing, 104(6), 1233–1254.
21. Sivani, T., & Mishra, S. (2022). Wearable Devices: Evolution and Usage in Remote Patient Monitoring System. In Connected e-Health: Integrated IoT and Cloud Computing (pp. 311–332). Springer International Publishing, Cham.
22. Alwashmi, M. F. (2020). The use of digital health in the detection and management of COVID-19. International Journal of Environmental Research and Public Health, 17(8), 2906.
23. Pace, P., Aloi, G., Gravina, R., Caliciuri, G., Fortino, G., & Liotta, A. (2018). An edge-based architecture to support efficient applications for healthcare industry 4.0. IEEE Transactions on Industrial Informatics, 15(1), 481–489.

4 Prospective of Internet of Medical Things in Revolutionizing Connected Healthcare

Kratika Kansal, Samikshya Sarangi, Saakshi Smriti, and Khaled Shaalan

4.1 INTRODUCTION

The Internet of Medical Things (IoMT) is part of the Internet of Things (IoT), commonly known as the Healthcare IoT, which represents a network of medical devices, software, treatments, and services that utilize network technology to transmit real-time information. An illustration of such a "device" in an IoMT system is a pulse rate monitor that transmits the patient's data to the medical center's cloud-based software, allowing the doctor to access it during emergencies [1, 2].

The IoT encompasses the connectivity and data exchange among physical devices or "things" using the Internet. It has experienced consistent expansion since Ashton's initial proposal in 1999, resulting in approximately 10 billion interconnected IoT devices today and projected to reach 25 billion by 2025. Technically, it involves enhancing data exchange and storage in secure cloud servers, focusing on the interaction equipment that facilitates network communication. Many product/device innovations make them "intelligent" by incorporating software capable of introducing new functionalities or enabling new features/apps. The IoMT empowers rural patients to utilize telemedicine for monitoring, diagnosing, and treatment, connecting them with caregivers or doctors.

The IoMT is a network of medical devices and applications that can be connected to medical information systems using connected devices. It can reduce unnecessary hospital visits and treatment burden by connecting patients to their doctors and allowing medical information to be sent in network security. According to Frost & Sullivan, the global IoT market was valued at $22.5 billion in 2016; It is expected to reach $72.02 billion by 2021 with a YBBO of 26. IoT business strictly includes smart equipment such as equipment and medical/life care equipment for use in physical therapy, home or community, treatment center illness or hospital, and related to real-time, telemedicine and other services.

 DOI: 10.1201/9781032624891-4

4.2 ARCHITECTURE OF IoMT

The architecture of IoMT combines medical devices, sensors, connectivity, data management, analytics, security, and integration to create a robust ecosystem for connected healthcare. By leveraging these components, IoMT aims to enhance patient monitoring, enable remote care, support personalized medicine, and drive improvements in healthcare outcomes.

- The perception layer consists of a range of intelligent medical devices that collect various health data.
- The connectivity layer facilitates data transmission between the perception layer and the cloud, using connectivity technologies like networks and gateways.
- The processing layer involves cloud middleware or IoT platforms responsible for storing and managing data.
- The application layer provides end users with data analytics, reporting, and device control opportunities through software solutions.

The architecture of IoMT in Figure 4.1 combines medical devices, sensors, connectivity, data management, analytics, security, and integration to create a robust ecosystem for connected healthcare. By leveraging these components, IoMT aims to enhance patient monitoring, enable remote care, support personalized medicine, and drive improvements in healthcare outcomes.

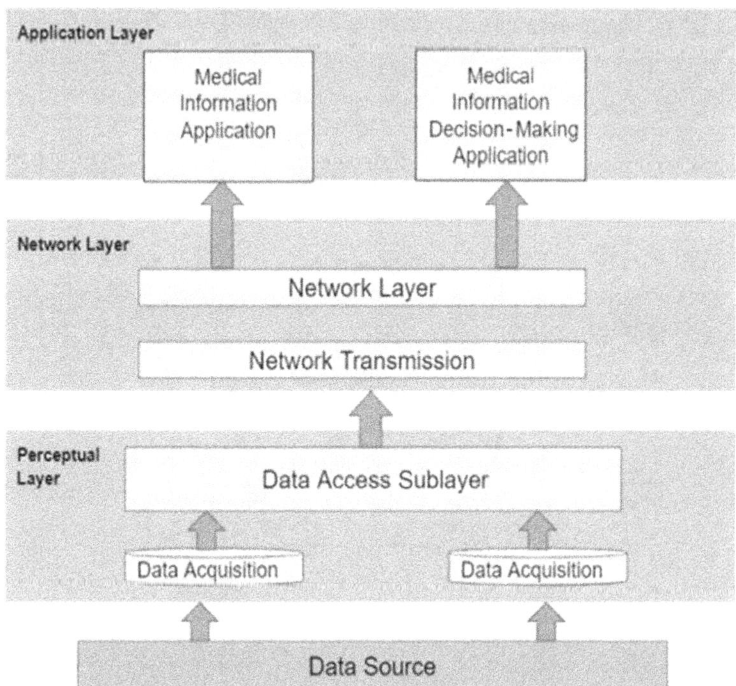

FIGURE 4.1 Architecture of IoMT.

4.3 EVOLUTION OF IoMT

Revenue from the IoT segment should reach approximately $66 billion in 2020, up 20% from 2019 due to the rapid growth of IoT in healthcare [3]. According to the 2018 Deloitte report, IoT markets are expected to be worth $158.1 billion by 2022. That's triple the amount compared to 2017 in Figure 4.2. Another 27% expect to consider using technology in the short term. IoT-based smart rehabilitation was recently introduced to reduce resource scarcity caused by the elderly. It can be seen as a subsystem within the framework of a smart city.

By interconnecting all available resources, it enables remote medical tasks like diagnosis, monitoring, and surgery to be performed over the Internet.

- Complete responsibility is assumed for the seamless continuation of healthcare services, spanning from the hospital to the community and ultimately to patients' homes [4, 5]. Wireless technology plays a significant role in tandem with monitoring equipment, with the latter serving as a network manager. This comprehensive system interlinks all accessible medical resources within the community, encompassing hospitals, clinics, doctors, nurses, ambulances, and medical equipment while also being accessible to patients. The core of this system consists of a server housing a central database. Expert personnel are tasked with data analysis, integration, identification of critical incidents, and the formulation of rehabilitation strategies. All aspects of this system are interconnected through the Internet, supported by RFID technology-based programs. The overall evolution of the IoMT is shown in Figure 4.3.

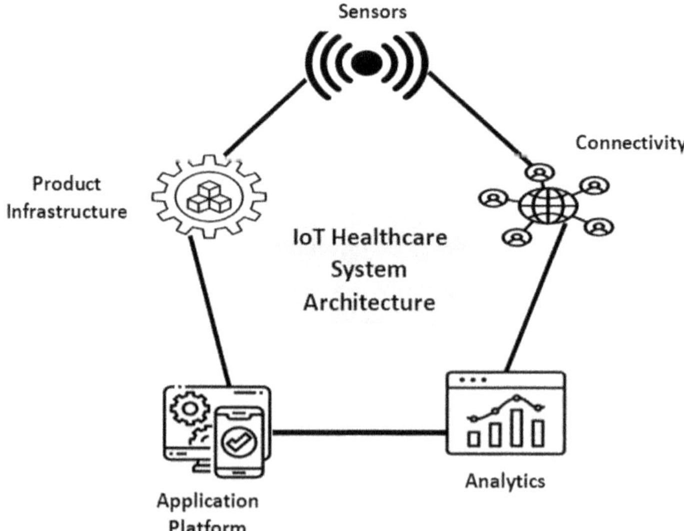

FIGURE 4.2 IoT healthcare system architecture.

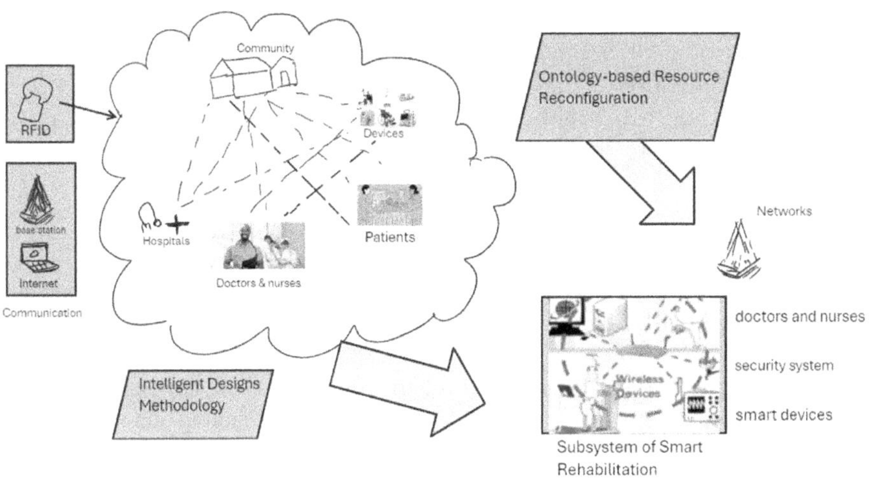

FIGURE 4.3 Evolution of IoMT.

A mechanized allocation system was developed to identify solutions that would meet the patient's unique criteria.

The concept of IoT in healthcare has gradually evolved, comprising three main components: Control, Hub, and Entities. Control involves doctors, nurses, and patients, accessing the system through end-user devices like smartphones, PCs, or tablets with specific permissions. Hub serves as the central part of the healthcare system, managing prescriptions, databases, data analysis, subsystems, and knowledge bases. Entities encompass all physical objects, including patients and human resources, connected via wide area networks (WAN), multimedia tech, or SMS. Additionally, non-networked devices used in rehabilitation are integrated into the smart rehabilitation system and made network-compatible. The proposed architecture's efficacy has been validated through pioneering exoskeleton applications.

4.4 FEATURES OF IoMT

In the healthcare domain, IoMT finds diverse applications, particularly in remote and self-health monitoring. Vital functions like heart rate, skin temperature, movement, and overall health conditions are monitored, along with nutrition status and rehabilitation for elderly or infected patients. These applications contribute significantly to increasing life expectancy and reducing morbidity and mortality rates [6, 7]. Treatment is getting more and more expensive and sometimes not worth it. IoT solutions can reduce service provider costs through the prevention of serious diseases, elimination of self-diagnosis, and provision of affordable healthcare; IoT brings numerous benefits. Analysts predict that the implementation of IoT in the US healthcare industry could result in annual savings of $300 billion. With the spread of COVID-19 in the world, more and more people are taking their health more and more seriously, resulting in increased demand for healthcare products.

4.5 FACTORS AFFECTING THE IoMT APPLICATION

There are various factors (Figure 4.4) that affect the IoT healthcare application. Some of them are listed below:

- Ongoing research plays a crucial role in advancing medical fields, such as intelligent gadgets and high-speed communication, enabling enhanced and expedited care options for patients.
- The integration of intelligent gadgets in healthcare services is essential, as IoT unlocks the potential of existing technologies, driving innovation in medical devices and services.
- Leveraging IoT technology, healthcare professionals gain access to extensive patient data, facilitating comprehensive analysis and enabling the delivery of superior patient care.
- IoT technology fosters transparent sharing of medical information, ensuring accurate and timely dissemination to patients. These results in reduced errors arising from miscommunication, improved preventive care, and heightened patient satisfaction.

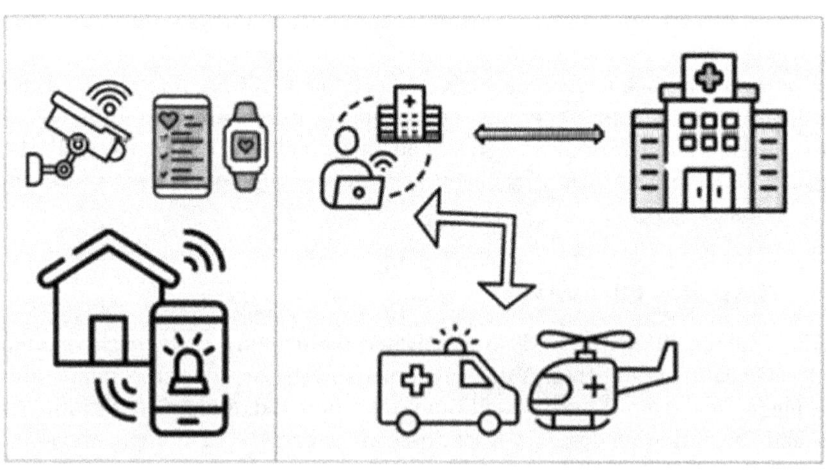

FIGURE 4.4 Factors affecting IoT healthcare application.

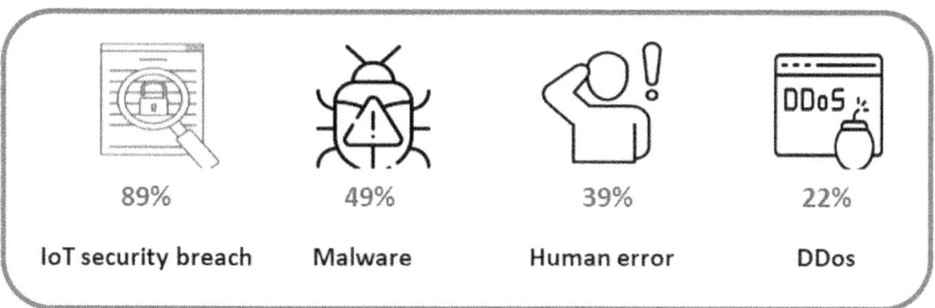

FIGURE 4.5 Challenges of IoT in healthcare.

4.6 CHALLENGES IN IoMT

With IoMT, most of the data collection tasks are reduced, but to improve pain knowledge, one needs to have some additional knowledge about:

- General body pain and response assessment. This indicates the need for an automated system with certain settings.
- Knowing the conditions that cause pain will help to avoid diagnosis.
- Data collected from medical, psychiatric, and Medical Internet of Things (MIoT) devices (including computers) will be useful in diagnosing patients. Because it is not possible to measure pain using either or both. Therefore, human-computer interaction will really help in automatic recognition [8].
- The most difficult problem for automatic pain recognition is the availability of data. If we consider facial pain, we know that pain is present and lasts only a few minutes [9–13]. So these kinds of things are hard to catch. Another advantage that exists in data is that it is multi-modal, annotated, and needs to be constructed with pain to evaluate details by other states.
- Information should be shared and progress should be made in this area. In the current context, several databases are available for research, including the BioVid and the UNBC-McMaster shoulder pain database. In the future, more data validation and evaluation are needed to find out how well the system works for other diseases, types of diseases, and for all medical professionals.
- The need for improved algorithms and IoMT tools to improve clinical operations [14].

Figure 4.5 outlines various challenges of IoT in healthcare.

4.7 SECURITY FOR HEALTHCARE SYSTEMS

The IoT plays an important role in many medical applications, from chronic disease management on one end to disease prevention on the other. This requires sensors to collect data about the body and employing gateway devices and cloud infrastructure facilitates data analysis and storage, followed by wireless transmission of the analyzed data to medical professionals for further examination and assessment [15]. Implementing these innovative methods enhances healthcare accessibility and quality while concurrently decreasing overall costs. However, incorporating novel technologies in healthcare without adequate consideration for security compromises patient confidentiality, making their privacy susceptible to breaches and potential cyberattacks. A person's body knowledge is very powerful. Modern healthcare requires comprehensive healthcare with physical interaction between doctors and patients, and this can be achieved through the IoT host. It uses eight Wireless Medical Sensor Networks (WMSN).

Wireless medical sensors can be mobile and compact and can combine various wireless communication technologies (Mica2, MicaZ, Telos, etc.). Wireless medical sensors collect/generate a lot of data that needs to be protected against security attacks. By using security algorithms/technologies, we can prevent a lot of bad data from occurring during transmission to remote locations [16]. Therefore, safety is important for medical use.

For ethical and legal reasons, the success of medical practice depends on the safety and privacy of the patient. Some Healthcare Safety Applications Based on WMSN:

- **Remote Monitoring:** It can be used to collect patients' health information between sensors, use complex algorithms to analyze the data, and then send it over the wireless link to the medical device. Professionals can provide appropriate health advice. It is shown in Figure 4.6.
- **Body Tracking for the Elderly:** Body Sensor Networks (BSN) measuring movement/speed, vital signs, temperature, blood pressure, and heart rate and mobile devices collect, visualize, and document work [17].

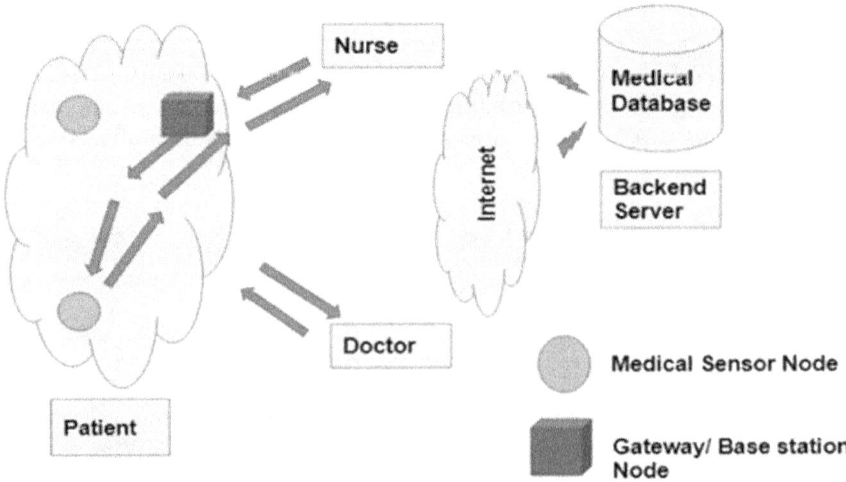

FIGURE 4.6 Healthcare architecture for patient monitoring.

- **Patient Self-Care:** The Body Area Network (BAN) network in diabetic patients can facilitate insulin injection from the pump when insulin levels drop [18, 19].
- **Disease Management:** It can be used for patient care with integrated patient care and remote care of patients with diseases such as pneumonia, heart and diabetes.

4.8 BENEFITS OF IoMT IN HEALTHCARE

IoT for healthcare is helping hospitals better care for their patients. While the rapid growth of the population will not help control the growing number of diseases, aging, and other health problems, the introduction of IoT medical solutions will pay off. There is no doubt that IoT and healthcare go hand in hand. Some crucial use cases of IoMT are shown in Figure 4.7. Some of the most important benefits of IoT are listed below.

- **Simultaneous Observation and Surveillance** IoT in the medical industry helps doctors to treat heart failure, diabetes, pain, asthma, heart disease, etc. It enables it to monitor patients in real time for emergencies such as remote patient diagnosis and clinical parameters tracking.

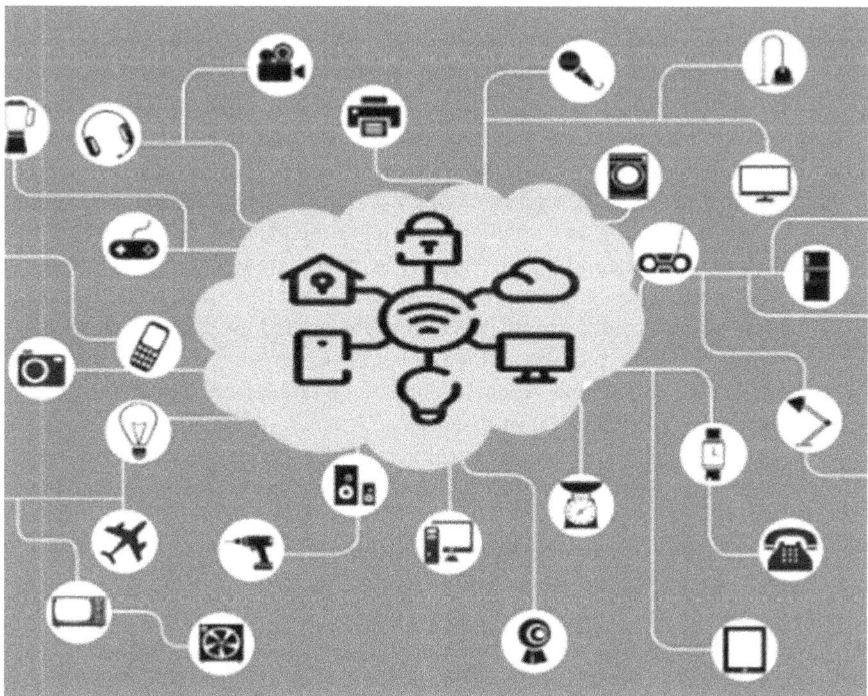

FIGURE 4.7 Real-life IoMT use cases.

For example, a patient's vital signs can be monitored through real-time observation and real-time surveillance, and information can be instantly shown to their doctor. This is especially useful in emergencies where every second counts [20]. Another example is clinical trials, where data from many patients can be collected and analyzed simultaneously. This helps speed up the process of finding new treatments and curing diseases.

- **End-to-End Connectivity and Affordability** In healthcare applications, the IoT provides better connectivity and uses new technologies to improve connectivity and information sharing. Bluetooth, Wi-Fi, etc. With these technologies, tracking and identification of the virus is easier and takes less time [21, 22]. For example, the IoT can connect different devices and systems in hospitals to provide better care. In addition, IoT can help reduce the cost of care by improving quality and improving patient outcomes. The IoT can also assist in remote monitoring of patients with chronic diseases and ultimately reduce readmissions. Similarly, the use of smart drugs and consumables can help improve medication adherence and prevent side effects.
- **Real-Time Data Analysis and Real-time Data Distribution** The benefits of IoMT include collecting a large amount of information about patients' medical history. IoT devices seamlessly transmit data to other devices [23–25]. Analyzing such large amounts of personal data is impossible, but IoT medical devices can do it. IoT medical devices can collect, analyze, monitor, transmit, and receive data with the help of the cloud.

  The amount of data is large, cannot be stored on the server, and requires a cloud library. What can help greater adoption and efficiency of data storage and transmission is the IoT blockchain. This can help IoT and healthcare collaboration prove its value in the healthcare industry [26–28].
- **Assisting the Elderly** One broad area that will particularly benefit from the use of IoT healthcare solutions is helping the elderly. By providing the elderly with devices that can monitor their vital signs and provide medication reminders, caregivers can provide more care while reducing the risk of hospitalization or other health problems [29, 30]. In addition, IoT devices are used to monitor losses and notify supervisors immediately in an emergency. For example, Apple has integrated fall detection into the Apple Watch, which can detect if the user has fallen.

  As the population ages and healthcare needs increase, IoT healthcare solutions are becoming more and more important in ensuring that the elderly receive care.
- **Real-Time Tracking and Real-Time Alerts** Consider how many people could be saved with emergency alerts sent by patients. This is possible because of IoMT. Smart devices in the medical profession helped the medical information of the patients to be recorded in a timely manner and sent to the doctor [31]. When there is a threat, the doctor will first be notified and will offer the appropriate aid.

Consider a heart attack patient who is fitted with a device to monitor heart rate. If the device detects an abnormal heartbeat, it can send real-time notifications to the patient's doctor. This will allow physicians to take prompt action and perhaps save lives.

- **Check-up on the Go** IoT in healthcare has been used for some major projects in the healthcare IoT industry. From monitoring patients to helping them recover, the applications for IoT are vast and varied. Below are some of the medical IoT applications [32]. While the transportation and logistics industry is rapidly adopting IoT for more efficient fleet management, the medical industry is not far behind in medical devices using IoT. Let's see when and where IoT technology can be used in real life.
- **Fall Detection and Fall Prevention** Elderly individuals are at a higher risk of experiencing falls and the resulting injuries, such as harm to the head or ankle. A variety of IoT solutions have been tailored to target this issue. For instance, Active Protector's Tango smart belt is outfitted with sensors capable of detecting falls and delivering immediate safeguarding [33]. The belt synchronizes with the relevant software app, enabling it to promptly notify medical personnel or nursing staff in the event of a fall, as well as record and exhibit motion data on a phone or computer (Figure 4.8).
- **Sleep Monitor** Numerous sleep-tracking devices and software options are accessible to aid in monitoring sleep, recognizing crucial indicators, and enhancing sleep quality. For instance, Apple and Samsung smartwatches come equipped with sensors that observe heart rate and respiration. The information provides a rough overview of sleep duration, intensity, and phases. Since the device is synchronized with the smartphone, the data can be used for in-depth analysis and shared with doctors.

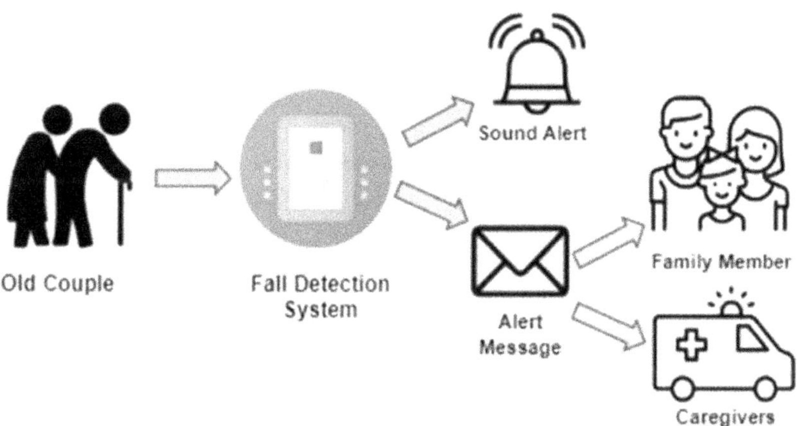

FIGURE 4.8 Fall detection system.

- **Management of Hospital Assets and Upkeep of Equipment** IoT makes the concept of smart hospitals a reality. Hospitals can receive a signal about the location of equipment such as defibrillators with tracking devices connected to medical equipment, so it can be quickly transported to where it is needed, such as an emergency room. Or they may know when stocks are running low to replenish.
- **Diabetes Data Monitoring and Reporting** The corporation also possesses exclusive software for overseeing and generating reports about diabetes data. Notably, there exist uninterrupted glucose monitoring systems, such as Dexcom, which aid individuals with type 2 diabetes in regulating their health and blood sugar levels without necessitating constant manual input. This setup encompasses a wearable gadget alongside a water-resistant sensor positioned beneath the skin's surface. The sensor tracks interstitial fluid and wirelessly transmits glucose readings every five minutes to a receptor, smartphone, or smartwatch.
- **Remote Patient Monitoring** Private Healthcare Software Development Company The company mainly uses IoT for remote patient monitoring. Medical IoT devices can measure the blood pressure, pulse, body temperature, etc., of patients outside the hospital. It is designed to collect health metrics. These algorithms can help identify key symptoms and recommend treatment or simply generate alerts.
- **Reducing Waiting Time** Patient contentment holds significant significance within healthcare, and diminishing periods of waiting stands as a means to augment patient contentment. The IoT can contribute to the reduction of waiting duration through diverse approaches [34]. As an illustration, IoT-empowered patient registration can expedite the enrollment procedure. Moreover, IoT-linked devices can be utilized to trace the real-time whereabouts of both patients and personnel, thereby enhancing the movement of patients within the vicinity. IoT holds the potential to heighten the patient encounter and elevate satisfaction levels by mitigating wait times.
- **Keeping Track of Hardware Maintenance** One of the most crucial elements of implementing IoT in the healthcare sector is the monitoring of hardware. Envision a medical facility with numerous pieces of medical apparatus. It's practically unfeasible for staff to recall the most recent maintenance date for each individual piece of equipment. In IoT systems, each device can be outfitted with a sensor that transmits data to a central database [35]. This data can generate reports that aid staff in staying informed about the servicing needs of any equipment. This not only guarantees the proper upkeep of all equipment but also diminishes the likelihood of malfunctions. Within medical institutions, where even a brief span of time can lead to severe ramifications, such a system has the potential to save lives.
- **Tracking Employees and Patients** Hospitals have large buildings, so it is impossible to keep track of the whereabouts of every employee or doctor at

any given time. The same is true for all patients. It is easy to follow patients and staff with IoT technology [36]. This technology is also employed for the surveillance of hospital assets to ensure security. It stands as an excellent method for monitoring items or individuals without incurring additional expenses or exerting extra energy.

- **Drug Management** By employing IoT devices, people can promptly receive notifications when it's time to take their prescribed medicines. Data collected from these devices can also be utilized to supervise compliance with medication schedules and identify possible issues connected to drugs [37]. Moreover, IoT technology has the capacity to monitor the storage and transportation of pharmaceuticals, ensuring proper storage conditions and providing protection against tampering. By enhancing the efficiency and effectiveness of pharmaceutical monitoring, IoT offers the potential to improve patient outcomes and reduce healthcare costs.
- **Identification of Chronic Diseases** IoT medical technology can identify the chronic diseases a patient suffers from. How it works: enter patient symptoms and IoT medical devices compete with available data to identify disease. Wearables like the Fitbit are good heart rate, blood sugar, and blood pressure monitors [38]. Medical application development for wearable devices and mobile applications allows people to be more health conscious and know about their diseases.
- **Healthcare Charting** Doctors spend a lot of time and effort educating their patients. It will be interesting to see how the IoT (Figure 4.9) is used and doctors can call up important information about patients via voice commands.

This health document comprises medical background, population characteristics, diagnoses, medications, therapy strategies, prescriptions, immunization timetables, sensitivities, examinations (X-ray, cardiology, radiology, urine, blood, etc.), and findings. To illustrate, Augmedix aids in generating health records, allowing physicians to concentrate on patient well-being.

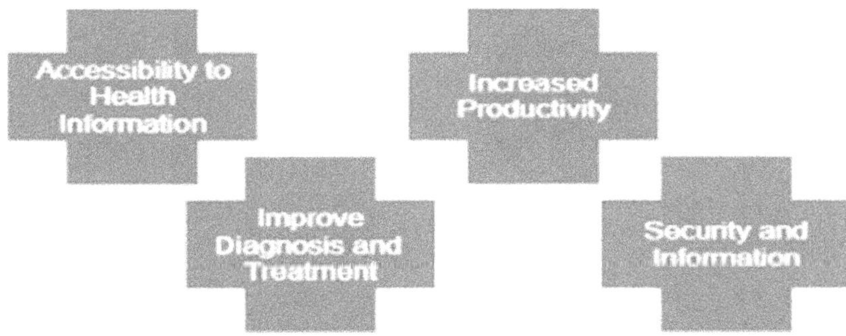

FIGURE 4.9 Benefits of medical charting.

4.9 FUTURE SCOPE OF IoMT

The futuristic trend scope is shown in Figure 4.10. The IoT holds significant promise, extending beyond just the healthcare sector. Numerous medical IoT enterprises are engaged in novel initiatives, leveraging this technology to advance the field of medicine. According to Mordor Intelligence, the IoT's influence on healthcare is projected to amass a market value of $89.6 billion by 2026, a catalyst for the burgeoning adoption of IoT in healthcare. In spite of the challenges and limitations posed by the IoT, these impediments will not impede its technological evolution. The demand for IoT within the healthcare realm is substantial and stands to substantially benefit the industry [39]. Its potential impact spans across global patient populations, bridging the gap between medical practitioners and patients. Evidently, the IoT has already exerted a profound influence on healthcare and will continue its expansion.

The medical field predominantly focuses on IoT advancements, marking a juncture where medical IoT applications could expedite patient treatment and reduce costs. Giants like Google and Apple are diligently advancing the amalgamation of IoT and healthcare, soon integrating iOS and Android devices into medical interactions.

In the foreseeable future, IoT will enable real-time monitoring of patients' vital signs, digitally recording comprehensive treatment data to mitigate ongoing inquiries, especially concerning patients afflicted by COVID-19. Healthcare will witness enhancement through novel technologies, compelling medical professionals to embrace these innovations. IoT, a mature and sophisticated technology with extensive applications, epitomizes precision medicine, providing an exceptional platform to analyze invaluable data, insights, and diagnostics. It harbors future potential in streamlining medical inventory management, guaranteeing timely access to appropriate medical resources.

IoT-enabled smart devices will operate autonomously, preserving data within both private and public clouds. Even software components will reside in the cloud, optimizing analysis and retrieval efficiency. This transformative innovation in information technology stands poised to fortify intelligent healthcare within the context of the healthcare 4.0 paradigm.

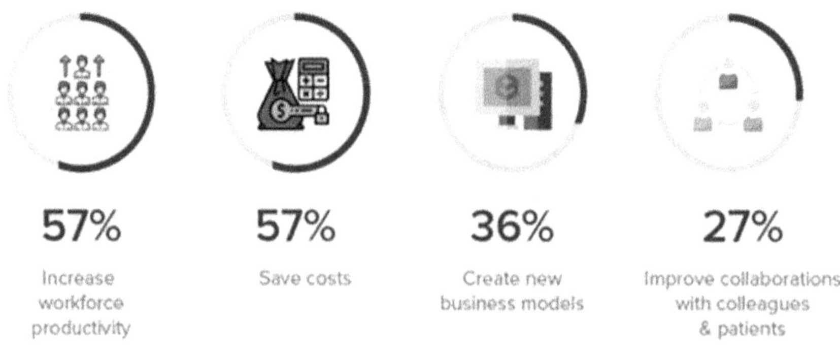

FIGURE 4.10 The future outlook of IoT in healthcare.

4.10 CONCLUSION

IoT is used for quality disease control, emergency medicine, better patient care, healthcare, blood pressure monitoring, health screening, measurement and control systems, heart rate monitors, and hearing aids. It provides continuous and reliable monitoring of COVID-19 patients and provides better self-awareness in healthcare. IoT devices can support digital storage of COVID-19 patients' personal health information and connect to different databases. These systems can help reduce data processing. It minimizes errors and delivers timely results with informed decision making.

Medical devices and connections using this technology are getting smarter and more efficient during the COVID-19 pandemic. Therefore, these technologies can provide up-to-date information and expand communication to improve patients' quality of life. In the future, this technology will advance in better treatment of patients and will be applicable to any COVID-19 outbreak.

In the current situation, information technologies have opened the door to innovations in our daily lives. Among these information technologies, IoT is a new technology that offers better and better solutions in healthcare such as accurate medical information storage such as joint and disease causes.

IoT sensor-based technology has the potential to reduce the risk of surgery in critical situations and help respond to the COVID-19 outbreak. In healthcare, IoT focuses on helping treat different cases of COVID-19. It makes the surgeon's job easier by reducing risk and improving overall performance. Using this technology, doctors can detect changes in vital signs of COVID-19 patients. Such a knowledge-based program opens the door to new medical applications as it improves the treatment system in the hospital and adapts to the best information path to match outcomes in the world.

Medical students are now better trained in disease research and better informed for their future careers. Proper use of IoT can help solve different health problems such as speed, cost, and complexity. It can be easily adjusted to monitor calorie intake and treatment of COVID-19 patients such as asthma, diabetes, and arthritis. This digital health management system can improve the overall performance of the health system during the COVID-19 pandemic.

REFERENCES

1. K. Christensen, G. Doblhammer, R. Rau, and J. W. Vaupel, "Aging populations: The challenges ahead," The Lancet, vol. 374, no. 9696, pp. 1196–1208, 2009.
2. D. Yach, C. Hawkes, C. L. Gould, and K. J. Hofman, "The global burden of chronic diseases: Overcoming impediments to prevention and control," Journal of the American Medical Association, vol. 291, no. 21, pp. 2616–2622, 2004.
3. A. Darkins, P. Ryan, R. Kobb, L. Foster, E. Edmonson, B. Wakefield, and A. E. Lancaster, "Care coordination/home telehealth: The systematic implementation of health informatics, home telehealth, and disease management to support the care of veteran patients with chronic conditions," Telemedicine and e-Health, vol. 14, no. 10, pp. 1118–1126, 2008.
4. A. G. Ekeland, A. Bowes, and S. Flottorp, "Effectiveness of telemedicine: A systematic review of reviews," International Journal of Medical Informatics, vol. 79, no. 11, pp. 736–771, 2010.

5. I. Lee, and O. Sokolsky, "Medical cyber physical systems," in Proceedings of the 47th Design Automation Conference. ACM, 2010, pp. 743–748.
6. W. Wolf, "Cyber-physical systems," Computer, vol. 3, no. 3, pp. 88–89, 2009.
7. E. Lee, "Cyber physical systems: Design challenges," in 11th IEEE International Symposium on Object Oriented Real-Time Distributed Computing. IEEE, 2008, pp. 363–369.
8. E. A. Lee, "CPS foundations," in Proceedings of the 47th Design Automation Conference. ACM, 2010, pp. 737–742.
9. P. J. Ramadge, and W. M. Wonham, "The control of discrete event systems," Proceedings of the IEEE, vol. 77, no. 1, pp. 81–98, 1989.
10. E. A. Lee, and H. Zheng, "Operational semantics of hybrid systems," in Hybrid Systems: Computation and Control. Springer, 2005, pp. 25–53.
11. A. J. Van der Schaft, and J. M. Schumacher, "Complementarity modeling of hybrid systems," IEEE Transactions on Automatic Control, vol. 43, no. 4, pp. 483–490, 1998.
12. P. J. Antsaklis, J. A. Stiver, and M. Lemmon, "Hybrid system modeling and autonomous control systems," in Hybrid Systems. Springer, 1993, pp. 366–392.
13. M. L. Bujorianu, and N. Piterman, "A modeling framework for cyber-physical system resilience," in Cyber Physical Systems. Design, Modeling, and Evaluation. Springer, 2015, pp. 67–82.
14. R. R. Rajkumar, I. Lee, L. Sha, and J. Stankovic, "Cyber-physical systems: The next computing revolution," in Proceedings of the 47th Design Automation Conference, ACM, pp. 731–736, 2010.
15. A. Cardenas, S. Amin, B. Sinopoli, A. Giani, A. Perrig, and S. Sastry, "Challenges for securing cyber physical systems," in Workshop on Future Directions in Cyber-Physical Systems Security, 2009.
16. C. Neuman, "Challenges in security for cyber-physical systems," in DHS: S&T Workshop on Future Directions in Cyber-Physical Systems Security, vol. 7, 2009.
17. N. Kottenstette, G. Karsai, and J. Sztipanovits, "A passivity-based framework for resilient cyber physical systems," in Proceedings of the 2nd International Symposium on Resilient Control Systems. IEEE, 2009, pp. 43–50.
18. Q. Zhu, and T. Başar, "Robust and resilient control design for cyberphysical systems with an application to power systems," in Proceedings of the 50th IEEE Conference on Decision and Control and European Control Conference. IEEE, 2011, pp. 4066–4071.
19. K. Parmar, and D. C. Jinwala, "Hybrid secure data aggregation in wireless sensor networks," in Cyber Physical Systems. Design, Modeling, and Evaluation. Springer, 2015, pp. 116–131.
20. R. Mitchell, and I.-R. Chen, "Behavior rule specification-based intrusion detection for safety critical medical cyber physical systems," IEEE Transactions on Dependable and Secure Computing, vol. 12, no. 1, pp. 16–30, 2015.
21. M. Ghorbani, and P. Bogdan, "A cyber-physical system approach to artificial pancreas design," in Proceedings of the 9th IEEE/ACM/IFIP International Conference on Hardware/Software Codesign and System Synthesis. IEEE Press, 2013, pp. 1–10.
22. P. Bogdan, S. Jain, K. Goyal, and R. Marculescu, "Implantable pacemakers control and optimization via fractional calculus approaches: a cyber-physical systems perspective," in Proceedings of the 2012 IEEE/ACM Third International Conference on Cyber-Physical Systems. IEEE Computer Society, 2012, pp. 23–32.
23. K. K. Venkatasubramanian, E. Y. Vasserman, V. Sfyrla, O. Sokolsky, and I. Lee, "Requirement engineering for functional alarm system for interoperable medical devices," in Computer Safety, Reliability, and Security. Springer, 2015, pp. 252–266.
24. A. Banerjee, K. K. Venkatasubramanian, T. Mukherjee, and S. K. S. Gupta, "Ensuring safety, security, and sustainability of mission-critical cyber–physical systems," Proceedings of the IEEE, vol. 100, no. 1, pp. 283–299, 2012.

25. P. Dong, Y. Han, X. Guo, and F. Xie, "A security and safety framework for cyber physical system," in 7th Conference on Control and Automation. IEEE, 2014, pp. 49–51.
26. S. Schupp, E. Ábrahám, X. Chen, I. B. Makhlouf, G. Frehse, S. Sankaranarayanan, and S. Kowalewski, "Current challenges in the verification of hybrid systems," in Cyber Physical Systems. Design, Modeling, and Evaluation. Springer, 2015, pp. 8–24.
27. P. Kumar, D. Goswami, S. Chakraborty, A. Annaswamy, K. Lampka, and L. Thiele, "A hybrid approach to cyber-physical systems verification," in Proceedings of the 49th Annual Design Automation Conference. ACM, 2012, pp. 688–696.
28. R. A. Thacker, K. R. Jones, C. J. Myers, and H. Zheng, "Automatic abstraction for verification of cyber-physical systems," in Proceedings of the 1st ACM/IEEE International Conference on Cyber-Physical Systems. ACM, 2010, pp. 12–21.
29. G. Frehse, "PHAVer: Algorithmic verification of hybrid systems past HyTech," International Journal on Software Tools for Technology Transfer, vol. 10, no. 3, pp. 263–279, 2008.
30. M. Pajic, Z. Jiang, A. Connolly, S. Dixit, and R. Mangharam, "A platform for implantable medical device validation," in Proceedings of the 9th ACM/IEEE International Conference on Information Processing in Sensor Networks. ACM, 2010, pp. 418–419.
31. A. Arrieta, G. Sagardui, and L. Etxeberria, "Test control algorithms for the validation of cyber-physical systems product lines," in Proceedings of the 19th International Conference on Software Product Line. ACM, 2015, pp. 273–282.
32. Z. Jiang, M. Pajic, and R. Mangharam, "Cyber–physical modeling of implantable cardiac medical devices," Proceedings of the IEEE, vol. 100, no. 1, pp. 122–137, 2012.
33. L. C. Silva, M. Perkusich, F. M. Bublitz, H. O. Almeida, and A. Perkusich, "A model-based architecture for testing medical cyber physical systems," in Proceedings of the 29th Annual ACM Symposium on Applied Computing. ACM, 2014, pp. 25–30.
34. M. U. Sanwal, and O. Hasan, "Formally analyzing continuous aspects of cyber-physical systems modeled by homogeneous linear differential equations," in Cyber Physical Systems. Design, Modeling, and Evaluation. Springer, 2015, pp. 132–146.
35. J. C. Jensen, D. H. Chang, E. Lee, et al., "A model-based design methodology for cyber-physical systems," in 7th International on Wireless Communications and Mobile Computing Conference. IEEE, 2011, pp. 1666–1671.
36. E. A. Lee, and S. A. Seshia, Introduction to Embedded Systems: A Cyber-Physical Systems Approach. Lee & Seshia, 2011.
37. E. Lee, and D. G. Messerschmitt, "Synchronous data flow," Proceedings of the IEEE, vol. 75, no. 9, pp. 1235–1245, 1987.
38. J. Eker, J. W. Janneck, E. Lee, J. Liu, X. Liu, J. Ludvig, S. Neuendorffer, S. Sachs, Y. Xiong, et al., "Taming heterogeneity-the Ptolemy approach," Proceedings of the IEEE, vol. 91, no. 1, pp. 127–144, 2003.
39. C. M. Woodside, J. E. Neilson, D. C. Petriu, and S. Majumdar, "The stochastic rendezvous network model for performance of synchronous client-server-like distributed software," IEEE Transactions on Computers, vol. 44, no. 1, pp. 20–34, 1995.

5 A Comparison Analysis of Cryptographic Methods in Sustainable Healthcare

Tapaswini Tripathy, Anjana Mishra, and Rukaiya Khan

5.1 INTRODUCTION

Currently, the biggest issue with cloud service applications is security [1]. The English word "cryptography" has its roots in the Greek words "Kryptos," which means "hidden," and "graphein," which means "to write" [2]. It's a system for secure communication that prevents third parties from reading private dispatches. Cryptology is about creating protocols that cover the data and prevent it from being accessed by third parties. There are four important aspects of Information Security: (i) Confidentiality, (ii) Non-repudiation, (iii) Data integrity, and (iv) Authentication.

There can be numerous types of attacks possible on defended health information stored on the cloud, e.g., if a patient's credit card information is addressed by a hacker, then he may lose all his money. Also, if the complaint information of a celebrity is blurted out then he/she may lose their career. That's why defended/sensitive information requires protection. All medical data is currently controlled and kept online on a global scale. The information can be used by medical experts, cases for their comprehension, governmental agencies, insurance firms, etc. With electronic health records (EHR), which are always available online, the medically related data can be protected. It includes information on X-ray images, examination images, treatment methods, medical customs, and patient details. The issue with all of these sensitive documents of this nature is how securely they can be stored, as well as who may access the data and examine it. Data security is absolutely necessary for any database that contains digital data in order to protect the data from any unauthorized users. EHR are a common tool used nowadays to convert patient records to electronic format and store them on centralized data servers [1]. Keeping EHRs secure, the patient data may be electronically saved on a local computer, a shared server, or cloud storage [3].

Ciphers have been used for encryption and decryption regularly before authentication and integrity checks. Asymmetric and videlicet symmetric cryptosystems are the two different forms of cryptosystems. In symmetric systems, a message is encoded using a public key and decoded using a private key; in asymmetric systems, both operations call for the use of the secret key (the same key). In symmetric systems, data manipulation is brisk as compared to asymmetric systems as they make use of shorter crucial lengths. Asymmetric systems enhance further

 DOI: 10.1201/9781032624891-5

secure communication. Another method is to use cryptographic quantum hashing. Cryptographic hashing has several useful applications [4].

In all modern paradigms, health monitoring has emerged as a major problem. A UN assessment estimates that by 2050, 22% of the world's population will be made up of weak individuals who are susceptible to contracting numerous diseases. The large data collected from medical devices such as sphygmomanometers and glucose machines should only be shared with authorized persons. And this process has escalated since COVID-19. While working with medical data we must consider the fact that data should be both secured and preserved. It should be secure as about 91% of Medical companies have had data breaches that have, on average, cost them more than $2 million. Apart from that, patients' card details are also at stake because of low privacy. It should be preserved because it can be used for research work, education, diagnosis (recent studies about Parkinson's disease suggest techniques for diagnosing it by improving the automation detection), and treatment of the patient further. One such method—EHR technology; the old paper record paradigm has been replaced by EHR technology, which comes in many forms, including diagnostic reports, pictures, and vital sign signals. It may similarly include a patient's medical background. (This data is centralized and doctors can access the data.) Data, such as demographic information, information about physical exams, lab test results, treatment plans, and medications is all extremely private. It increases data upkeep costs, availability, and sharing. Because critical patient data are shared over a big network, further caution is required, as the loss of these data would jeopardize appropriate diagnosis. When patient information is sent electronically, such information's security, integrity, and secrecy are of utmost importance. A novel research technique for managing multimedia information called digital watermarking (DWM) which is digital watermarking gradually integrates data which is a watermark, into a signal of the host (cover), such as a picture, piece of music, or piece of video. Digital watermarks are used to identify an image uniquely and assert its originality or content. Medical data management and dissemination issues can be solved using DWM techniques, which have the potential to become an all-purpose tool that offers alternatives and/or complementary solutions. The process of DWM involves using a region growth (RG) technique; we start by dividing the supplied tumor image's region of interest (ROI) component. The Secure Hash Algorithm (SHA)-256 is then used to encrypt the ROI. The elliptical curve cryptography is utilized to encrypt the EHR (emergency cardiovascular care [ECC]) method in a similar way. We combine the picture and EHR data and compress it using an AC technique to boost security. Eventually, the original image contains the compressed bit stream. The extraction procedure proceeds in the same manner. The process of watermarking combines dispersed watermark bit embedding in the embedding region with lossless data compression and encryption techniques. According to Mishra [5] in a different study, a security strategy should specifically outline the guidelines for creating, getting access to, and maintaining the integrity of patient e-health data as well as the scope of obligations for each responsible party.

The main methods of data protection have been cryptography and steganography [6]. Although they have diverse goals, they are classified as separate methods of data security. The goal of steganography is to conceal the existence of sensitive information in computer files. While cryptography obscures the importance of a message. Cryptography does not disguise the existence of a message. To increase the security of medical data, this research uses least significant bit (LSB) and 3DESto develop a whole combined system of steganography and cryptography. There are two processes involved.

5.1.1 Triple Data Encryption Standard

For a 192-bit key length, three 64-bit keys are needed. Simply put, we enter all 192 bits. The user-supplied key is then divided into three sub-keys by the Triple-DES DLL, each of which is padded as necessary to a length of 64 bits. Triple DES uses the same encryption process as traditional DES but repeats it three times. With the first key, data is first encrypted, then decrypted, and then encrypted again with the third key. Due to the possibility of meet-in-the-middle attacks, 3DES's robust security is only 112 bits. 3DES is a fairly safe algorithm. It uses a cryptic 168 key that is broken down into three 56-bit keys for decryption.

5.1.2 Least Significant Bit

In picture steganography, the LSB is a common strategy. It deals with the secret information being encoded by manipulating the LSB in the cover image. It is well-known for its capacity for handling a lot of data.

The cloud technology is used to process different types of data globally. In the healthcare sector, cloud infrastructure is now the only option that can be used to monitor and connect Internet of Things (IoT) devices. Connecting IoT devices to cloud infrastructure allows for the transfer of computationally and energy-intensive jobs, which lessens the stress on these devices and extends their battery life. The configuration of these systems, their security, and the infrastructure that can process these data, however, are significant drawbacks. Another significant problem is that this volume of data causes a lot of network traffic and is not available when it is needed, rendering it useless. To solve this, Fog computing comes into the picture. Between the IoT device and the cloud server, there is a node layer. Moreover, it also contributes to cloud scalability. Fog computing can reduce reaction latency by up to 50% for real-time applications. Fog computing can support IoT devices and apps more efficiently, but data security is still a major worry. IoT devices share sensitive data and are directly connected to the internet. Thus even a little fault could result in significant data loss. Many researchers are focusing on the infrastructure of IoT devices. But if they make a sophisticated device it would lead to high battery consumption and in turn lead to low efficiency. They are also thinking of encrypting the data, but decryption and encrypting will be highly computationally. To gain efficiency, these cryptographic operations are transferred to fog nodes. Fog nodes, on the other hand, must provide accurate access control as well as convenient, manageable, and easy communication.

But according to our research, the most effective and secure technique is certificate-based incremental proxy re-encryption. In this study, we'll talk about (certificate-based incremental proxy re-encryption scheme [CB-PReS]) for sharing e-healthcare data in fog computing. The escrow problem was likewise overcome in this case.

The conventional cryptosystems have extraordinarily high communication and computing costs due to the usage of standard cryptographic techniques like Rivest-Shamir-Adleman (RSA), which uses keys with a key size of 1024 bits. Bilinear pairing is 14.42 times worse than the hyperelliptic curve and 13.65 times worse than RSA. The proxy re-encryption strategy can considerably increase speed when numerous parties need to share encrypted data. When updating EHR data, we occasionally have to start over in order to calculate the hash value. Every time we wish to make a little adjustment to a significant chunk of the EHR data, we must start over from scratch. Because of this, incremental cryptography is required to reduce the expense of starting from scratch with new hash values.

5.1.3 Watermarking Model

The strategies are listed in Ref. [7], starting with the segmentation of medical images. The most important component of medical imaging is the ROI. Given that it is the most crucial component of the medical image, it shouldn't be changed. The author of this paper used the RG approach to segment the ROI area of the image. Considering Figure 5.1, we have added 256 × 256 pixels as the input images. The picture used as input is initially used to extract the ROI. Regarding a location known as a seed, the input image is segmented using the projected RG technique. Managing the first seed spots is the primary objective of RG segmentation. The segmentation solution depends greatly on the selection of the seed point, which is RG's beginning point.

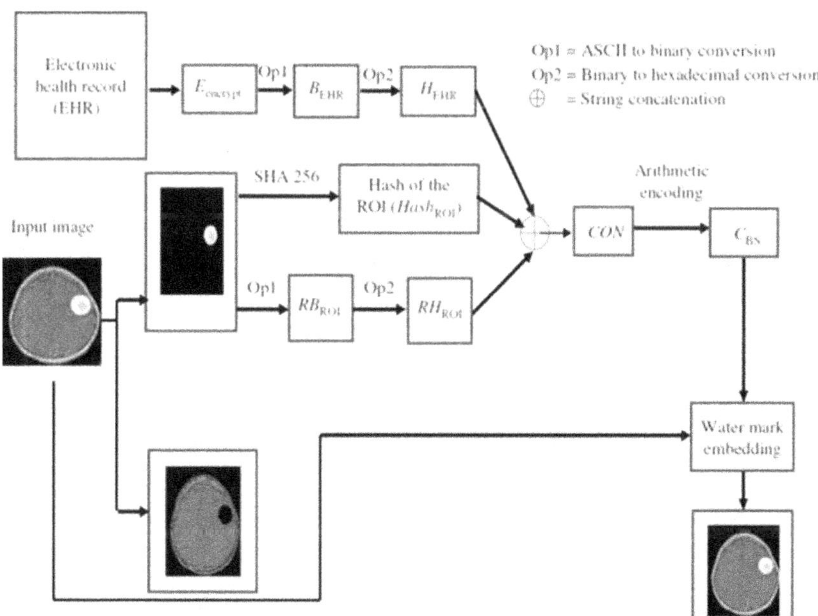

FIGURE 5.1 Watermark embedding system. (Source [6].)

The next stage involves hashing the ROI. The ROI region is removed from the input image during the segmentation stage of the RG method. After segmentation, a hash value is calculated for the ROI. This work generates a 64-character (256-bit) message digest by computing the ROI hash using SHA-256. This approach generates a unique code for any input using a one-way function. For authentication, ROI's intended hash value is used. Despite concentrating on only one ROI in this study, the proposed method can be applied to many ROIs.

The elliptic curve over finite fields' algebraic structure serves as the foundation for the next cryptographic technique, called ECC. It is compatible with public-key cryptography, which requires that each user have a set of keys—a public key and a private key—as well as a set of actions linked to the keys—in order to perform cryptographic operations.

A four-step process is used in the design to validate the user. Connection establishment is the first phase, followed by account creation, authentication, and data update. Given that this method's computing speed is rather slow when compared to other linear methods, we picked ECC. Another advantage is that because of its sub-exponential time difficulty, it is difficult to crack. Before being sent to the cloud, sensitive data is passed to an encryption algorithm, which encrypts it. Users can explain sensitive information by using the key and the information of owner's consent. The next step is to apply the compression algorithm AC to a bit stream. Statistical coder AC is an expert in lossless data compression [1, 9, 14]. The objective of AC is to design a method for producing code phrases of the ideal length. The average code length is quite close to the minimum recommended by data theory. The AC assigns a range to each symbol, the size of which replicates the likelihood of that symbol occurring. The code word for a symbol is an arbitrary rational number that falls inside the conforming interval. A rational integer that is always entered within the range of each symbol serves as the representation for the entire collection of data.

The primary contribution of this study is a strong and resourceful medical picture and record watermarking solution for an E-healthcare application that can address all four concerns. This approach uses encryption and lossless data compression to include an EHR and an image hash in the medical image, protecting it from damaging outbreaks. The ROI is extracted from the input image using an RG technique that accurately segments the image. The proposed approach ought to improve patient data security while avoiding any distortion. The suggested technique must be resistant to the numerous attacks that a malicious party can use to tamper with the incorporated watermark.

5.1.4 Overview of Advanced Encryption Standard

Data security is given the utmost significance since, by automating payment collection and improving patient satisfaction, it lowers fraud for payers and providers. The science of limiting unauthorized access to sensitive information is known as cryptography, and it does so through upholding data integrity and authentication. Because of the hashing technique, it is much more important to make sure that transmitted messages are unchanged. The notions of fingerprints, biometric identity, and iris recognition are all products of artificial intelligence. It describes how to

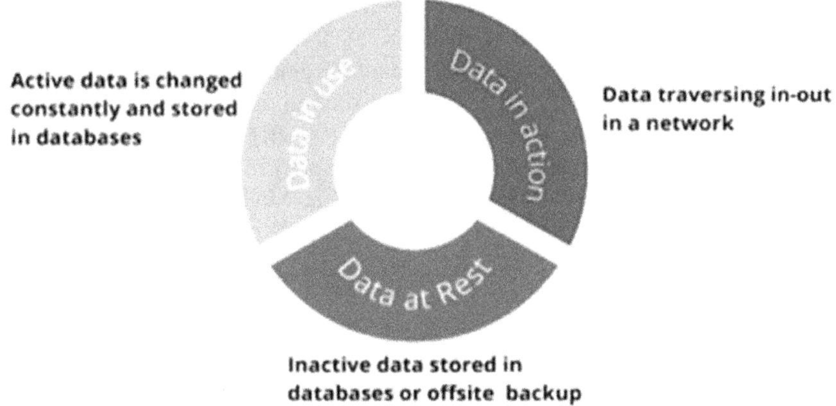

FIGURE 5.2 Three stages of data.

handle and safeguard electronic health data much more securely using the Advanced Encryption Standard (AES) algorithm and Blockchain (BC). Data must be protected the least bit times; the three stages of information are represented in Figure 5.2—(1) data in action, (2) data in use, and (3) data at rest. The data that moves over multiple networks, between systems, and between different points is referred to as the information in motion. Daily updates and modifications are made to the information in use. Large amounts of knowledge are at rest, and organizations like enterprises, governments, and other groups are beginning to prioritize this issue. The data is retained inactive and unused for a long time. Maximum information theft happens to backup data. As a result, encryption is necessary even at the most basic levels.

The security in the hardware device is implemented to protect long-term data storage from unsafe and malicious users or data breaches. The biometric technique is one such hardware security application that is utilized in this chapter to stop rogue logging in of the users, logging out, or meddling with rights. Verifying a user's identity is the process of authentication. The two stages are identification and true authentication. During the identification stage, any person's identity is sent to the security system in the form of user identity. Before providing permission, the secure system scans all of the abstract objects and locates the real user. When the user provides the system with an indication to support the specification, this is done. The authentication process entails using the user's own documentation to verify the user's identity. Encryption is the method of encoding a message or piece of data so that only those with the right access may read it.

The method creates a pseudo-random encryption key. Asymmetric encryption and symmetric encryption are the two types of encryption used. The encryption and decryption keys used are same in symmetric. To maintain safe communication, users who are conversing utilize the same key. Asymmetric encryption enables the receiving team to read the communications even when the encryption key is made public information since the decryption key, which is considered to be the private key, does so. Data that is at rest is frequently encrypted using the techniques of AES or RSA. AES was utilized for data encryption, and keys with key sizes of 128, 196, or 256 bits were used. The authors employed an RSA 1024-bit key to encrypt AES keys in order to double-protect data and keys [8]. The primary focus will be on the particular security issues posed by cloud computing employed in the healthcare sector and the support provided by the ABE in resolving the regulatory requirements in the healthcare sector [8]. The proposed study on ABE ensures data availability, availability, confidentiality, authentication, and integrity in the multi-level hierarchy [8]. One major advantage, particularly in medical research, is the ease with which healthcare practitioners can add or remove any order [9].

5.1.5 3DES Method

Patient's health data is stored and transmitted electronically by the internet; the medical industry is not safe from cyberattacks like other sectors such as banking, academia, and finance. Patient data theft and intrusion have a direct influence on the services offered by healthcare institutions and put patients' lives in danger. This work uses both steganography and encryption techniques to increase the security of medical data. Common DES cipher is used three times by the triple DES algorithm. It is given a 168-bit secret key that is broken up into three 56-bit keys [10].

Data concealment and Encryption are the two main techniques utilized in this paper's methods to safeguard medical data, whereas the opposite is applied in the other way to recover the information. Before utilizing LSB to embed the ciphertext from the 3DES into an image carrier, the patients' information is first converted into ciphertext. The retrieving stage uses the stego picture, which is the securing stage's output, as an input. The data retrieval process starts with LSB, which takes the stego picture's encrypted data and decrypts it using 3DES. The analysis indicates that the findings of this investigation are consistent with the intended outcome. In conclusion, this study reveals how to increase data security in medical or healthcare organizations by combining cryptography (algorithm of 3DES) and steganography (Encoding technique of LSB). This study's demonstration of a two-layer security strategy was motivated by the devastation caused by a cyber-attack on health-related data. According to the study's findings, a dual-layered security system offers more protection and makes successful cyberattacks more challenging. In reality, medical information can be hidden from other medical information. This means that non-sensitive medical data in a picture format can be used as a cover for more sensitive medical data. Healthcare is a very important industry that deals with people's lives and should be safeguarded; thus in the future, a quicker and more secure approach should be investigated. However, a security system that is too sluggish might cause more damage than good. To boost the security level of the encryption and decryption operations, the best key will be chosen using hybrid swarm optimization, also known as grasshopper and particle swarm optimization in elliptic curve cryptography [11].

5.1.6 Access Control

To protect patient privacy and the confidentiality of medical data and records, solid security architecture and policies are needed. Access control is a security risk in the shared computer environment since information is kept in databases and transferred through heterogeneous file systems in networked settings, where duties and privileges differ depending on the system's use and the Organization to which it belongs. Because of this, users' access to some resources must be restricted by allowing or disallowing them access as necessary.

The three different methods of access control are technical, logical, and physical. Cryptography-based access control is a conceptually based control method for sharing resources and gaining access to crucial components of a healthcare Web system. Cryptography-based access control is a brand-new approach to access-based control developed for information systems. It outlines an implicit access control strategy that entirely depends on encryption to protect the privacy and accuracy of data kept by the system. It is designed to function in hazardous circumstances where a lack of global awareness and control is a distinguishing feature. Access control was developed using non-cryptographic methods. These methods are typically broken down into three categories: Discretionary Access Control (DAC), Mandatory Access Control (MAC), and Role-Based Access Control (RBAC) [15]. The basic purpose of access control implementation is to restrict who has access to what data and how it can be utilized.

Given their inability to improve the workflow of the healthcare workforce, access control strategies haven't always been effective from a usability aspect when used in modern healthcare information systems. The result of it is that, in order to accommodate the needs of its drug use, these systems have to plan on providing deviation from the standard access control procedures. From the standpoint of information security, exceptions are undesirable since they lead to a loss of control over the input's information. The purpose of the work that is being presented is to examine mechanisms and assess how closely they adhere to the standards from which it is claimed that they diverge in order to gather data for the creation of an advanced access control model for healthcare operations.

5.1.7 CB-PREs

In this study, we present a straightforward incremental proxy re-encryption technique for e-healthcare data transport in fog computing. Each user in a certificate-based system has the capacity to verify the other users' public keys. Using 256-bit and 160-bit keys, respectively, recently suggested I-PRE systems carry out expensive Bilinear pairing and elliptic curve computations. The block modification results of this method are compared with those of the previously proposed I-PRE techniques in terms of turnaround time using an 80-bit key and the hyperelliptic curve technique. The outcomes demonstrate that our approach is unquestionably more efficient than the prior suggested approaches. By utilizing the concepts of fog computing, we are able to offer data integrity and secrecy while simultaneously solving the latency problem. Figure 5.3 illustrates several IoT device levels that let IoT devices cope with resource limitations by sending difficult and resource-intensive cryptographic activities to fog nodes. In the future, we'll create a system based on organizations that will benefit a lot of individuals.

IoT device security and privacy have sparked serious concerns. Given these issues, immediate security measures are required. IoT devices have limited resources, making

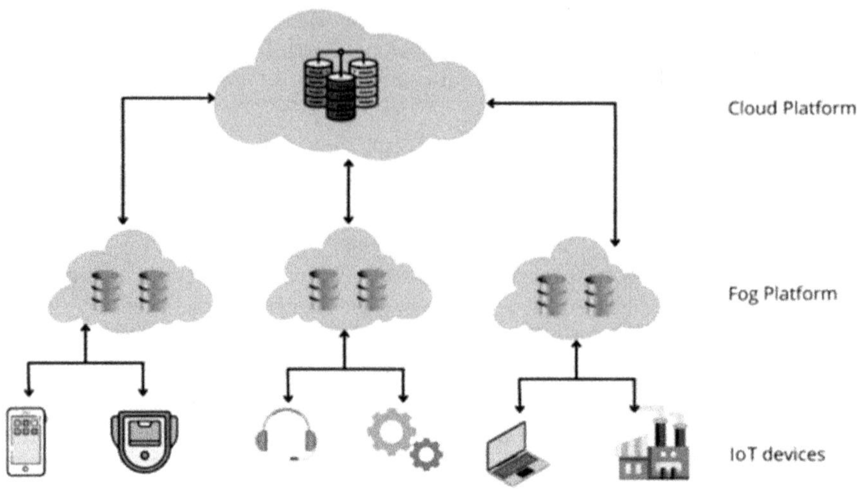

FIGURE 5.3 Different IoT levels of devices.

resource-intensive and sophisticated security tasks impossible to implement. This reduces the battery life of the gadget and results in greater processing expenses and real-time applications with significant latency that need quick replies [12]. As a result, rather than completing these complicated security tasks on resource-constrained IoT devices, we can avoid these issues by outsourcing them to the fog. Because of classic cryptographic techniques like RSA, which employs keys with a 1024-bit size, the communication and computing costs of the old cryptosystems are extremely high. IoT device security and privacy have been a source of substantial worry. These problems necessitate quick security measures. Because IoT devices have limited resources, they are unable to perform resource-intensive and advanced security duties. This decreases the battery life of the device, raises processing costs, and significantly slows down real-time applications that require quick replies. As a result, rather than executing these complex security activities on resource-constrained IoT devices, we may outsource them to the fog and avoid these concerns. The previous crypto system's communication and computing costs are extraordinarily expensive due to classic cryptographic approaches like RSA, which has a 1024-bit key size.

5.2 LITERATURE REVIEW

The author has defined a multilayer technique for e-health services in accordance with ISO 17799. He divides the material into three categories: top-secret, extremely confidential, and proprietary data. The symmetric encryption techniques 3DES and hash value function have been introduced [13]. Layer 1 has a key size of 193 bits, layer 2 has a key size of 129 to 192 bits, layer 3 has a key size of 112 to 128 bits, and layer 4 has a key size of 80 to 111 bits. However, their research is limited to a single algorithm, 3DES. For encryption and decryption, just one algorithm is used.

In Ref. [12], the author proposes an E-healthcare cloud computing using certificate-based incremental proxy re-encryption. As a result, earlier PRE schemes suffer from overhead and delay issues. This method lowers the cost of computation and communication for IoT devices with limited resources. To make our method easier, we substitute bilinear pairs for 160-bit keys and 1024-bit keys, respectively, and hyperelliptic curves for elliptical curves. The idea of incremental cryptography serves as the foundation for the block-based data modification approach. By utilizing certificate-based proxy re-encryption, this method also tackles the key escrow problem. He has also given us a security model and an analysis of our plan. The security features provided by this system include integrity, secrecy, unforgeability, and anti-replay attacks.

According to Ref. [7], the RG, SHA-256, ECC, and AC algorithms have a reduced level of processing complexity since they supply authentication and recovery data and recover the ROI by simple mathematical calculations. The suggested approach maintains the quality of the watermarked image with an average PSNR of 42.23 dB, an embedding capacity of 72,384 bits, extraction accuracy of 98 percent, and an NC of 1. The results of the experiments also show that the suggested strategy improves watermark picture quality and embedding performance. The proposed technique could be implemented in medical information systems in the future to guarantee medical picture integrity, system authentication, and confidentiality.

Table 5.1 presents a succinct analysis of the existing literature survey of the relevant works being undertaken.

TABLE 5.1
Existing Literature Analysis

References	Underlying Principle	Strength	Weakness
[6]	Medical or healthcare organizations can increase data security by implementing double-layer security, which combines steganography (LSB image encoding) and cryptography (3DES encryption algorithm)	The findings of this study suggest that a dual-layered security system provides greater security and makes successful cyberattacks more difficult. It is possible for medical data to be concealed from other medical data. As a result, medical data that is in an image format and does not contain any sensitive information can be used to disguise sensitive medical information.	The combined method's only drawback is its slow operation speed, yet it outperforms 3DES and LSB in terms of security reliability.

(Continued)

TABLE 5.1 *(Continued)*
Existing Literature Analysis

References	Underlying Principle	Strength	Weakness
[12]	An incremental proxy re-encryption strategy based on certificates has been developed by the author for e-healthcare data sharing	The author is able to guarantee the security and secrecy of data while also addressing the latency issue by utilizing fog computing principles. Complex and resource-intensive cryptographic functions are offloaded from IoT devices to fog nodes in order to lessen the impact of resource constraints.	When adopting cloud infrastructure, secure EHR storage and sharing is a major concern. We cannot validate any user's public key with certificateless cryptography, which is a major shortcoming of certificateless cryptographic techniques.
[7]	Algorithms such as RG, SHA-256, ECC, and AC	Suggested method has a lower computational complexity since it generates authentication and recovery data using basic mathematical computations while maintaining image quality.	The overall process is time consuming.
[14]	AES with double hashing	Artificial intelligence is used to help confirm the identity of the person accessing the database.	Data security—as data could be stolen by anyone.
[15]	Cryptography-based access controls, PKI access control model	In addition to enhancing certification and online authentication, PKIs are becoming increasingly cost-effective.	Provides the key holder access permissions so that they can grant access to the resource.

5.3 METHODOLOGY

5.3.1 Water Model

The goal of this study is to provide a hybridized compression algorithm and encryption technique-based lossless medical image watermarking solution. To protect private messages from prying eyes, privacy apps frequently employ watermarking. In the proposed system, two stages are involved: (i) extraction and (ii) embedding. Both the patient information and the medical imaging data are watermarked in this instance. The subsections that follow include descriptions of the embedding and extraction techniques.

The embedding procedure is based on a combination of compression and encryption techniques. The embedding process is depicted in the diagram below.

1. Take into account the 256 × 256 pixel input image I. First, we use the RG technique to segment the ROI area (IROI) from the input image.
2. After segmenting the data, we use SHA-256 to build the ROI hash function ($Hash_{ROI}$).
3. Then, we convert $Hash_{ROI}$'s binary value (B_{ROI}) to its hexadecimal equivalent, H_{ROI}.
4. As soon as possible, we also translate the IROI into binary format and encode the binary picture as a hexadecimal number.
5. It is important to note that the EHR is another component of the input. The EHR is encrypted using the ECC method, and it contains information such as the patient reference number, patient's age, patient's name, doctor's name, and date of addition; for this we use the ECC method.
6. The Encrypt data is then transformed into B_{EHR} binary data. For analysis purposes, we also translate the binary data into a corresponding hexadecimal value., abbreviated H_{EHR}.
7. We combine the picture data and the EHR after the encryption procedure. H_{ROI}, H_{EHR}, and RH_{ROI} are combined to create CON_I.
8. We apply the AC approach to compress CONI in order to enhance the embedding process. You can get CBS's compressed bit feed here.
9. Then, using the procedures below, we create the first random matrix R. The incoming image's pixel values are added together and given the name I_{seed}.

$$I_{seed} = \sum_{i=1}^{n}\sum_{j=1}^{n} I_{ij}$$

With the aid of I_{seed}'s development of a pseudo-random matrix:

$$R = PRMG[R_{seed}]_{(2\times2)}$$

10. The random matrix R is created using the supplied image's size. Then, with R, we create the ideal random matrix RM by carrying out the subsequent actions:
    i. The generated random matrix R is denoted as R_t after being multiplied by 2 after being multiplied by 0.5.

    $$R_t = (R - 0.5) \times 2$$

    ii. Then, using the R_t matrix as a seed value, the pseudo-random matrix generator generates the desired random matrix RM.

    $$RM = PRMG[R_t]_{(2\times2)}$$

11. Then, we include CBS in the original image I. In the end, the watermarked picture IW is acquired. Below is a description of the embedding procedures.
    i. The random matrix RM is multiplied by the embedding strength and connected to the original image I by setting the watermark bit to 0.
    ii. When the bit of the watermark is set to 1, no operation is carried out.
12. Steps 10 and 11 are repeated until the pixels are implanted.

5.3.1.1 Process of Extraction

This is accomplished by, in contrast to how embedding is done, extracting the compressed bit CBS from the dubious watermarked image IW during the extraction phase and comparing it to the original image I as well as the data EHR. To find the original information, the extraction method starts by following the same steps as the embedding process. The extraction operation's input receives the embedded watermark image IW first.

1. To begin the extraction procedure, use steps 8 and 9 from the previous paragraph to create a random matrix RM. According to the preceding paragraph, the PRMG begins with seed Iseed for every iteration and produces the initial random matrix R.
2. The correlation coefficient R^{Cor} between the watermarked image IW and the generated random matrix [RM] is then calculated using the following formula:

$$R^{Cor} = \frac{\sum_{m}\sum_{n}\left(I_{W}^{mn} - \overline{I_{W}}\right)\left(B_{mn} - \overline{B}\right)}{\sqrt{\left(\sum_{m}\sum_{n}\left(I_{W}^{mn} - \overline{I_{W}}\right)^{2}\right)\left(\sum_{m}\sum_{n}\left(B_{mn} - \overline{B}\right)^{2}\right)}}$$

3. R_Z is the result of dividing the estimated correlation coefficient value R^{Cor} by two.
4. To change the watermark image's size, repeat steps 1–3. After that, save the RZ values as a vector VRZ.
5. By dividing the vector by the number of nodes, find the mean VRZ value.

$$\overline{V\,R_Z} = \sum_{i=1}^{k} V\,R_Z^{i} \big/ k, \text{where } k \left| V\,R_Z \right|.$$

6. To identify the watermark picture pixels, a comparison is done between the elements of the vector VRZ and the mean value. The watermark image pixel is zero if the element value is greater than the mean value. If not, it is 1. The equation reads as follows:

$$E_{BS}(x, y) = \begin{cases} 0, & V\,R_Z^{i} > \overline{V\,R_Z} \\ 1, & \text{Otherwise} \end{cases}, \text{where } n = \left| V\,R_Z \right|$$

7. E_{BS} is a bit stream that needs to be decompressed. Obtain the original bit stream D_{BS} using the arithmetic decoder approach.
8. Extract H_{ROI}, H_{EHR}, and RH_{ROI} from the original bit stream D_{BS}.
9. Convert H_{EHR} to B_{EHR}, which is the bit stream representation. Then, as Encrypt, transform B_{EHR} back to its original form.
10. To retrieve EHR, decrypt Encrypt using K using the ECC technique.
11. Calculate the hash for H_{ROI} in the same way to get the original ROI image.

5.3.2 Advanced Encryption Standard

5.3.2.1 Biometrics in Industries

Biometrics is a component of security in any industry since it allows for the numerical analysis and measurement of a person's unique physical and behavioral features. Biometrics can be used to identify any individual and provide proof of identification and control over the person under observation. It might be challenging to break into a system 166. With modernized cyber security and biometrics, cryptography is being used in the healthcare sector. The technology analyses a person's unique characteristics, such as speech patterns, iris patterns, and fingerprint patterns. The behavioral category includes face recognition, hand/palm, iris identification, fingerprints, and DNA, whereas the physiological category includes fingerprints, iris identification, hand/palm, and DNA. Behavioral categories include keystrokes, signatures, and voice patterns, as shown in Figure 5.4.

5.3.2.2 Voice Print

As the population increases, people are more accustomed to biometrics, and they need a safe means to settle payments in and around the workplace. One such biometric that

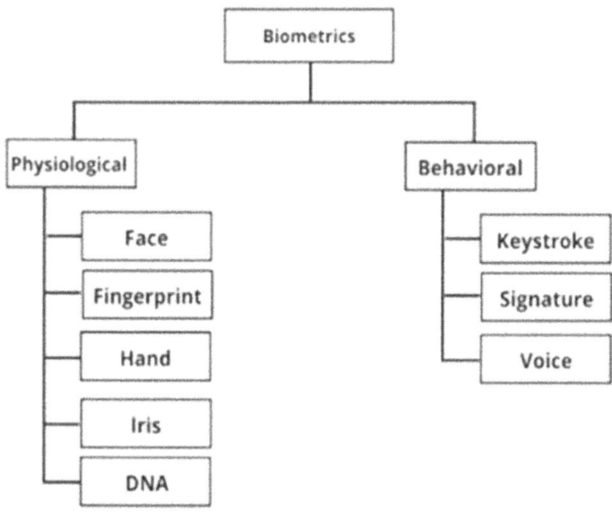

FIGURE 5.4 Types of biometrics for human identification.

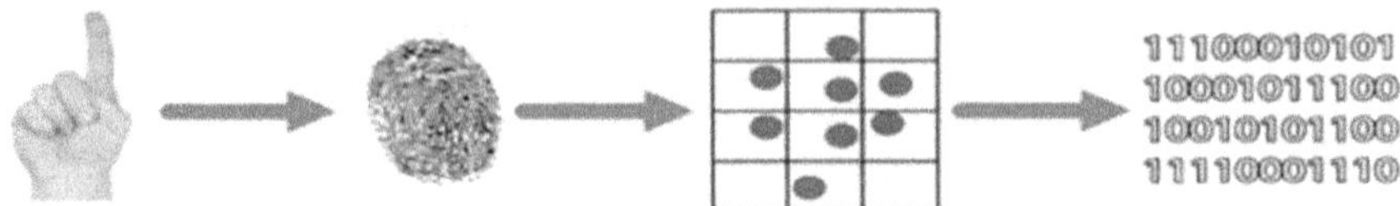

FIGURE 5.5 The representation by 1s and 0s of fingerprints.

is gaining acceptance in a number of sectors, including healthcare, finance, and education, is voice authentication. In order to identify and authenticate a speaker, voice recognition software maintains notes of their rhythm, accent, nasal route, and vocal tract structure [14]. It describes a voice recognition system that records voices by examining and storing name, age, address, and a number of hidden sounds in addition to speech and breathing patterns. Along with other login details, the voice print is encrypted and stored in the user's Active Directory authentication data. When someone signs up for voice authentication calls, their voice is compared to the voice print that has been kept in the active directory, which speeds up the verification process. This voiceprint recognition system (VRS) is also known as Speaker Recognition Technology.

5.3.2.3 Face Recognition and Fingerprints

Based on the acquired image quality, the biometric input for fingerprint and facial identity discovers accurately displayed results. The scanning of fingerprints for biometric purposes and subsequent storage of the data as a matrix of 1s and 0s as shown in Figure 5.5. With the regular implementation of security needs, this matrix is maintained for potential use in the future. The data is recorded, encrypted, and then stored in the database using the AES technique. A three-step technique is used to recognize a person's face. Identifying a person in the image by starting with the topic picture. The method establishes the location of the subject's head and eyes. A matrix of the person's facial traits serves as the basis for the creation of a face signature.

5.3.3 3DES Model

The methodology for this investigation combines steganography and cryptography. Examples include the LSB steganography technique and the 3DES encryption algorithm (both of which are seen in Figures 5.6 and 5.7. The approach utilized includes the following two important steps to protect medical data in text format.

a. In the first stage, 3DES is used to encrypt patient data in plain text and produce ciphertext. This stage necessitates the use of a secret key.

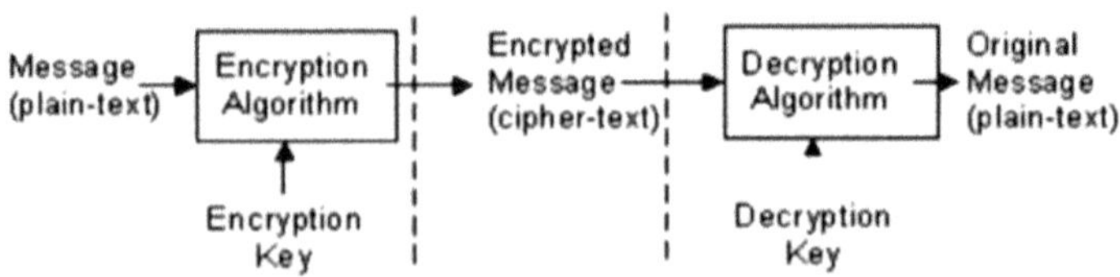

FIGURE 5.6 The encryption scheme.

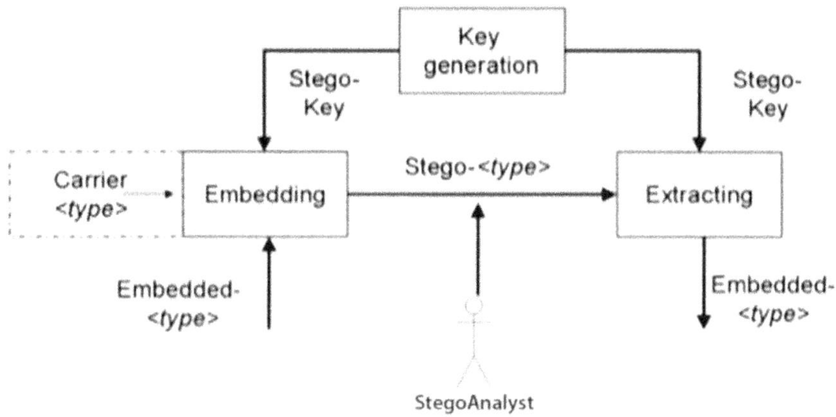

FIGURE 5.7 Conceptual view of steganography scheme (source [6]).

b. The outputs of the first stage will be the input for the second phase, which will use LSB to embed them in the cover picture and create a stego image as the output.

The stages involved in retrieving data for the stego picture are primarily two. (a) The ciphertext must first be extracted from the stego image in order to obtain the protected data. (b) The 2nd stage in getting the secure data involves decrypting the ciphertext using the 3DES method. A secret key that matches the encryption key must be used for this step. Figure 5.6 shows the encryption approach.

5.3.3.1 Secure Phase

In this stage, the health of the patient information is secured. The interface allows medical professionals to choose which patient records should be encrypted and which cover picture should be used to conceal the data. For input selection, utilize the first "Selection of File/Data" and "Selection of the Cover Image" buttons, respectively. The Conceptual view of steganography scheme using the 3DES encryption algorithm is shown in Figure 5.7.

The reverse of the secure phase is the retrieved phase. It aids in the retrieval of secure medical information stego generated from images during the safe phase. It has two buttons that are used to pick the required input: "Select Secured File/Data" and "Select Cover Image."

5.3.4 Access Control

Cryptographic-based access controls are an innovative technique to enforce access control (hierarchical or distributed). A class key or node key should be created for each type of resource, and all users who fall under that class should have access to it. A user must supply the source's key in order to access any resources. We will contrast the given key and the resource key. Access to the resource is either given if the key matches the resource key or is refused in the other case. Users of the parent class have access to the resources of its children's classes, according the hierarchical access control. For web-distributed systems where the data and the resources are scattered and moved across all the networks, cryptography-based access eliminates the requirement for an access matrix to maintain access information for each topic and object. Additionally, the availability of encrypted sources in domains that are public is made possible while preserving access control, thanks to the data security offered by cryptography.

This article offers a thorough analysis of access control, covering traditional access control, a common overview of algorithms (which also includes the access control model), the current access control model, and a wide range of algorithms (including cryptography access control-based algorithms). Utilizing suite B [15], this study suggests a novel approach for combining cryptographic access control based on role-specific access and hierarchical access control for a single entity. The security approach employed between transactional entities is dispersed and public-key infrastructure (PKI) based, whereas the model is on the user entity (for example, a neighborhood hospital or medical facility).

5.3.4.1 PKI—Evaluation of Access Control Model

PKI is now only used in healthcare for issues of certification involving payments of healthcare, and it is enforced online rather than by the healthcare institution. In addition, unlike our method, the current PKI is predicated on single-person access rather than grouped based or cross-certification. The suggested model, which was built on PKI, has the ability to deliver the following qualities in comparison to earlier RBAC models or other models, depending on the certification and authentication. The concept supports cross-certification, group certification, and access.

Non-repudiation is guaranteed by utilizing a digital signature over the internet using private key encryption (no other solution does this). Using public key encryption, emails are private and secure. Due to the need to maintain an expensive PKI for dispersing and managing public keys and digital certificates for all healthcare providers, certain techniques, such as RSA, offer a secure solution but are not feasible for secure EHR storage [16]. Signatures in software encourage the usage of smart cards for authentication. Encrypt your files. Web authentication and encryption (Secure Sockets Layer) are used to provide e-health support (not supported by other models). The support for—IPSec and VPN authentication using a port (802.1X) (no other model supports this). For the purpose of key management, key distribution, and also authentication, the approach employs an NSA-recommended suite.

Unlike earlier PKI architectures mentioned in Figure 5.8, our solution is completely based on group certifications, authentications, and authorization, with all the laboratories in part forming a group and all laboratories in two different hospitals organizing subgroup certification and subgroup authority. With all of the advantages, it may be considered that the PKI access control method may significantly advance e-health. The processing speed offered by the RSA and the largest prime number used are the two most important drawbacks. A fast solution can be an accelerator that

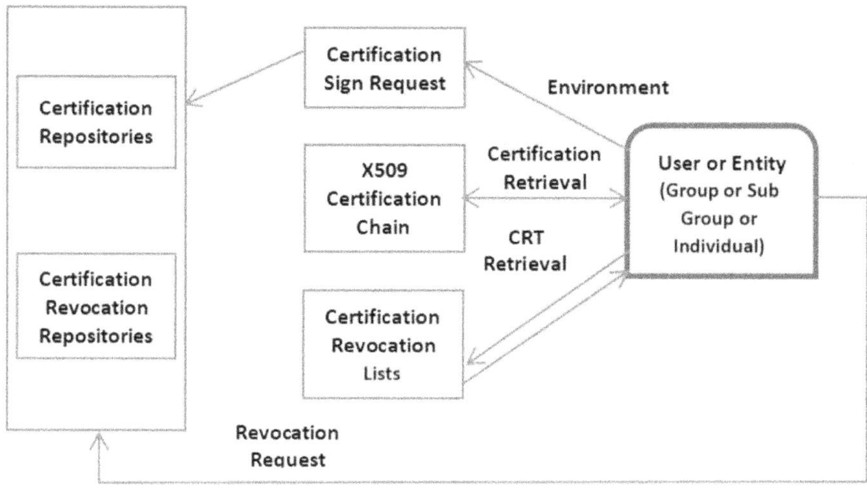

FIGURE 5.8 PKI entities.

uses chains in the remainder of the algorithm. A more sophisticated approach in the future would be to make PKI access control using elliptic and curve cryptographic methods. **Figure 5.8** shows a public-key infrastructure showing certification databases, certification chain, and entities involved.

Due to the lack of some standards being tested and released, this solution is not yet suitable for usage. When measuring the use of the RSA, such a solution will provide: Obtaining information takes less time, and there is less space available to complete tasks. PKI will be a fantastic answer because it is becoming increasingly affordable while also improving certification and online authentication. Since it hasn't yet been shown to be a cost effective solution, 78 cryptographic access con trol is still in question. Additionally, it is anticipated that the market will adopt a well-liked solution that has won the support of a third party. Since certain businesses are prepared to use it, encryption access control will be a suitable option, but as Suite B becomes the de facto norm, more and more healthcare companies will adopt and embrace it.

5.3.5 CB-PREs

The author of the study suggests using an incremental proxy re-encryption method based on certificates for fog computing. Our approach resolves the computation and communication issues of earlier PRE schemes, which were caused by cloud computing and the usage of pricey cryptography methods. This method helps IoT devices deal with resource limitations by offloading complicated and resource-intensive cryptographic operations to fog nodes. We show that our technology, which is needed for real-time devices, has lower communication costs than earlier PRE systems. In order to do the resource-intensive tasks required for the re-encryption process, it is treated as if each fog node were a proxy node.

i. **System Configuration:** This procedure is carried out by a certificate authority (CA), which chooses to obtain a hyperelliptic curve; we need to set up a finite field Fq of order q and a security parameter (E). The curve's order q generating point, which CA selects as a divisor, is an integer. Then, CA calculates the master public key as MPk using a master secret key that it randomly selects from a range of (1, 2, …, q−1). A number of public encryption, decryption, and proxy re-encryption parameters were finally released by CA.

ii. **Generation of Public and Private Keys**: In this phase, the algorithm is executed by each participant (the sender, the recipient, and the certificate authority). Prior to calculating X +,.(c), and c.(+ c), the participant randomly chooses three numbers, such as 1, 2, …, q1, and c 1, 2, …, q1. The participant computes the private and public key pairs with the identification. Both the private and public keys are calculated for each participant. The public is shown the public key of each participant.

iii. **Certificate Generation** It takes as input (IDp, Pk) the participant's public key Pk, identity IDp, and public parameters. In this phase, the participant's identity (IDU), public key (Pk), and public parameters (IDp, Pk) are inputs that the CA uses to create a certificate (CertU) for each participant (both sender and recipient). It generates the certificate by the CA using the following steps: CA accepts the participant's public key P_k and computes its hash, such as H_{PU} = h1 (PK||IDP)+MPk, after which it digitally signs H_{PU} using its private key, for example, S = K_{CertA}. (H_{PU}).

iv. **Key Generation for Re-encryption:** If User A wants to communicate data with User B, User A can use this procedure to generate a re-encryption key, such as RAB = Kb/Ka, and send it to the neighborhood fog proxy server anonymously.

v. **Encryption:** The user breaks a file F into z blocks, each of which contains d bits, except for the final block, which is encrypted with his public key. This is done in order to outsource the file to the fog node.

vi. **Re-Encryption of the Proxy:** User B asks the proxy server to re-encrypt the file before user A uploads it to the fog node. The second-level ciphertext (CB C2) of user B is replaced by user A's first-level ciphertext (CA C1) once the proxy server selects a new nonce during the process of re-encryption. The proxy server first determines whether user B has access rights to the access control list before re-encrypting the uploaded file and assigning it a Nonce value.

vii. **Decryption:** In this instance, user B gets the total number of blocks ("z"), the second-level ciphertext ("C, CB"), and the final hash value ("MACfinal") from the server. User B then uses both CB's private key and CB's public key to unlock the file. If the computed hash function matches the value of the final hash function (MACfinal), the integrity of the FILE is verified; otherwise, the original file has been altered by an outsider.

5.4 CONCLUSION

Today's healthcare information systems include access control measures, but they have not been entirely effective in terms of usability and have not supported the working processes of healthcare workers. Therefore that action can be done as soon as feasible in the event of questionable behavior; the system should generate real-time notifications. These can undoubtedly be avoided with better methods, steps, tools, etc., used in the adoption of cloud computing [17–19]. Because of this, the systems were forced to rely on access control methods that were not conventional in order to satisfy user requests. The lack of control over the data flow caused by exceptions makes them hazardous from the standpoint of information security. Data security is the main concern that needs to be addressed. When adopting cloud infrastructure, secure EHR storage and sharing is a major concern. We cannot validate any user's public key with certificateless cryptography, which is a major shortcoming of certificate cryptographic techniques. Internal medical organization data has been computerized and is now further integrated into the medical information system as a result of the advancement and development of information technology [20].

A combined method can cause a drawback that may slow operation speed. The overall process may be time-consuming. But a dual-layered security system provides greater security and makes successful cyber-attacks more challenging. In reality, all medical information can be concealed within other information. This means that the non-sensitive medical data in a picture format can be used to cover the more sensitive medical-related data. These can undoubtedly be avoided with better methods, steps, tools, etc., used in the adoption of cloud computing. Efficiency, encouraging self-care, and data management are some of the advantages we discovered, and they will help the hospital information system [21–23]. It is also feasible to offer data integrity and secrecy while simultaneously solving the latency issue by using fog computing concepts. Fog nodes are used to offload complicated and resource-intensive cryptographic operations, which helps IoT devices that have limited resources. The whole validation and verification process will be improved by using AI and cloud computing. It aids in confirming the legitimacy of the individual attempting to access the database. It may be improved and made more secure by using multilayer approaches.

5.5 FUTURE WORK

Protecting patient-sensitive data is a particularly challenging process due to security issues. A thorough assessment of the literature is being used to determine which techniques have been presented. Finding new techniques was quite challenging. Despite the fact that many encryption algorithms have been developed and utilized successfully (RSA, AES, Rijndael, RC6, DES, 3DES, IDEA, RC4, Blowfish), choosing the right one to ensure safe storage is still a difficult problem [20, 21]. Implementing multi-layer encryption techniques can be much more helpful in securing healthcare information. Also, key management issues are resolved with this cost-effective method, provided with new opportunities for researchers to improve their level of anonymity [22].

Future innovation goals include the following:

- Randomly choosing an encryption algorithm
- Encryption speed will rise, and more industry standards algorithms will be included
- Multilayer algorithms based on patient imaging data will be used
- Also the speed of encryption can be increased

REFERENCES

1. P. Chinnasamy, and P. Deepalakshmi, "Design of secure storage for health-care cloud using hybrid cryptography," in *2018 Second International Conference on Inventive Communication and Computational Technologies (ICICCT)*, 2018.
2. P. K. Sahoo, S. Mishra, R. Panigrahi, A. K. Bhoi, and P. Barsocchi, "An improvised deep-learning-based mask R-CNN model for laryngeal cancer detection using CT images," *Sensors (Basel)*, vol. 22, no. 22, p. 8834, 2022.
3. M. Meingast, T. Roosta, and S. Sastry, "Security and privacy issues with health care information technology," *Conference Proceedings of IEEE Engineering in Medicine and Biology Society*, vol. 2006, pp. 5453–5458, 2006.
4. S. K. Mohapatra, S. Mishra, H. K. Tripathy, and A. Alkhayyat, "A sustainable data-driven energy consumption assessment model for building infrastructures in resource constraint environment," *Sustainable Energy Technologies and Assessments*, vol. 53, 2022.
5. S. Mishra, H. K. Thakkar, P. Singh, and G. Sharma, "A decisive metaheuristic attribute selector enabled combined unsupervised-supervised model for chronic disease risk assessment," *Comput. Intell. Neurosci*, vol. 2022, p. 8749353, 2022.
6. P. Dutta, and S. Mishra, "A Comprehensive Review Analysis of Alzheimer's Disorder Using Machine Learning Approach. Augmented Intelligence in Healthcare: A Pragmatic and Integrated Analysis," pp. 63–76, 2022. https://doi.org/10.1007/978-981-19-1076-0_4
7. P. Aparna, and P. V. V. Kishore, "An efficient medical image watermarking technique in e-healthcare application using hybridization of compression and cryptography algorithm," *Journal of Intelligent Systems*, vol. 27, no. 1, pp. 115–133, 2018.
8. S. Suman, S. Mishra, K. S. Sahoo, and A. Nayyar, *Vision Navigator: A Smart and Intelligent Obstacle Recognition Model for Visually Impaired Users. Mobile Information Systems*. 2022.
9. C. Krishnan, and T. Lalitha, "Securing healthcare data using attribute based encryption techniques in cloud environment," *Ejmcm.com*. [Online], 2021. Available: https://ejmcm.com/article_8294_ec86cece114e0d90b2bc077e9701fa57.pdf. [Accessed: 24 May 2023].
10. S. Chakraborty, K. S. Sahoo, S. Mishra, and S. M. N. Islam, "AI driven cough voice-based COVID detection framework using spectrographic imaging: An improved technology," in *2022 IEEE 7th International conference for Convergence in Technology (I2CT)*, 2022.
11. M. Elhoseny, K. Shankar, S. K. Lakshmanaprabu, A. Maseleno, and N. Arunkumar, "Retraction note: Hybrid optimization with cryptography encryption for medical image security in internet of things," *Neural Comput. Appl*, vol. 35, no. 4, pp. 3573–3573, 2023.
12. J. Hassan, D. Shehzad, I. Ullah, F. Algarni, Md. U. Aftab, Md. A. Khan, and M. I. Uddin "A lightweight proxy re-encryption approach with certificate-based and incremental cryptography for fog-enabled e-healthcare," *Security and Communication Networks*, vol. 2021, pp. 1–17, 2021.
13. H. A. Shah, "A multilayer encryption model to protect healthcare data in cloud environment," *Edu.pk*. [Online], 2023. Available: https://thesis.cust.edu.pk/UploadedFiles/MCS173006.pdf. [Accessed: 24 May 2023].

14. P. Jayanthi, and M. Iyyanki, "Cryptography in the healthcare sector with modernized cyber security," in *Quantum Cryptography and the Future of Cyber Security*, IGI Global, Hershey, PA, 2020, pp. 163–183.
15. W. A. Al-Hamdani, "Cryptography based access control in healthcare web systems," in *2010 Information Security Curriculum Development Conference*, 2010.
16. S. Alshehri, S. P. Radziszowski, and R. K. Raj, "Secure access for healthcare data in the cloud using ciphertext-policy attribute-based encryption," in *2012 IEEE 28th International Conference on Data Engineering Workshops*, 2012.
17. F. Howarth, "Why is medical data so difficult to protect?," *Security Intelligence*, 03 March 2016. [Online]. Available: https://securityintelligence.com/why-is-medical-data-so-difficult-to-protect/. [Accessed: 24 May 2023].
18. C.-H. Liu, Y.-F. Chung, T.-S. Chen, and S.-D. Wang, "The enhancement of security in healthcare information systems," *Journal of Medical Systems*, vol. 36, no. 3, pp. 1673–1688, 2012.
19. A. Fatima, and R. Colomo-Palacios, "Security aspects in healthcare information systems: A systematic mapping," *Procedia Computer Science*, vol. 138, pp. 12–19, 2018.
20. K. Abouelmehdi, A. Beni-Hessane, and H. Khaloufi, "Big healthcare data: Preserving security and privacy," *Journal of Big Data*, vol. 5, no. 1, 2018.
21. H. K. Tripathy, S. Mishra, S. Suman, A. Nayyar, and K. S. Sahoo, "Smart COVID-shield: An IoT driven reliable and automated prototype model for COVID-19 symptoms tracking," *Computing*, vol. 104, no. 6, pp. 1233–1254, 2022.
22. S. Raghuwanshi, M. Singh, S. Rath, and S. Mishra, "Prominent cancer risk detection using ensemble learning," in *Cognitive Informatics and Soft Computing*, Singapore: Springer Nature Singapore, 2022, pp. 677–689.
23. A. Mohanty, and S. Mishra, "A comprehensive study of explainable artificial intelligence in healthcare," in *Augmented Intelligence in Healthcare: A Pragmatic and Integrated Analysis*, Singapore: Springer, 2022, pp. 475–502.

6 Integration of Quantum Computing in Healthcare Using Machine Learning Models

Tridiv Swain

6.1 INTRODUCTION

Image-assisted diagnosis could be considerably improved by quantum computing by improving medical imaging processing tasks like edge detection and picture matching. It is also possible to investigate the application of single-cell approaches in already-in-use diagnostic procedures. Nanotechnology has the potential to revolutionize the development of treatments by utilizing quantum uncertainty. It can also enable in clinical trials by providing realistic time with virtual human replication, hasten comprehensive genetic testing and analysis, enable hospital data migration with no disruption, support preventive healthcare measures, and improve clinical information security, hasten comprehensive genetic testing and analysis, enable hospital data migration with no disruption, support preventive healthcare measures, and improve clinical information security.

Nondeterministic computing and traditional machine learning (ML), two of the most fascinating areas of modern research, are combined in quantum automation. It looks into the possibility of applying findings and methods from one field to settle disputes in another.

Traditional computational models are reaching their limits in contemporary ML systems due to the ongoing accumulation of data. When it comes to ML tasks, quantum processing may be advantageous. The development and application of software with quantum properties that can outperform conventional computers in performing ML tasks is the main goal of quantum learning algorithms. It is plausible to predict that supercomputers will be able to outperform quantum systems in the area of computational capacity for learning tasks, even though quantum algorithms may not excel at constructing complex patterns that are difficult for conventional systems.

Internet data interchange is essential to the public health system because it improves connectivity and streamlines service delivery. The idea that services are available everywhere is used by smart healthcare to develop communication across the actual and virtual worlds.

By ensuring that systems are current, arranging healthcare information in a logical framework, and quickly obtaining and accessing patients' prior data, medical experts are able to produce excellent medical results. There is considerable interest

DOI: 10.1201/9781032624891-6

in the possible use of nuclear ML with gate-based innovation as a workable strategy in the future as healthcare develops quickly.

6.2 LITERATURE REVIEW

According to studies [1], numerical simulation is severely hampered for quantum interactions with only a small number of particles because the equivalent memory required to maintain or change the core wave equation is greater than the capacity of even the most powerful conventional computers. This shows that the confirmation and design of novel quantum devices and experiments are intrinsically limited to tiny system sizes. It is unknown how the full potential of massive quantum systems may be attained.

Algorithms and optimization techniques are used in the research [2] to look for optic computation chip devices that can conduct particular changes among both input and output states. Finding circuits that produce the necessary qubit in the most basic scenario of a single-bit state is the technique's main goal. The technique creates circuits that imitate the actions of the intended linear shift in more complicated circumstances with various input and output connections. The network architecture makes use of a continuous quantum neural network made up of several optical gate layers. The Strawberries Fields optoelectronic quantum-based simulator's TensorFlow back end is used to improve the configurable variables of these gates.

Figure 6.1 presents the quantum state model in quantum computing. The most recent work in the research [3] demonstrates how to use quantum random access coding (QRAC), an essential technique for converting binary data structures into quantum variations, to translate discrete qualities with fewer quantum bits. They quantitatively show how it may be used in equations to classify quantum data to improve efficiency when detecting real-world datasets, suggesting that it could be useful in cognitive algorithms for learning on nearby quantum systems.

In the research [4], the researcher presents a better method for installing computational quantum applications on a platform for cloud computing that streamlines

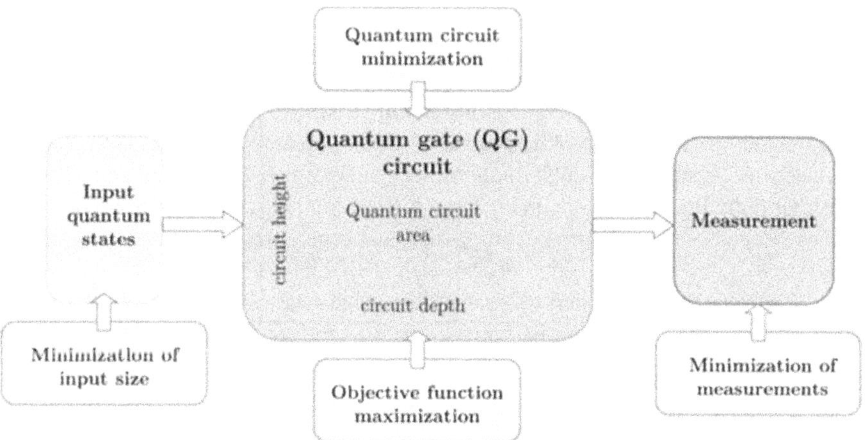

FIGURE 6.1 Model of quantum state in quantum computing.

data movement between servers using a message-passing protocol in order to speed up quantum computing.

In this research paper [5], the researchers propose a quantum walk algorithm designed to enable decentralized quantum computing in a virtual network. The protocol utilizes a quantum walk as a traditional process variable to facilitate distributed quantum operations. The study focuses on the quantum walk model, which extends the concept to discrete time and considers the connection of a quantum walker device within network devices through directed graphs and quantum registers. The protocol effectively represents distributed quantum computing by separating hardware design from quantum information flow through channels. The distribution of the control system is translated into network transmission of the walker system, while the coin operator, which provides instructions, facilitates the exchange between the control and data planes and the quantum registers.

The investigators perform a thorough analysis in this work [6] where they carefully review, group, and assess articles, tools, techniques, and systems that support the use of quantum computers from both quantum computing and its practical standpoint. They shed light on the accessibility of quantum technology and the quantum information layers, including the existence of a Circuit Simulator. Also highlighted are open-source tools like Cirq, TensorFlow Quantum, and ProjectQ, among others, that make it easier to create quantum applications for Python using a robust yet approachable language. The researchers then evaluate the situation as it stands, point out problems that need to be fixed, and make suggestions for future studies. They think that as a result of the recent emergence of numerous paradigms, methods, and systems, improving current tools would benefit from the collaborative work of the quantum research community.

Researchers present an ideal framework for defining distributed policy measures that run an evolving network with gates acting on qubits in different nodes in this publication [7]. A programming logic planes quantum walk protocol can be used to explain the fault-tolerant operations in the quantum network. For choosing qubit assignment and channel configurations for cognitive control data flows, they suggest an integer programming method. Due to the complexity of the issue, our proposal is limited to circuits with two-qubit regulated gates. This method can be used to examine how channel usage relates with node energy and circuit size in terms of bandwidth demand.

In this article [8], researchers look at the digital system needed for Measurement-Based Quantum Computing (MBQC)-based photo-detectors to handle not-gates and conduct exact arbitrary one-qubit rotations. Understanding the synchronization restrictions that digital systems place on analog structures and quantum devices is the main goal of the study, especially in the setting of a state generating system. By doing operational simulations and reviewing linear models with a Xilinx field-programmable gate array (7 series), the researchers validated the design features. As a result, they were able to determine the system's photonic clock rate and set an appropriate ceiling on the bandwidth at which sophisticated analysis coding can be used. The created and tested system is openly accessible and may be utilized to build more sophisticated systems that make use of modern photonic quantum computing methods. To achieve the demanding specifications of an optical quantum computer, the researchers underline the need to jointly develop the quantum states and the conventional control mechanism.

QRAC is used in this study [9] to effectively transform such discontinuous features into a finite number of qubits for VQC. We use computer modeling to demonstrate the limitations and potential of various encoding strategies. We demonstrate how QRAC can speed up VQC training by reducing its parameters and the amount of qubits used for mapping. By conducting tests on real-world database categorization utilizing a simulator and actual quantum hardware, we demonstrate the QRAC's effectiveness in VQC.

The study [10] looked into the effects that different interruption scenarios, noise inaccuracy parameters, and federal network phase counts have on the correctness of algorithm outputs. The IBM Quantum Lab's infrastructure, which consists of superconductor quantum servers and simulators, was used for the research. Due to a variety of issues, including the complexity of the operating surroundings, computing instabilities, and the finite number of qubits accessible, the outputs received from the quantum-based the server side frequently have low quality.

Researchers in the study [11] created a lauded single photon source utilizing a superior silicon microring resonator. They later created low-loss quantum photonic devices that allowed for the integration of spatial evaluation, Bell projection, or merging activities, and the generation of entangled states. In the study [12], researchers develop and show a technique for reducing software crosstalk noise in the NISQ system. Our study shows that software crosstalk reduction is doable and can greatly increase the reliability of noisy quantum machines. Through a back-end connection to the IBM Quantum Experience cloud service, researchers in the research [13] ProjectQ, a free and open-source initiative for quantum computing, can build quantum computations and apply them on real quantum hardware.

Figure 6.2 shows the model incorporating quantum Fourier transform (QFT) considering noise and comparing the gate noise strength among single qubit gate, two qubit gate, phase damping, etc.

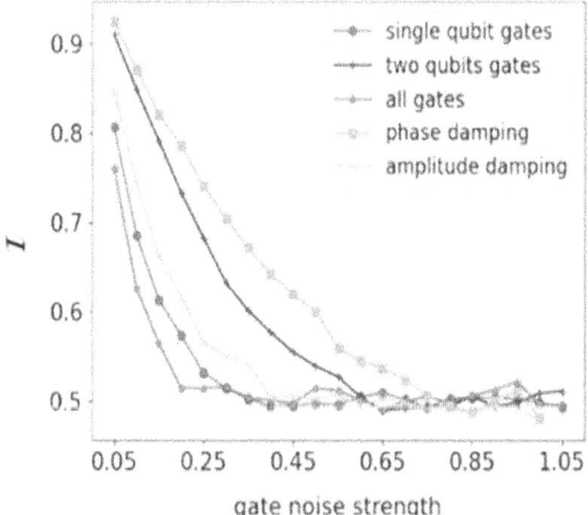

FIGURE 6.2 Model incorporating quantum Fourier transform (QFT) considering noise.

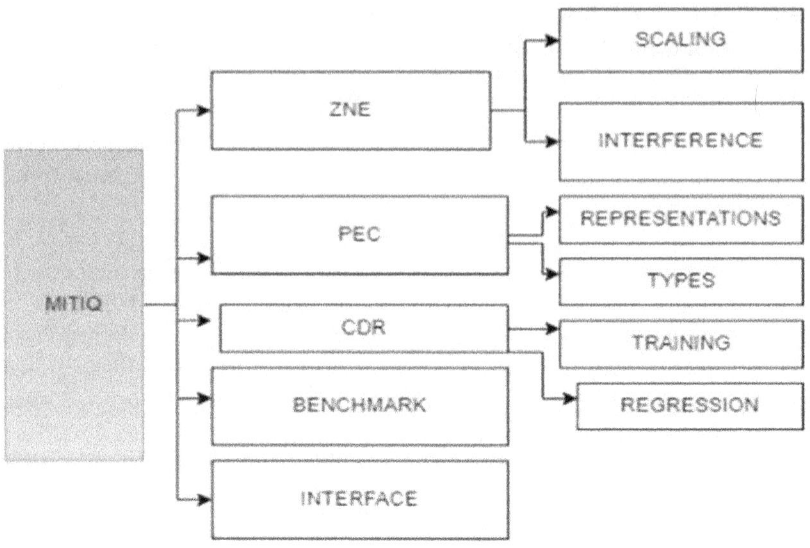

FIGURE 6.3 Model of quantum interface in quantum computing.

In the research [14], researchers used practical and theoretical demonstrations to show how error mitigation may enhance the results of a chaotic quantum information processing system. Then, they carefully combed through the library, focusing on the specific Mitiq modules relevant to different error-mitigating strategies, such as Clifford data regression analysis, zero-noise extrapolations, and statistical error cancellation. A quantum interface is shown in Figure 6.3.

The research [15] examined how to create a set of libraries for quantum simulation in computers using hardware acceleration through the OpenCL platform. Quantum computer modeling is a crucial step in developing and evaluating novel quantum algorithms, despite being time-consuming for a large number of qubits (relative to hardware).

6.3 PROPOSED MODEL

Quantum computation and traditional ML, two of the most fascinating areas of modern research, are combined in quantum algorithms. It looks at the relationship between quantum computing and ML and how advancements and approaches from one field could be used to address problems in the other. Current ML approaches are quickly pushing the limits of traditional numerical simulations as a result of an increasing number of data. In this aspect, quantum processing capacity may provide an advantage in ML initiatives. The study of developing and deploying quantum software that does ML more quickly than conventional computers is known as the field of quantum learning algorithm.

However, due to the exponential growth in complexity with an increasing number of photons, the proposed method is constrained to small-scale systems. Therefore, although photonic hardware capabilities continue to advance, there is currently no robust computational approach that can effectively harness the extensive resources of these systems. Additionally, photonic quantum advantage tests are reaching a stage where conventional equipment is no longer capable of performing the computations required.

The transition from classical bits to quantum qubits has the potential to revolutionize the healthcare system by enabling rapid drug development and in silico drug testing using high-performance graphics cards.

We foresee that developing optoelectronic hardware with unpredictable systems will become a viable scenario there in consideration with future due to recent significant advancements in the production of quantum artificial intelligence computers in healthcare. Nevertheless, in addition to quantum systems, the optimization techniques presented here may serve as useful benchmarks. While optical setup refinement is primarily concerned with estimating its features for a specific end quantum state, the former is mostly concerned with calculating the efficiency for an unidentified beginning configuration. The proposed model is shown in Figure 6.4.

TOPOLOGICAL OPTIMIZER: By satisfying previously set criteria and minimizing a predefined cost function, topology optimization is a computer function for optimizing the spatial distribution of material inside a specific region.

Variational optimization has been offered as a means to address optimization issues more quickly and broadly than traditional approaches allow.

DIGITAL QUANTUM COMPUTER: The objective of experimental quantum computing is to enhance the capabilities of the current quantum processors in order to realize some of the many potential applications of quantum computers on actual physical devices.

Now let's discuss qubits, the fundamental building blocks of quantum computers. These are computational systems that grow enormously beyond the typical ones and

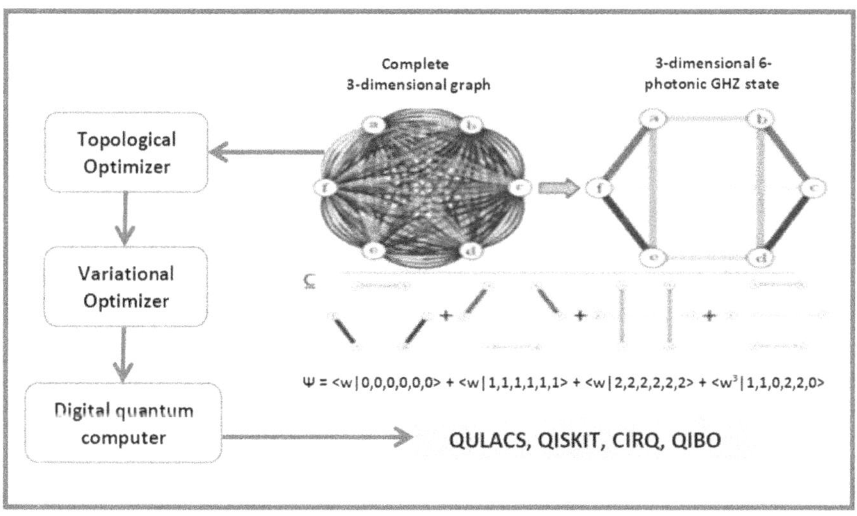

FIGURE 6.4 Proposed model for quantum optimizer for healthcare security

zeros and may accept a wide variety of quantum values. For instance, a system with 2 components may execute 4 simultaneous calculations, while a system with 3 qubits can perform 8, and a system with 4 qubits can accomplish 16.

Consider the Qubit Representation

Take a look at the picture above, where a bit is represented by the letters A-B and can have a value of 0 or 1. On the other hand, the sphere representation shows that the qubit can accept a variety of values that are represented on the sphere's surface. Each point is coupled with a latitude-longitude combination that stands for the values 0 or 1, respectively, and the phase.

The use of parameterized components inside a completely differentiable framework when modeling elector-optic structures on a distributed quantum chip is a major benefit. Effortlessly carrying out quantum electronic operations like quantum teleportation, quantum sensing, and experiments to confirm basic quantum physics concepts is the goal. There are various benefits to improving the optical transmission setup utilizing a widely used gate-based dynamic technique. Due to particular situations, the reliability of a real-world goods state is investigated instead of the intricate nature of an intertwined state.

According to the concepts of finite difference quantum eigensolvers (VQEs), which were first proposed for variational approximation of the eigenstates of a particular Hamiltonian, the optimization process contains the nondeterministic component. In this study, the accurate reflection of a given target state, which can be expressed as the expected value, is maximized using a variational approach.

The Hamiltonian H = |ΨihΨ| is determined by, and the number of quantifiable components (tensor products of Pauli matrices) changes correspondingly. FΨ = |hΨ||Φi|2 = hΦ|H|Φi.

6.4 BENEFITS OF THE MODEL

1. Quantum computers are incredibly efficient and rapid. They can perform computations that today's data centers would take decades, if not millennia, to complete.
2. Quantum computer calculations are highly promising for evaluating or modeling exceedingly complex processes with large amounts of data. Natural science disciplines, in particular, see significant promise in addition to digital marketing. Quantum computers could help us comprehend the interactions of specific particles, components, and processes in living cells in greater depth. However, there are possible medical applications.
3. When dealing with such a vast amount of data, modern computers and supercomputers are prone to errors, impacting performance. Furthermore, computational activities like assessing the effects of medications at the molecular level are too complex for traditional computers to handle. Instead, quantum computers are better suited for such activities since they can process large amounts of data more quickly.

6.5 FUTURE CHALLENGES

Due to their susceptibility to environmental disruptions, current quantum computers are highly vulnerable and need to be housed in expensive freezers maintained at temperatures close to absolute zero. Moreover, the existing quantum devices with 70 qubits fall significantly short of the 1 million qubits necessary to achieve the economic viability of quantum computers.

Quantum computers are incredibly difficult to design, build, and operate. As a result, they are hampered by faults like interference, breakdowns, and lack of quantum integrity, which is crucial to their operation but breaks before any nontrivial code can complete.

Providing and allocating resources for quantum services to service customers is a major challenge in quantum computing environments.

6.6 QUANTUM HEALTHCARE APPLICATIONS

Quantum computing has been used in a range of applications in the healthcare sector [16–18]. The amount of drug trials, disease databases, Electronic Health Information (EHRs), and implanted device observations have all grown. The growth of healthcare data plays a vital role in tackling the triple aim of enhancing patient care, reducing costs, and improving clinical management, along with boosting healthcare staff satisfaction. However, healthcare decision-makers face the challenge of making ongoing judgments based on data provided by complex systems. Recent research indicates significant advancements in providing relevant information and insightful ideas to healthcare personnel. Industry developments are promoting online experiences that promote healthy and preventive habits, while new data is expanding the capabilities of traditional computer systems. Quantum technology has the ability to offer healthcare practitioners a wide range of applications, including healthcare planning, quick diagnostics, personalized treatment, and price optimization. Additionally, the usage of unpredictable entanglement and conventional modeling techniques for storing people's beings grows as exposure to health-related information sources increases.

Although quantum technology has the ability to significantly improve healthcare, the majority of early-period computing technology secrets were confidential, underscoring the necessity of developing flexible tactics and collaborating with the sector. Specific computer technologies won't be able to match the exponential improvements that quantum computing will bring to healthcare [19–21].

The preceding represents some of the most significant functions of quantum computing in wellness. The applications of quantum indeterminate computing in healthcare are listed below:

1. Regenerative health care and development: A key component of medical research is the ability to recreate intricate responses at the nanoscale, thus which is made possible by quantum computing. This development has enormous potential for a range of medical applications, such as monitoring,

counseling, regeneration medicine, and diagnosis. The usage of AI methods to assist in patient diagnosis is growing. The majority of current ML approaches are focused on recognition of patterns, in which numerous ML algorithms are trained using a vast amount of patient data, leading to the creation of a computer-assisted diagnosis system. Quantum computing significantly accelerates the handling of this data compared to conventional computing techniques.

2. Radiotherapy: Radiotherapy is the use of radiation, a cancer treatment method that utilizes radiation beams to eliminate cancerous cells and inhibit their growth, requires precise calculations to target cancerous areas without affecting healthy cells. To achieve the necessary accuracy in radiography, which involves complex and precise simulations to find optimal solutions, powerful computers are used, posing a significant optimization challenge. The utilization of quantum computing in simulations offers a wide range of possibilities, enabling multiple simulations to run simultaneously and accelerating the development of an optimal strategy. This allows for faster and more efficient execution of radiography procedures.
3. DNA sequencing and analysis at breakneck speed: Over the past 20 years, genomics and genetics have undergone significant advancements. It is expected that the project called the Human Genome Project, which started in 1990 and on which a lot of money was spent, will present all of its findings in 2006. As a result, over 2000 genetic screenings for human disorders are presently available, and directly with consumers genetic testing companies let you order them online. These tests help medical professionals diagnose illnesses and tell patients about their genetic vulnerability to disease. Quantum ML is expected to significantly advance the discipline, allowing for faster whole-genome sequencing and more thorough and timely research.
4. Clinical studies using computer simulation: In silico experiments test a particular treatment without the need of humans, animals, even just one cell, a professional judgment, or a medicine, yet their effects may be meticulously recorded. A pharmacological simulation is a custom simulation model that is used in research or to examine the effects of a drug, device, or intervention. Comprehensive simulations like the HumMod, which includes over 1500 formulas and 10,000 natural processes in which mucus secretion, blood vessel tissue, electrolytes, steroids, metabolism, and skin galvanic response are all factors, have the potential to significantly enhance the development of "virtual characters" thanks to quantum computing. Additionally, it would enable "live" clinical trials using as many virtual participants as possible and components customized to the preferences of the testers. Figure 6.5 denotes the vital applications of quantum computing.

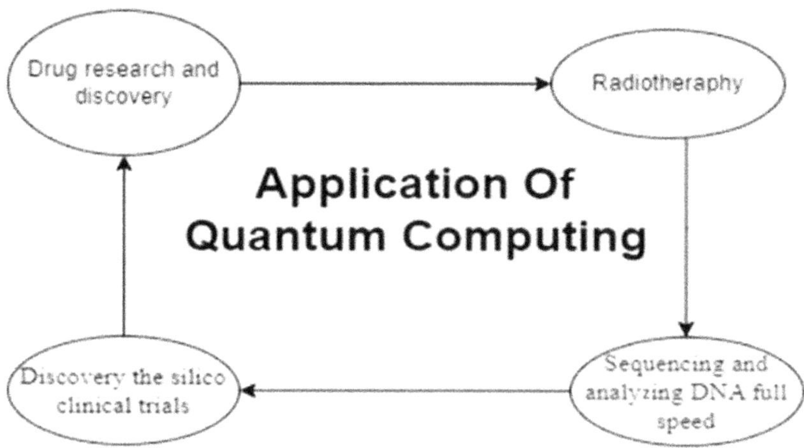

FIGURE 6.5 Applications trending in quantum computing.

6.7 QUANTUM COMPUTING REQUIREMENTS IN HEALTHCARE

Quantum computing helps to reduce processing time in numerous areas of health care. The specifications of the use of quantum computers in healthcare could not be generalized because they differ in the area of quantum computing employed. For example, drug discovery needs in vaccine development schemes Therefore, for efficient deployment of quantum computing applications in healthcare, various issues must be considered.

The generic resource requirements for quantum computing are shown in Table 6.1.

TABLE 6.1
Requirements for Quantum Computing in Healthcare Sector

Requirements	Causes	Solutions
Computational power	1. Existing approaches have less processing capability. 2. Higher computational cost computational complication. 3. High issue proportions. 4. Integration is difficult.	1. Quantum computation multivariate areas. 2. Larger difficulties are effectively represented. 3. Interference of quantum waves. 4. Quantum computing's astonishing performance.
Fault-tolerance	1. Inability to tolerate faults. 2. Entangled quantum properties. 3. Mistakes in qubits. 4. Absence of a quantum rectification algorithm.	1. Using an auxiliary qubit to detect qubits. 2. Detection of logical mistakes. 3. Error-detection code. 4. Relative error is limited.

(Continued)

TABLE 6.1 *(Continued)*
Requirements for Quantum Computing in Healthcare Sector

Requirements	Causes	Solutions
Scalability	1. Inadequate scalability. 2. Lack of adaptability. 3. Insufficient assistance for increased computational volume. 4. A scarcity of virtualization environments.	1. Domain adaptation techniques. The application of neural Boltzmann machines. 2. Quantum theory transfer-learning methods. 3. Computing applications based on FPGAs.
Quantum ML	1. Prolonged execution time. 2. A scarcity of resources. 3. Increased intricacy. 4. Increased operational overhead.	1. Technologies based on quantum computing. 2. Reduce the computational effort. 3. Faster response times. 4. Effective implementation.
Deployment of quantum gates	1. No replication prohibition. 2. Issues with linking architecture. 3. Problems of optimization algorithms. 4. No error—correcting code.	1. Application of gate-model quantum systems. 2. Gated-model computing. 3. Shor's factoring technique is third. 4. Permutation procedure performance.
Physical implementation	1. Expensive implementation. 2. A scarcity of resources. 3. Inadequate knowledge. 4. Reduced revenue.	1. Evolution of physical systems. 2. Economical solutions. 3. Manpower development. 4. Economical approaches.

6.8 RESULT ANALYSIS

We used TEQUILA, a Python program created to utilize various quantum computing techniques in ML, to analyze the data model. TEQUILA facilitates the quick and flexible development, testing, and implementation of novel quantum computations in fields like electrical engineering and others. It utilizes abstract expectation values that can be combined, modified, compared, and optimized. Once evaluated, these abstract data structures can be assembled to run on state-of-the-art quantum simulators or interfaces.

Pseudo-code for Tequila implementation:

1. Define variable 'a' using Tequila: a = tq.variables("a")
2. Construct a unitary operator 'U' using Tequila gates: U = tq.gates.Ry(angle= (-a**2).apply(tq.numpy.exp) * pi, target=0) U += tq.gates.X(target=1, control=0)
3. Create a QubitHamiltonian 'H' from a string representation: H = tq.QubitHamiltonian.from_string("-1.0*X(0)X(1)+0.5Z(0)+Y(1)")
4. Define an expectation value 'E' using 'H' and 'U': E = tq.ExpectationValue(H= H, U=U)
5. Compute the gradient of 'E' with respect to 'a': dE = tq.grad(E, "a")

6. Define the objective function 'Objective' as the sum of 'E' and the exponential of the negative squared 'dE': Objective = E + (-dE**2).apply(tq.numpy.exp)
7. Minimize the objective function using the "phoenics" optimization method: Result = tq.minimize(method="phoenics", objective=Objective)

For Measuring Fidelities

1. Fidelity can be calculated as the squared magnitude of the overlap between two quantum states: $F = |<\Phi(\theta)|\Psi>|\text{^}2$
2. Fidelity can also be expressed as the expectation value of the Hamiltonian 'H' with the state '$\Phi(\theta)$': $F = <\Phi(\theta)|H|\Phi(\theta)>$
3. This can be written as the expectation value of 'H' using the unitary operator '$U(\theta)$': $F = <H>U(\theta)$

The process flow chart in Figure 6.6 shows how a quantum problem is defined using a Hamiltonian, how a quantum state is transformed using quantum circuits, how expectation values are calculated, how an objective function is created, how

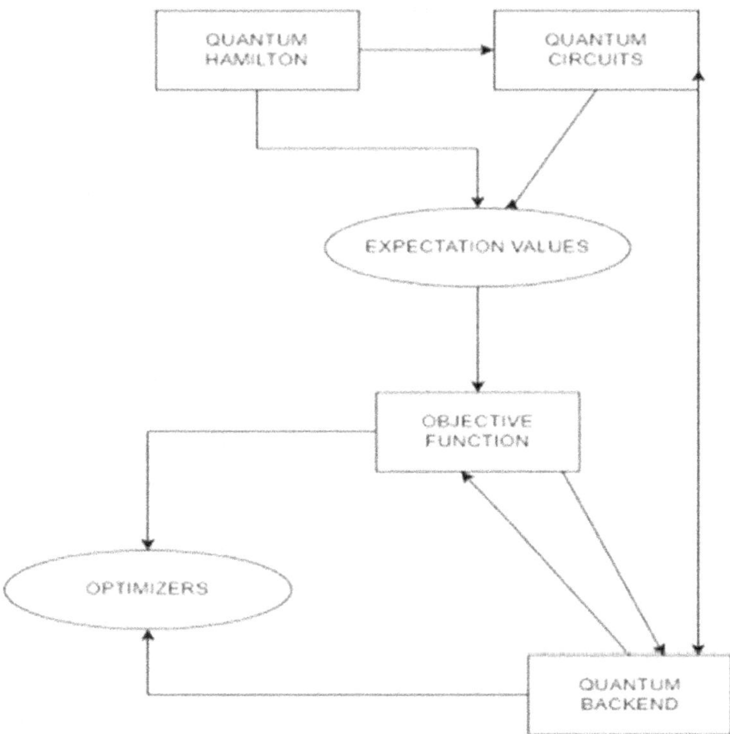

FIGURE 6.6 Model for quantum circuits for hardware in healthcare

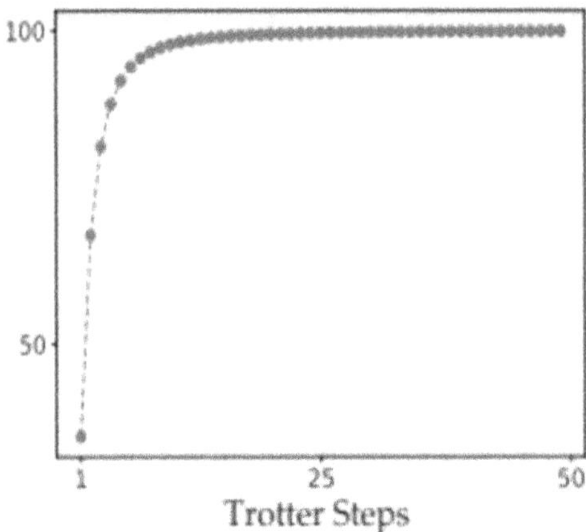

FIGURE 6.7 Accuracy of the machine learning model in quantum computing.

TABLE 6.2
Requirements to Run the Quantum Algorithm

Function	Configuration
CPU	16 Core
Memory	64G
Network bandwidth	1.2 Gbit/s
Hard disc capacity	20 G
Number of network cards	1
Operating system	Ubuntu 18.04 64-bit

quantum optimizer are used for optimizing the objective function, and how the solution is ultimately refined using classical optimizers.

We obtained the following hyperbolic graph in Figure 6.7 after applying the aforementioned technique utilizing the ML paradigm, and it showed that the number of trotting steps was increasing exponentially.

As a result, this is discovered to be more accurate, with an accuracy of 98.9%, and is suitable for models created by ML utilizing TEQUILA.

The above Table 6.2 shows the requirement for the system to go along with the algorithm to work in healthcare field.

6.9 CONCLUSION

Researchers considered quantum computing options from the perspective of healthcare systems throughout this study. They discussed novel application areas where advanced computational operations could be aided by quantum computing. They discussed the most crucial requirements for the application of quantum computing systems in the field of healthcare. On the other hand, using combinations with traditional algorithms should not be discouraged but rather encouraged to get the best of both worlds. Comparing using our solution to dealing with photonic equipment directly in healthcare has a number of benefits. It is fair to expect that quantum technology will perform better than conventional algorithms in computational duties given the intrinsic limits of classical systems to effectively construct unexpected patterns. When we employ TEQUILA as its packaging since it's faster, this method becomes more effective and yields more accurate results, increasing our accuracy to 98.9%. The system requirements are the only obstacle we currently have; if we can do so, calculating accuracy will be easier. The ML algorithm may be trained to predict the output more accurately, swiftly, and efficiently as the dataset changes in the coming months, increasing the safety of the data.

6.10 FUTURE SCOPE

The study of quantum computation and related disciplines of study are expanding quickly. The field of quantum algorithms has a lot of room for development, and different algorithms' usefulness will increase over time. Healthcare image processing, including operations like identifying edges and visual matching, can be improved by quantum computing. These improvements would make image-aided diagnosis much better. Additionally, single-cell strategies may be used to present diagnostic techniques.

REFERENCES

1. Kottmann, J. S., Krenn, M., Kyaw, T. H., Alperin-Lea, S., & Aspuru-Guzik, A. (2021). Quantum computer-aided design of quantum optics hardware.
2. Arrazola, J. M., Bromley, T. R., Izaac, J., Myers, C. R., Brádler, K., & Killoran, N. (2018). Machine learning method for state preparation and gate synthesis on photonic quantum computers.
3. Thumwanit, N., Lortaraprasert, C., Yano, H., & Raymond, R. (2021). Trainable Discrete Feature Embeddings for Quantum Machine Learning.
4. Huang, Z., Qian, L., & Cai, D. (2022). A quantum computing simulator scheme using MPI technology on cloud platform.
5. de Andrade, M. G., Dai, W., Guha, S., & Towsley, D. (2021). A quantum walk control plane for distributed quantum computing in quantum networks.
6. Upama, P. B., Farukt, M. J. H., Nazim, M., Masum, M., Shahriar, H., Uddin, G., Barzanjeh, S., Ahamed, S. I., Rahman, A. (2022). Evolution of Quantum Computing: A Systematic Survey on the Use of Quantum Computing Tools.
7. de Andrade, M. G., Dai, W., Guha, S., & Towsley, D. (2021). Optimal Policies for Distributed Quantum Computing with Quantum Walk Control Plane Protocol.
8. Scott, J. R., & Balram, K. C. (2022). Timing Constraints Imposed by Classical Digital Control Systems on Photonic Implementations of Measurement-Based Quantum Computing.
9. Yano, H., Suzuki, Y., Itoh, K. M., Raymond, R., & Yamamoto, N. (2021). Efficient Discrete Feature Encoding for Variational Quantum Classifier.
10. Wang, J., Zhang, M., Lai, J.-s., Zhao, W.-y., & Zhang, H.-y. (2021). Analysis on noise impact in algorithm-based quantum computing benchmark.
11. Ding, Y., Llewellyn, D., Faruque, I. I., Bacco, D., Rottwitt, K., Thompson, M. G., Wang, J., & Oxenlowe, L. K. (2020). Quantum Entanglement and Teleportation Based on Silicon Photonics.

12. Murali, P., McKay, D. C., Martonosi, M., & Javadi-Abhari, A. (2020). Software Mitigation of Crosstalk on Noisy Intermediate-Scale Quantum Computers.
13. Steiger, D. S., Häner, T., & Troyer, M. (2018). ProjectQ: An Open Source Software Framework for Quantum Computing.
14. LaRose, R., Mari, A., Kaiser, S., Karalekas, P. J., Alves, A. A., Czarnik, P., Mandouh, M. E., Gordon, M. H., Hindy, Y., Robertson, A., Thakre, P., Wahl, M., Samuel, D., Mistri, R., Tremblay, M., Gardner, N., Stemen, N. T., Shammah, N., & Zeng, W. J. (2022). Mitiq: A software package for error mitigation on noisy quantum computers.
15. Kelly, A. (2018). Simulating Quantum Computers Using OpenCL.
16. Rasool, R. U., Ahmad, H. F., Rafiq, W., Qadir, J., & Qayyum, A. (2021). Quantum Computing for Healthcare: A Review.
17. Sivani, T., & Mishra, S. (2022). Wearable Devices: Evolution and Usage in Remote Patient Monitoring System. In Connected e-Health (pp. 311–332). Springer, Cham.
18. Mohanty, A., & Mishra, S. (2022). A Comprehensive Study of Explainable Artificial Intelligence in Healthcare. In Augmented Intelligence in Healthcare: A Pragmatic and Integrated Analysis (pp. 475–502). Springer, Singapore.
19. Patnaik, M., & Mishra, S (2022). Indoor Positioning System Assisted Big Data Analytics in Smart Healthcare. In Connected e-Health (pp. 393–415). Springer, Cham.
20. Sahoo, P. K., Mishra, S., Panigrahi, R., Bhoi, A. K., & Barsocchi, P. (2022). An improvised deep-learning-based mask r-CNN model for laryngeal cancer detection using CT images. Sensors, 22(22), 8834.
21. Mishra, S., Thakkar, H. K., Singh, P., & Sharma, G. (2022). A decisive metaheuristic attribute selector enabled combined unsupervised-supervised model for chronic disease risk assessment. Computational Intelligence and Neuroscience, 2022. https://doi.org/10.1155/2022/8749353

7 Enhancing Communication by Using Sign Language Recognition

Souryadipta Das and Oindrila Ajha

7.1 INTRODUCTION

Human survival relies on interaction, a basic yet efficient method of exchanging ideas, feelings, and thoughts. However, a significant portion of the global population faces limitations in this aspect. Many individuals struggle with speech impairments, hearing difficulties, or both. Deaf mutism, or deaf-mute condition, can manifest in children who are unable to grasp language due to hearing impairment [1–3]. These conditions are widespread across the world. According to the World Health Organization (WHO), approximately 278 million people were deaf globally in 2005. It's crucial to address communication barriers that hinder social interactions and daily life for the growing deaf community. Sign language serves as the primary mode of communication for deaf and hard-of-hearing individuals worldwide, effectively bridging the gap with those who can hear. Sign language interpreters assist by converting sign language to spoken language, easing communication with individuals who have visual impairments [4]. However, the shortage of interpreters and the flexible nature of sign language necessitate technological support.

Sign language uses gestures, facial expressions, lip reading, nods, and posture to convey ideas. Body-worn modules like sensory gloves are effective tools for interpreting sign language. These gloves incorporate conventional or optical sensors attached to the user's glove to translate hand movements into motorized gestures, enabling body position detection [5]. Vision-based techniques estimate features such as palm, finger, and joint angles for recognition. This approach involves capturing signs through photos or videos and processing them using image-processing software. Intelligent sign language recognition (SLR) systems find applications in diverse fields, from hand tracking to gaming, robotics, augmented intelligence, and communication systems.

Despite significant progress, developing intelligent alternatives for sign language interpretation holds potential [6]. This analysis focuses on survey articles in the realm of intelligent SLR models, aiming to explore the use of predictive models and control in bridging communication gaps for visually impaired individuals.

Our research aims to pioneer the use of sign language to address information sharing challenges faced by the visually impaired, enhancing their integration into

DOI: 10.1201/9781032624891-7

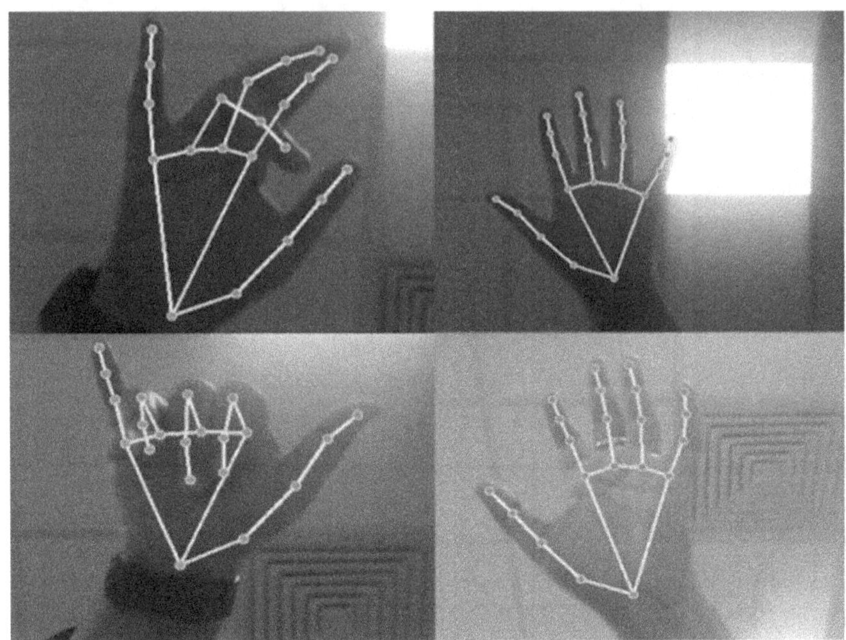

FIGURE 7.1 Gesture recognition and its applications.

society [7, 8]. If extended to language and everyday expressions, this technology could not only expedite communication for the deaf community but also foster autonomous understanding, ultimately aiding their overall development. Figure 7.1 shows a sample representation of gesture control and its scope.

7.2 RELATED WORKS

An important field where gesture management finds application is SLR. Numerous comprehensive studies have detailed applications and techniques in this realm over the past two decades. However, irrespective of the approach adopted, certain distinct challenges frequently emerge when dealing with SLR. The true test lies in crafting effective solutions that navigate the complexities and obstacles posed by the inherent intricacies of the problem. In their investigations into sign formation, sharing, hand associations, various sign types, lexical abnormalities, unnormalized sign mapping, and other aspects of sign language models, [9], as well as [10], delve into these subjects. Furthermore, researchers [9] introduce a novel model for sign language identification, presenting a framework that encompasses stages such as sign determination, sign selection, and identification of linkages among signs. Every phase could have a quite complicated model design. Parton (2006) provides a summary of how methods used in many branches of machine intelligence address SLR and mappings. SLR system design is a cross-disciplinary endeavor that may incorporate robots, augmented intelligence, machine vision, cognitive learning, augmented analytics, multi-vector animated vision, image analysis, and intelligence-driven system-assisted control.

In Futane, authors [11, 12] most recently compared several SLR techniques. Out of the potential methods mentioned in their study, like glove-enabled methods, image-driven approaches, and gesture analysis, we think that visually analytical methods denote a very normal approach to building a manual-system prompt and give importance to relevant issues. Here, hand motion segmentation, monitoring and processing of hand movements, and detection are the approaches.

Communication among the user executing the signs and processing part should come first when creating systems for SLR. In this interface, glove-based or vision-based solutions may be used. First, researchers in [13] as well as [14] give in-depth descriptions of the gloves, tools, and sensors utilized in several HGR applications. The authors of these two papers go over several applications for data blinkers. The authors of the investigations use colored gloves as markers. In [15] system for mobile sign detection, several sensors are used.

The pattern recognition and classification stage of these systems has been implemented using a variety of strategies. Architectures based on neural networks (NN) are typically used (2012), as in [16–19]. SVM (2013) has been utilized by Yang and Lee.

On the other hand, Hidden Markov Models (HMM) have been used in many works for classification of the hands, as in [20–24].

This study's organizing idea is based on our novel conceptual model of the essential components of a hand gesture detection system.

It includes the following:

The depth-based hand gesture identification process starts with the acquisition of clear or high-resolution images, which depends on the sensor being utilized.

The collected image sequence is subjected to hand localization using tracking and segmentation techniques.

Finally, the segmented hand images and their tracked trajectories utilization are classified using McNeill's gesture kind classification, which was developed from data sharing studies.

The technique of recognizing a group of postures and gestures from a given gesture set is known as gesture classification, and the focus of this analysis is on its components.

7.3 PROPOSED MODEL

A flowchart that illustrates the proposed methods for extracting gestures and converting into text is shown in Figure 7.2.

A novel conceptual model for hand gesture recognition systems, shown in Figure 7.2, served as the structure's foundation. The first step in recognizing hand gestures with depth-based technology is to take depth photographs, which depends on the type of sensor being utilized. Then, in Section II, the acquired image sequence is analyzed for hand localization using tracking and segmentation techniques such as OpenCV or clustering or OpenNI framework.

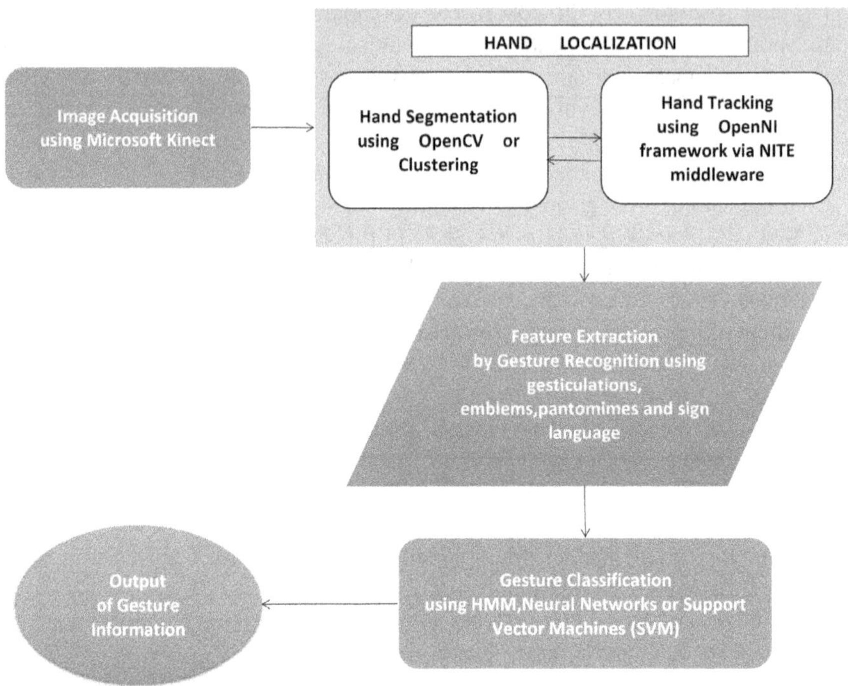

FIGURE 7.2 Block diagram of proposed method.

Then, in Section III feature extraction takes place which is a valuable step in creating a database for sign recognition. In order to efficiently and effectively characterize the various visual aspects of manual alphabet letters, both global visual features and local visual features are extracted to establish similarity between letter images. Finally, using McNeill's gesture type taxonomy from the communication literature [25–27], the segmentation-based hand scans or the monitored trajections are categorized as a specific gesture or posture in Section IV. The survey especially focuses on the factors that go into classifying gestures, which form as the procedure to identify a series of specified postures. It does not go into depth with 3D hand pose estimate, which seeks to recreate a whole 3D representation of the hand's posture and is depicted in gray. The applications reported so far are covered in Section IV, and the conclusions are discussed in Section V.

7.3.1 Image Acquisition

Various image-capturing devices are employed for categorizing signage images, including cameras, webcams, and the Kinect. Microsoft developed the Kinect primarily for full-body tracking. The Kinect features a QVGA depth (320 × 240) display, a camera, and a VGA (640 × 480) video camera, generating a 30-frame-per-second (fps) image stream. Microsoft provided a dedicated Kinect SDK, offering users access to depth and video feeds along with unique body tracking techniques tailored for the

Kinect. This system is widely utilized due to its efficiency, providing simultaneous color and depth video streams. It simplifies the differentiation between background and actual drawn images and facilitates the extraction of 3D trajectories from hand movements. However, one downside of the Kinect is its considerably high cost.

7.3.2 Hand Localization

Hand segmentation and hand tracking are two subproblems of hand localization, which is a key component of gesture recognition.

Hand segmented method is the challenge of detecting the pixels of an image belonging to a hand, while hand monitoring is the issue to determine the position of a hand in a set of photos.

7.3.3 Hand Segmentation

Hand segmentation is the division of an image into segmented, meaningful areas. The benefit of depth cameras over color cameras for gesture identification can be very apparent when doing hand segmentation [28]. It is normal to just utilize a depth limit to separate the hands in use cases in which the person faces the camera holding hands in front of themselves for posturing.

Prior to recognition, the input image must first be processed using segmentation. To obtain the hand area, a camera-captured image is divided into segments. Use of a clever edge detector is one of the segmentation techniques. The hand area in this image was located using the face detector available in OpenCV, which is used to identify boundaries from images.

By determining the boundary of hands and figuring out the centroid point of hands, skin assessment should be integrated with hand motion tracing.

Another approach to distinguish between the head and the face is to consider that the head is more static and bulky as compared to face.

It lists several hand segmentation techniques that have been discussed in various studies along with their segmentation accuracy.

Two other segmentation methods that are described in the literature include cluster analysis and zone-wise development. While region expanding begins with a seed part within the intended site and looks for related parts to expand and fill it, clustering combines neighboring points into contiguous regions [29]. Area growth is effective for segmentation because it tightly relates the expanding zone to the hand alone, unlike free-moving hands in depth images that are prone to have depth discontinuities at their borders.

7.3.4 Hand Tracking

Hand tracking is a helpful step before dynamic gesture detection since it can capture both temporal and geographic information. Kinect is specifically designed for whole-body motion tracking and OpenNI. The architecture (via NITE middleware) and the Microsoft Kinect SDK employ each hand node to generate completely articulated 20-point body tracing.

7.3.5 Feature Extraction Method

It may take dynamic movement of the hands, face, fingers, or complete body to recognize sign language. Hand gestures alone feature a huge variety of shapes, motions, and textures. For the feature to handle the variety of these variances, it must be reliable and effective. Even when features are extracted using geometric approaches, they are not always available and dependable due to self-occlusion and ambient lighting. It is also stressed how crucial it is to choose the best feature extraction technique [30]. After suitable feature extraction technique and recognition algorithm have been identified, resilience can be attained.

Since the input to a classifier is generated from this step, the chosen feature might have an impact on the success or failure of an experiment in the area of human-computer interaction utilizing hand gestures. The work explains the general processes of the feature extraction method that are visible.

7.3.6 Gesture Recognition Methods

Once the location and structure of hand movement is known, a prediction model that gives estimations of a specific posture being held can be used as an input. This section discusses the classification methods used as well as the kind of gestures and postures discovered by the articles that were assessed.

7.3.7 Gesture Types

Gestures can be divided into four basic categories: pantomimes, emblems, gesticulations, and sign language. Automatic sign language detection for the deaf is being tested, coupled with the use of gestures, emblems, and pantomimes to develop new types of participation, to help a group of users in this situation communicate naturally [31]. Finger counting gestures are categorized as symbols in McNeill's taxonomy of gestures because everyone can grasp their verbal equivalent and because spoken and gestural forms are frequently used interchangeably in everyday circumstances.

Gestures used to navigate menus are regarded as pantomimes rather than verbal equivalents because they take the place of speech.

7.3.8 Gesture Classification

Traditional prediction-based techniques or specific functional algorithms that leverage selected attributes derived from the depth image's extracted hand attributes are capable of performing gesture categorization.

For the classification of adaptive postures, HMMs are a commonly employed choice due to their effectiveness in classifying data with temporal characteristics. For the classification of static postures, similar to the previous case, straightforward k-Nearest Neighbors (k-NN) classifiers are frequently utilized owing to their strong classification rates and uncomplicated architecture. Additionally, Neural Networks and Support Vector Machines (SVMs) are prevalent in gesture recognition, often requiring less dataset filtering [32].

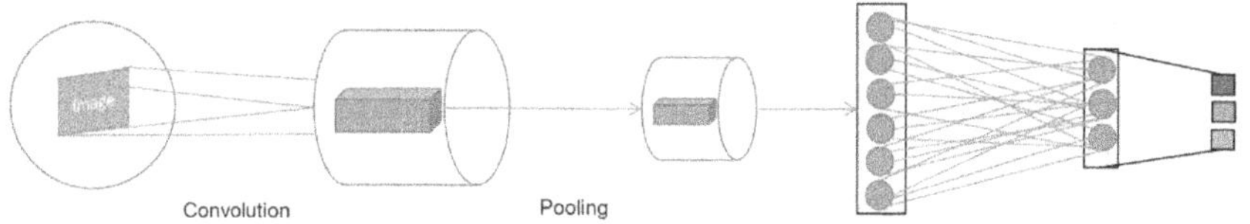

FIGURE 7.3 Block diagram for convolutional neural network in SLR.

Convolutional Neural Network is a kind of deep learning model which uses values to differentiate between different characteristics in an image after receiving an input image and assigning values to each feature in the image. Applications for the convolution neural network include voice recognition, scene labeling, face identification, picture classification, and natural language processing.

A supervised learning model using non-probabilistic learning methods is the SVM. It is a well-liked method of learning pattern recognition for classification regression analysis. It can be used to resolve non-linear regression and pattern classification issues, but it excels at resolving challenging pattern classification issues. SVM uses differentiation between two or more data classes to conduct classification. To do this, an ideal hyperplane that divides all categories is defined. Figure 7.3 shows the basic framework for convolutional neural network in SLR.

7.4 SCOPE AND USE CASES

The range of scope for gesture detection techniques that were covered in the articles was more constrained than the variety of methods themselves. The three areas of robot motion control, SLR, and interactive displays/tabletops/whiteboards accounted for 75% of the applications. Notably, all implementations beyond the three major groups were discovered in publications employing the Kinect as the depth sensor, and all but one of these used the OpenNI/NITE hand tracking algorithms to localize the hands.

Users of the gestures determination models were urged in 23 publications to move ahead of depth sensor from a specific distance, with the hands positioned such that they could be quickly recognized by the system [33]. All gadgets, with the exception of two, were used indoors under artificial lighting.

There hasn't been much research done on the new depth-based systems' limits or on using depth cameras for gesture detection in circumstances that are challenging for previous systems.

Despite the fact that several studies use the Kinect (22 papers) and the OpenNI/NITE hand tracing alternative for cheap and straightforward hand localization that can be utilized for gesture detection, this method has certain constraints. Additionally, while using the NITE skeletal tracking technique, the user must stand in a calibration posture for about ten seconds before body tracking can begin.

The Kinect/OpenNI/NITE approach is therefore really only suitable for utilities that need face-forward communication while the user is sitting or standing inside and in an indoor setting.

There are several possible applications for depth-based gesture recognition. Using such systems in complete darkness or low light scenarios, as well as in environments with a lot of debris that could appear as noise in a depth image, are examples of these circumstances [34, 35]. A user who is lying down may present a technological challenge for the hand local based approaches applied to depth cameras.

Advantages of the proposed model are:

- Low sensitivity to noise.
- Reduce redundant characteristics and large dimensionality of data. Therefore, the efficiency of model is improved.
- Reducing the number of functions helps solve the problem of data overfitting.
- Translation, scaling, and rotation invariant.
- Computational complexity is small.
- Reliable technology.
- Capture highly distinctive edge or gradient structures in local images.
- Near real-time performance.
- Invariant to scaling and lighting transforms.

Disadvantages of the proposed model are:

- Proper evaluation of the covariance matrix is difficult.
- Poor affine transformation and noise immunity.
- Local features cannot be identified because just the frequency's order of magnitude and not its precise location is known.
- It performs poorly when the lighting changes.
- A deep scanning strategy that covers the entire region of interest requires a lot of processing.
- High dimensionality of feature descriptors.

7.5 CONCLUSION

Among the analyzed 37 studies, 37 distinct techniques were employed for hand localization, with an additional 11 techniques dedicated to gesture categorization. Among these investigations, 24 showcased real-world instances. The evaluation of a gesture recognition system encompassed applications from a total of 8 distinct categories. Notably, 3 categories accounted for 75% of the papers studied. Out of the various types of depth sensors utilized, the Kinect emerged as the predominant choice, being employed in 21 of the publications. Within the realm of Kinect-based research, 8 articles utilized the hand-tracking libraries provided by the Kinect, with a predominant focus on applications over localization and classification techniques. The most commonly used methods for hand segmentation were depth thresholding and area growth. Kalman filters and mean shift were the prevailing choices for hand tracking, with some researchers opting for the NITE body- and hand-tracking module within the OpenNI framework. Gesture categorization techniques encompass a range of approaches, including HMMs, k-NN, Artificial Neural Networks, SVMs, and Finite State Machines. It is evident that gesture classification relies on fundamental machine learning algorithms, while hand localization and segmentation involve more specialized procedures. Additionally, commercially available alternatives such as Prime Sense's NITE module for the OpenNI framework have been replacing specialized hand identification and tracking methods. The current landscape of applications remains somewhat limited, with few discussions on the comparative advantages of depth cameras versus pixel cameras in gesture identification. Furthermore, the evaluation of depth-based gesture detection limitations within the designed use cases is still lacking. Many applications, aside from those pertaining to SLR, tend to revolve around light-hearted user interfaces for consumer products. There remains a dearth of applications focused on determining utility postures that can harness the potential of depth information in challenging scenarios.

Despite the shift toward encompassing use cases rather than localized and categorization approaches in recent studies, the advent of the Kinect has spurred a renewed interest in depth-based gesture recognition. Within the pool of 18 articles not involving the Kinect, a range of hand tracing techniques and 11 distinct gesture categorization methods were explored, albeit falling into 1 of 3 primary categories. Among the 22 studies involving the Kinect, a narrower range of 7 methods were employed for body positioning-based monitoring, 7 techniques for gesture categorization, and 8 categories of use cases. Eight of these articles specifically detailed applications employing the NITE skeleton and hand monitoring device. In sum, this analysis outlines the landscape of hand localization and gesture classification techniques prevalent in gesture determination studies. It is evident that the actual implementations employed to validate these methods display limited variation. The study underscores the need for applications that leverage depth information in challenging scenarios, along with use cases that validate the capabilities of depth sensory units – such as resistance to noise in depth images and hand detection amidst minimal movement or nearby objects. These sought-after applications encompass hand identification and gesture determination under low light conditions or with occlusions.

REFERENCES

1. Neha V. Tavari, P. A. V. D., "Indian sign language recognition based on histograms of oriented gradient," International Journal of Computer Science and Information Technologies, vol. 5, no. 3, pp. 3657–3660, 2014.
2. NMANIVAS. Gesture recognition system, 2014. https://github.com/nmanivas/Gesture-Recognition-System
3. S. Padmavathi, M. S. Saipreethy, V., and V. Valliammai. Indian sign language character recognition using neural networks. Recent Trends in Pattern Recognition and Image Analysis, RTPRIA, vol. 1, pp. 40–45, May 2013.
4. S. Goyal, and S. S. Ishita Sharma, "Sign language recognition system for deaf and dumb people," International Journal of Engineering Research Technology, vol. 2, no. 4, pp. 382–387, April 2013.
5. SCHAKENBERG. Schakenberg code for bag of visual words on GitHub, 2016. https://github.com/shackenberg/Minimal-Bag-of-Visual-Words-Image-Classifier
6. X. Teng, B. Wu, W. Yu, and C. Liu, "A hand gesture recognition system based on local linear embedding," Journal of Visual Languages & Computing, vol. 16, pp. 442–454, April 2005.

7. J. P. Wachs, M. Kölsch, H. Stern, and Y. Edan, "Vision-based hand-gesture applications," Communications of the ACM, vol. 54, pp. 60–71, 2011.
8. S. Mitra, and T. Acharya, "Gesture recognition: A survey," Systems, Man, and Cybernetics, Part C: Applications and Reviews, vol. 37, pp. 311–324, 2007.
9. Bossard, B., Braffort, A., & Jardino, M. (2003, April). Some issues in sign language processing. In *International Gesture Workshop* (pp. 90–100). Berlin, Heidelberg: Springer Berlin Heidelberg.
10. Caridakis, G., Karpouzis, K., Drosopoulos, A., & Kollias, S. (2010). SOMM: Self organizing Markov map for gesture recognition. *Pattern recognition letters, 31*(1), 52–59.
11. Ajmire, P. E., Dharaskar, R., & Thakare, V. M. (2012). Pattern Recognition Method for Study of botanical characteristics of Leaf. *Recent Trends in Computing" Proceedings published by International Journal of Computer Applications®(IJCA) ISSN*, 0975–8887.
12. Cooper, H. M., Ong, E. J., Pugeault, N., & Bowden, R. (2012). Sign language recognition using sub-units. *Journal of Machine Learning Research, 13*, 2205–2231.
13. Dipietro, L., Sabatini, A. M., & Dario, P. (2008). A survey of glove-based systems and their applications. *Ieee transactions on systems, man, and cybernetics, part c (applications and reviews), 38*(4), 461–482.
14. Parvini, F., McLeod, D., Shahabi, C., Navai, B., Zali, B., & Ghandeharizadeh, S. (2009). An approach to glove-based gesture recognition. In *Human-Computer Interaction. Novel Interaction Methods and Techniques: 13th International Conference, HCI International 2009, San Diego, CA, USA, July 19–24, 2009, Proceedings, Part II 13* (pp. 236–245). Springer Berlin Heidelberg.
15. Brashear, H., Starner, T., Lukowicz, P., & Junker, H. (2003, October). Using multiple sensors for mobile sign language recognition. In *Seventh IEEE International Symposium on Wearable Computers, 2003. Proceedings* (pp. 45–45). IEEE Computer Society.
16. Huang, Z. (1998). Extensions to the k-means algorithm for clustering large data sets with categorical values. *Data mining and knowledge discovery, 2*(3), 283–304.
17. Karami, A., Zanj, B., & Sarkaleh, A. K. (2011). Persian sign language (PSL) recognition using wavelet transform and neural networks. *Expert Systems with Applications, 38*(3), 2661–2667.
18. Sole, M. M., & Tsoeu, M. S. (2011, September). Sign language recognition using the extreme learning machine. In *IEEE Africon'11* (pp. 1–6). IEEE.
19. Karmokar, B. C., Alam, K. M. R., & Siddiquee, M. K. (2012). Bangladeshi sign language recognition employing neural network ensemble. *International journal of computer applications, 58*(16), 43–46.
20. Haberdar, H., & Albayrak, S. (2005, October). Real time isolated Turkish sign language recognition from video using hidden Markov models with global features. In *International Symposium on Computer and Information Sciences* (pp. 677–687). Berlin, Heidelberg: Springer Berlin Heidelberg.
21. Haberdar, H., & Albayrak, S. (2006, September). A two-stage visual Turkish sign language recognition system based on global and local features. In *International Symposium on Methodologies for Intelligent Systems* (pp. 29–37). Berlin, Heidelberg: Springer Berlin Heidelberg.
22. Zhang, Z. B., Zhu, J., Gao, J. F., Wang, C., Li, H., Li, H., ... & Yang, Z. N. (2007). Transcription factor AtMYB103 is required for anther development by regulating tapetum development, callose dissolution and exine formation in Arabidopsis. *The Plant Journal, 52*(3), 528–538.
23. Zaki, M. M., & Shaheen, S. I. (2011). Sign language recognition using a combination of new vision based features. *Pattern Recognition Letters, 32*(4), 572–577.

24. Auephanwiriyakul, S., Phitakwinai, S., Suttapak, W., Chanda, P., & Theera-Umpon, N. (2013). Thai sign language translation using scale invariant feature transform and hidden Markov models. *Pattern Recognition Letters*, *34*(11), 1291–1298.
25. A. Erol, G. Bebis, M. Nicolescu, R. D. Boyle, and X. Twombly, "Vision-based hand pose estimation: A review," Computer Vision and Image Understanding, vol. 108, pp. 52–73, 2007.
26. D. McNeill, Language and Gesture, vol. 2. Cambridge University Press, 2000.
27. K. K. Biswas and S. K. Basu. Gesture recognition using Microsoft Kinect®. In *The 5th international conference on automation, robotics and applications* (pp. 100–103). IEEE, 2011, December 2011.
28. C.-P. Chen, C. Yu-Ting, L. Ping-Han, T. Yu-Pao, and L. Shawmin, "Real-time hand tracking on depth images," in Visual Communications and Image Processing (VCIP), pp. 1–4. IEEE, 2011.
29. H. Du, and T. To, Hand Gesture Recognition Using Kinect. Boston University, 2011.
30. I. Oikonomidis, N. Kyriazis, and A. Argyros, Efficient Model-Based 3d Tracking of Hand Articulations Using Kinect. FORTH Institute of Computer Science, 2011.
31. S. Park, S. Yu, J. Kim, S. Kim, and S. Lee, "3D hand tracking using Kalman filter in depth space," EURASIP Journal on Advances in Signal Processing, vol. 2012, p. 36, 2012.
32. J. L. Raheja, A. Chaudhary, and K. Singal, "Tracking of fingertips and centers of palm using KINECT," in Computational Intelligence, Modelling and Simulation (CIMSiM), pp. 248–252, IEEE, 2011.
33. Z. Ren, J. Yuan, and Z. Zhang, "Robust hand gesture recognition based on finger-earth mover's distance with a commodity depth camera," in ACM International Conference on Multimedia, pp. 1093–1096, ACM, Melbourne, 2011.
34. M. Tang, Recognizing Hand Gestures with Microsoft's Kinect. Stanford University, 2011.
35. C. Yang, J. Yujeong, J. Beh, D. Han, and H. Ko, "Gesture recognition using depth-based hand tracking for contactless controller application," in Consumer Electronics (ICCE), pp. 297–298, IEEE, 2012.

8 Intelligent Ambulance Services Management

A Comprehensive Medical Service for Emergency Healthcare

Aradhana Behura

8.1 INTRODUCTION

Road traffic accidents lead to over 1.25 million fatalities worldwide annually, with India alone witnessing more than 200,000 deaths, a number that has been steadily rising since 2007. This concerning trend is primarily attributed to the inefficiencies within the existing Emergency Medical Services (EMS) in the country. The critical factor in reducing mortality rates after traumatic accidents is the timely provision of medical care, often referred to as the "golden hour." Unfortunately, in some Indian states, this crucial timeframe is compromised due to the inadequate state-funded EMS systems. The delay between an accident occurring and an ambulance arriving at the scene is a critical determinant of survival. Many accident victims may be unconscious and unable to call for help themselves. Moreover, in India, where emergency services rely on witnesses to report accidents, significant delays can occur. Ambulance drivers also face challenges in identifying accident locations and navigating through congested traffic. Post-accident follow-up care can take up to 48 hours. These delays are primarily attributable to human factors in the response process. To address these issues, the paper proposes an intelligent system designed to promptly detect accidents, dispatch the nearest ambulance, and guide it to the accident site, minimizing delays. This system aims to leverage technology to improve the efficiency of emergency responses and ultimately save lives. Before delving into the specifics of this proposed system, the paper provides a brief overview of relevant literature to contextualize the proposed approach [1–5].

A comprehensive solution for road traffic accident detection and ambulance management is crucial for improving response times and saving lives. Such a system can leverage technology and data to quickly identify accidents, dispatch ambulances efficiently, and provide real-time information to emergency services and healthcare providers [6–10]. Here's a detailed outline of a potential solution:

1. **Accident Detection:**
    - **Camera and Sensor Network:** Install a network of cameras and sensors at key locations on roads and highways to monitor traffic in real time.

DOI: 10.1201/9781032624891-8

- **AI-Based Image Recognition:** Implement AI algorithms to analyze camera feeds and detect anomalies such as accidents, collisions, or road blockages.
- **Connected Vehicles:** Integrate with modern vehicles equipped with sensors and communication systems to transmit accident data in real time.

2. **Data Fusion and Analysis:**
   - **Data Aggregation:** Collect data from various sources, including traffic cameras, sensors, connected vehicles, and social media reports.
   - **Machine Learning:** Use machine learning models to analyze and correlate data to verify accident occurrences and severity.
   - **Predictive Analytics:** Utilize historical data to predict accident-prone areas and times to proactively allocate resources.
3. **Alert and Notification System:**
   - **Automated Alerts:** When an accident is detected, automatically generate alerts to local emergency services, ambulance dispatch centers, and nearby hospitals.
   - **Public Alerts:** Send notifications to nearby drivers through mobile apps, electronic road signs, and social media to inform them about traffic disruptions.
4. **Ambulance Dispatch and Routing:**
   - **GPS Tracking:** Equip ambulances with GPS and real-time tracking systems for precise location monitoring.
   - **Algorithmic Dispatch:** Implement intelligent dispatch algorithms to select the nearest available ambulance.
   - **Traffic Data Integration:** Consider real-time traffic data to optimize ambulance routes for faster response times.
5. **Communication and Coordination:**
   - **Emergency Services Coordination:** Establish a central coordination center that communicates with police, fire departments, and other emergency services.
   - **Healthcare Integration:** Integrate with hospitals and medical facilities to streamline patient transfer and care.
6. **Mobile App for Public and First Responders:**
   - **Public Reporting:** Develop a user-friendly mobile app that allows the public to report accidents, providing location and basic details.
   - **First Responder Assistance:** Enable trained volunteers or off-duty medical personnel to respond to incidents and provide initial aid before ambulances arrive.
7. **Real-time Data Sharing:**
   - **Open Data Access:** Share accident and traffic data with government agencies, researchers, and developers to enhance road safety measures.
   - **Data Visualization:** Create dashboards and reports for stakeholders to monitor accident trends and response effectiveness.
8. **Integration with IoT and Smart Cities:**
   - **IoT Sensors:** Collaborate with smart city initiatives to integrate IoT sensors for real-time data sharing and monitoring.

    - **Traffic Management:** Work with traffic management systems to optimize traffic flow around accident sites.
9. **Training and Education:**
    - **Public Awareness:** Conduct awareness campaigns to educate the public about reporting accidents and providing first aid.
    - **Training for First Responders:** Offer training programs for volunteers and first responders to improve their ability to assist in emergencies.
10. **Continuous Improvement:**
    - **Feedback Loop:** Establish a feedback mechanism to gather input from emergency responders, hospitals, and the public to continually refine the system.

A comprehensive road traffic accident detection and ambulance management solution can significantly reduce response times, improve patient outcomes, and enhance overall road safety. It requires a collaborative effort among government agencies, healthcare providers, technology companies, and the public to achieve its full potential [7].

8.2 INTELLIGENT AMBULANCE MANAGEMENT SYSTEM

An Intelligent Ambulance Management System (IAMS) is a sophisticated solution designed to optimize the allocation, routing, and management of ambulance services. It leverages technology, data analysis, and automation to ensure efficient and timely responses to medical emergencies [11–16]. Here are the key components and features of an IAMS:

1. **Real-time Ambulance Tracking:**
    - **GPS and Location Services:** Equip ambulances with GPS devices and real-time location tracking systems to monitor their positions continuously.
    - **Status Updates:** Provide real-time updates on ambulance status, including availability, occupancy, and readiness.
2. **Emergency Call Handling:**
    - **Integrated Dispatch Center:** Establish a central dispatch center that receives emergency calls and communicates with ambulances.
    - **Call Triage:** Implement a system for call triage to assess the severity of the emergency and prioritize responses accordingly.
3. **Automated Dispatch:**
    - **Decision Support Algorithms:** Utilize intelligent algorithms to determine the nearest available ambulance and the optimal route to the emergency location.
    - **Dynamic Resource Allocation:** Adjust ambulance assignments in real time based on changing conditions and priorities.
4. **Traffic and Navigation Integration:**
    - **Real-time Traffic Data:** Integrate with traffic management systems and navigation tools to select the fastest and least congested routes.
    - **Traffic Prediction:** Use historical and real-time traffic data to predict congestion and suggest alternative routes.

5. **Electronic Health Records (EHR) Integration:**
    - **Access to Patient Information:** Enable ambulance crews to access essential patient information, such as medical history and allergies, before arriving at the scene.
    - **EHR Data Sharing:** Integrate with healthcare facilities to exchange patient data securely and seamlessly.
6. **Mobile Applications:**
    - **Ambulance Crew App:** Provide ambulance crews with a mobile app that includes navigation, patient data access, and communication tools.
    - **Public App:** Develop a mobile app for the public to request ambulance services and track their arrival.
7. **Communication and Coordination:**
    - **Interagency Collaboration:** Facilitate communication and coordination with other emergency services, hospitals, and law enforcement agencies.
    - **Two-Way Communication:** Enable two-way communication between dispatchers and ambulance crews for updates and instructions.
8. **Data Analytics and Reporting:**
    - **Performance Metrics:** Collect and analyze data on response times, patient outcomes, and resource utilization to identify areas for improvement.
    - **Reporting Tools:** Create dashboards and reports for stakeholders to monitor system performance.
9. **Resource Optimization:**
    - **Dynamic Resource Management:** Optimize ambulance deployment based on demand patterns, geographical areas, and historical data.
    - **Fleet Maintenance:** Implement maintenance schedules and alerts to ensure ambulance fleet reliability.
10. **Disaster and Mass Casualty Management:**
    - **Disaster Preparedness:** Develop protocols and resources for managing mass casualty incidents and disasters.
    - **Resource Mobilization:** Quickly mobilize additional ambulances and medical personnel during emergencies.
11. **Training and Simulation:**
    - **Training Programs:** Offer ongoing training for ambulance crews on the use of the system and emergency response procedures.
    - **Simulation Tools:** Provide simulation tools for practicing emergency scenarios and decision-making.
12. **Security and Privacy:**
    - **Data Encryption:** Ensure the security of patient data and communications through encryption and authentication measures.
    - **Compliance:** Adhere to healthcare data privacy regulations, such as HIPAA (in the United States) or GDPR (in Europe).

An IAMS enhances emergency response efficiency, reduces response times, and improves patient outcomes. It plays a critical role in modernizing EMS and ensuring that healthcare resources are allocated effectively during critical situations [17–21].

8.2.1 Smart Ambulance System in Countries

Smart ambulance systems are being implemented in various foreign countries to improve EMS and enhance the quality of healthcare. Here are some key features and examples of smart ambulance systems in foreign countries:

1. **United States:**
   - **Telemedicine-Equipped Ambulances:** Some regions in the United States have introduced ambulances equipped with telemedicine capabilities, allowing paramedics to consult with remote physicians in real-time, improving patient care during transit.
   - **Integrated EHR Systems:** Ambulances are integrated with electronic health record (EHR) systems, enabling seamless transfer of patient data to hospitals and ensuring continuity of care.
2. **United Kingdom:**
   - **GPS Navigation:** Ambulances in the United Kingdom use advanced GPS navigation systems to quickly reach accident scenes and hospitals, reducing response times.
   - **Emergency Alert Systems:** Smart ambulance systems are integrated with emergency alert systems that notify hospitals about incoming patients, enabling them to prepare in advance.
3. **Canada:**
   - **Community Paramedicine Programs:** In some Canadian provinces, paramedics provide preventive and follow-up care to patients at their homes, reducing the need for ambulance transport and hospital visits.
   - **Real-Time Data Sharing:** Ambulances share patient data, vital signs, and medical histories with hospitals in real time, ensuring that emergency departments are prepared for incoming patients.
4. **Germany:**
   - **Telemedicine Consultation:** German ambulances are equipped with telemedicine systems that allow paramedics to consult with specialized physicians for complex cases, improving the accuracy of diagnosis and treatment.
   - **Advanced Diagnostic Equipment:** Ambulances in Germany often carry advanced diagnostic equipment, such as mobile CT scanners, to enable early detection of critical conditions like strokes.
5. **Australia:**
   - **Integrated Communication:** Ambulances in Australia are integrated with a centralized communication system that coordinates the allocation of resources and ensures the closest available ambulance is dispatched to emergencies.
   - **Community Defibrillators:** Some regions have implemented smart systems that notify nearby trained volunteers of cardiac arrest cases, enabling them to reach the scene and provide defibrillation before the ambulance arrives.

6. **Singapore:**
   - **High-Tech Ambulances:** Singapore has introduced high-tech ambulances with advanced medical equipment and telemedicine capabilities to provide immediate care during transit.
   - **Smart Traffic Management:** Ambulances are equipped with systems that communicate with traffic lights to prioritize their passage through traffic, reducing delays.

These examples showcase the diversity of smart ambulance systems in foreign countries, emphasizing the use of technology, data integration, and telemedicine to enhance the efficiency and effectiveness of EMS. These systems not only reduce response times but also improve patient outcomes by ensuring that the right care is delivered promptly.

8.2.2 Disaster and Mass Casualty Management in Intelligent Ambulance

Intelligent ambulances play a crucial role in disaster and mass casualty management by providing a well-coordinated, efficient, and technology-driven response. Their ability to rapidly mobilize resources, communicate effectively, and provide advanced medical care is instrumental in saving lives and minimizing the impact of large-scale emergencies.

Disaster and Mass Casualty Management within the context of intelligent ambulances involves a comprehensive approach to handling large-scale emergencies and catastrophic events [22–28]. These ambulances are equipped with advanced technology and capabilities to respond effectively to such situations:

- **Rapid Deployment:** Intelligent ambulances can swiftly mobilize additional resources and personnel to the disaster site. Automated dispatch systems prioritize the allocation of ambulances based on the severity of injuries and casualties.
- **Triage Support:** These ambulances assist in the triage process by categorizing patients according to the seriousness of their injuries. This helps ensure that critical patients receive immediate care.
- **Data Sharing:** Intelligent ambulances facilitate real-time data sharing with hospitals and emergency response centers. This exchange of patient information and vital signs enables better resource allocation and tracking of patients' conditions.
- **Telemedicine:** Some intelligent ambulances are equipped with telemedicine capabilities, allowing paramedics to consult with remote medical experts. This ensures that patients receive expert guidance and care, even in challenging disaster scenarios.
- **Navigation and Routing Optimization:** Advanced navigation systems adapt to changing traffic conditions and road closures during disasters, ensuring ambulances reach affected areas quickly and efficiently.
- **Medical Equipment and Supplies:** Intelligent ambulances carry essential medical equipment and supplies tailored for disaster response, including

oxygen, trauma kits, and medications, ensuring that resources are readily available.

- **Interagency Coordination:** These ambulances facilitate communication and coordination between various emergency response agencies, such as fire departments, law enforcement, and search and rescue teams. This collaboration ensures a unified response to mass casualty incidents.
- **Public Communication:** Some systems can send mass notifications and updates to the public during disasters, providing critical information on how to seek assistance or stay safe.
- **Resource Tracking:** Intelligent ambulance systems track resources, medical supplies, and personnel during disaster response, ensuring efficient resource management and accountability.
- **Post-Disaster Analysis:** After the event, data collected by intelligent ambulances is invaluable for post-disaster analysis. It helps improve future disaster response strategies, resource allocation, and overall emergency preparedness.

In essence, intelligent ambulances are pivotal in disaster and mass casualty management by providing a coordinated, technology-driven response to large-scale emergencies. They enable rapid deployment of resources, efficient communication, advanced medical care, and data-driven improvements for future disaster responses, ultimately saving lives and minimizing the impact of catastrophic events [25, 29–35].

8.2.3 Telemedicine Support in Smart Ambulance

Telemedicine support in smart ambulances enhances the overall capabilities of EMS by providing access to expert medical advice and resources regardless of geographic location or the complexity of the medical condition. It improves patient outcomes, reduces response times, and ensures that patients receive the right care from the moment the ambulance arrives. Telemedicine support in smart ambulances is a cutting-edge feature that revolutionizes EMS by integrating telecommunication technology and healthcare. Here are the key aspects and benefits of telemedicine support in smart ambulances:

- **Real-Time Consultation:** Smart ambulances are equipped with secure telecommunication systems that enable paramedics to establish real-time video and audio connections with healthcare professionals at remote locations, such as hospitals or specialized medical centers.
- **Expert Medical Guidance:** Telemedicine support allows paramedics to consult with specialized physicians or medical specialists who can provide expert guidance on diagnosing and treating patients. This is especially valuable in complex or critical cases.
- **Pre-hospital Assessment:** Paramedics can conduct preliminary assessments of patients' conditions while en route to the hospital. Telemedicine enables remote medical experts to assess vital signs, review patient history, and provide immediate advice on treatment protocols.

- **Medication and Treatment Decision Support:** Remote healthcare professionals can assist paramedics in making crucial decisions regarding medication administration, interventions, and medical procedures, ensuring that patients receive the most appropriate care during transport.
- **Enhanced Diagnostic Capabilities:** Smart ambulances may be equipped with advanced diagnostic tools, such as portable ultrasound devices or mobile ECG machines, which can transmit real-time data to remote experts for interpretation and recommendations.
- **Reduced Time to Treatment:** Telemedicine support minimizes delays in receiving medical care by initiating treatment decisions and preparations while the patient is in transit, potentially saving critical minutes that can be life-saving.
- **Seamless Patient Handover:** Telemedicine facilitates the transfer of patient information, including vital signs, diagnostic results, and treatment plans, to the receiving hospital. This ensures that emergency department staff are well-informed and can provide continuity of care.
- **Multilingual Support:** In diverse regions or when language barriers exist, telemedicine can connect paramedics with healthcare professionals who can communicate effectively with patients and their families, improving patient understanding and comfort.
- **Continuous Monitoring:** For patients with chronic conditions or those requiring ongoing care, telemedicine allows for continuous remote monitoring, enabling healthcare professionals to intervene promptly if necessary.
- **Disaster Response:** During mass casualty incidents or disasters, telemedicine support enables on-site emergency responders to collaborate with remote medical teams, ensuring efficient triage, resource allocation, and patient care coordination.
- **Post-Disaster Follow-up:** After a disaster, telemedicine can be used to provide follow-up care to survivors, assess their health status remotely, and address any ongoing medical needs.

Telemedicine support in smart ambulances enhances the quality of emergency medical care, reduces response times, and extends access to specialized medical expertise. It is a critical component of modern EMS, ensuring that patients receive timely and appropriate care from the moment the ambulance is dispatched until they reach the hospital [36–41].

Smart ambulance management in case of road accident: Smart ambulance management during road accidents or heavy traffic situations is essential to ensure efficient and timely emergency response. Here's how smart ambulance management systems can address these challenges:

1. **Real-Time Traffic Monitoring:**
    - Utilize traffic management systems and data from GPS and sensors to monitor road conditions in real time. Smart ambulance systems can access this data to make informed decisions about ambulance routing and dispatch.

2. **Traffic Prediction Algorithms:**
    - Implement predictive algorithms that forecast traffic conditions based on historical data, events, and current traffic patterns. These predictions help ambulance dispatchers choose the fastest and least congested routes.
3. **Dynamic Resource Allocation:**
    - Smart ambulance systems can dynamically allocate ambulances based on traffic conditions. When heavy traffic is detected on a planned route, the system can reroute ambulances to alternative paths to minimize delays.
4. **Traffic Signal Interaction:**
    - Equip ambulances with technology that communicates with traffic signals. When an ambulance approaches, traffic lights can prioritize its passage, reducing intersection delays.
5. **Real-Time Communication:**
    - Establish real-time communication between ambulances and dispatch centers. This allows for continuous updates on traffic conditions and enables dispatchers to provide route adjustments as needed.
6. **Automated Decision Support:**
    - Implement automated decision support systems that factor in traffic conditions, accident severity, and ambulance availability to determine the most appropriate response plan.
7. **Public Notification:**
    - Use mobile apps or public alert systems to inform drivers about road closures or heavy traffic in the vicinity of an accident. This can help divert non-emergency traffic and clear the way for emergency vehicles.
8. **Alternative Transportation:**
    - In cases of extreme gridlock, consider using alternative transportation methods, such as drones or specialized emergency response vehicles capable of maneuvering through traffic.
9. **Data Analytics and Machine Learning:**
    - Leverage data analytics and machine learning to continually improve ambulance routing and traffic management algorithms. These systems can learn from past incidents to make more accurate predictions and decisions.
10. **Collaboration with Traffic Authorities:**
    - Collaborate with traffic management authorities to receive real-time updates and coordinate traffic flow for emergency vehicles.

Smart ambulance management during road accidents or heavy traffic conditions is essential for ensuring that critical medical care reaches patients as quickly as possible. By combining real-time traffic data, predictive algorithms, and advanced communication systems, smart ambulance management systems can navigate traffic challenges effectively and optimize response times, ultimately improving patient outcomes in emergencies [41–46].

8.3 ROLE OF MACHINE LEARNING IN CONGESTION HANDLING

Machine learning plays a significant role in traffic management on roads by leveraging data and algorithms to improve traffic flow, reduce congestion, enhance safety, and optimize transportation systems [47–50]. Here's how machine learning contributes to traffic management:

Machine learning techniques are instrumental in addressing various challenges in traffic management on roads. These techniques leverage data-driven insights to optimize traffic flow, reduce congestion, enhance safety, and improve transportation systems. Here are some of the key machine learning techniques used in traffic management:

8.3.1 Traffic Flow Prediction

Machine learning models, such as time series analysis and recurrent neural networks (RNNs), can predict traffic flow patterns based on historical data. These predictions help authorities plan for optimal traffic management strategies and resource allocation. RNNs are a class of artificial neural networks designed for processing sequential data. They are particularly well-suited for tasks involving time series data, natural language processing, and other sequential data applications. The fundamental component of an RNN is the recurrent layer, which allows the network to maintain a hidden state that captures information from previous time steps.

Traditional RNNs suffer from the vanishing gradient problem, which makes it challenging to capture long-range dependencies. To address this issue, variants of RNNs, such as Long Short-Term Memory (LSTM) and Gated Recurrent Unit (GRU), have been developed. These architectures include gating mechanisms that help the network better preserve and update information over long sequences. In summary, the RNN architecture is designed to process sequential data by maintaining a hidden state that captures information from previous time steps. It is a fundamental building block for various applications involving sequences, including time series forecasting, natural language processing, and speech recognition. More advanced variants like LSTM and GRU have improved the ability of RNNs to capture long-range dependencies in data [51–56].

LSTM is a type of RNN architecture that excels at modeling and predicting sequential data, making it particularly useful for traffic prediction on roads. Here's a brief overview of how LSTM is applied in traffic prediction:

8.3.2 Sequential Data Representation

Traffic data, such as traffic volume, speed, and congestion levels, can be considered as sequential data since it varies over time. LSTMs are well-suited to capture the temporal dependencies and patterns in such data.

8.3.3 LSTM Architecture

An LSTM network consists of multiple LSTM cells. Each LSTM cell maintains a hidden state, which acts as a memory that can capture relevant information from past time steps. The key components of an LSTM cell include:

- **Cell State (C_t):** Represents the internal memory of the cell, which can be updated or preserved based on the input and the previous cell state.
- **Hidden State (h_t):** Captures the output and also influences the next cell state. It carries information from past time steps to the current one.

Traffic data is preprocessed and organized into sequences. Each sequence contains historical traffic observations, and the goal is to predict future traffic conditions. At each time step, the LSTM model receives input features, which can include historical traffic data for that time step, as well as contextual information such as time of day, day of the week, and weather conditions. The LSTM model is trained using historical traffic data. The training process involves minimizing a loss function, such as mean squared error, by adjusting the model's weights and biases. The model learns to capture patterns and dependencies in the traffic data. Once the LSTM model is trained, it can be used for traffic prediction. Given a sequence of historical traffic data, the model predicts future traffic conditions, which may include traffic volume, speed, or congestion levels. The performance of the LSTM-based traffic prediction model is evaluated using metrics such as Mean Absolute Error (MAE) or Root Mean Square Error (RMSE). These metrics measure the accuracy of the model's predictions compared to the actual traffic data. If the LSTM model demonstrates good predictive performance during evaluation, it can be deployed in real-world traffic management systems. This allows traffic authorities to make informed decisions and take proactive measures to alleviate congestion and improve traffic flow. Traffic patterns can change over time due to various factors, so the LSTM model may require periodic retraining with updated data to maintain its accuracy. In summary, LSTM-based models are effective tools for traffic prediction on roads because they can capture complex temporal dependencies in traffic data. They are capable of providing valuable insights for traffic management, enabling authorities to optimize traffic flow and respond to changing traffic conditions effectively.

The GRU is used for traffic prediction on roads. It is similar to the LSTM network but has a more simplified structure. Here's a brief overview of how GRU is applied in traffic prediction:

1. **Sequential Data Representation:** Traffic data collected over time, including variables like traffic volume, speed, and congestion levels, is sequential in nature. GRU, like LSTM, is designed to handle such sequential data by capturing temporal dependencies and patterns.
2. **GRU Architecture:** A GRU network consists of GRU cells. Each GRU cell maintains a hidden state, similar to LSTM. The key mechanisms of the GRU architecture cell include:
   - **Update Gate (z_t):** Determines how much of the previous hidden state should be retained and how much should be updated with new information.

- **Reset Gate (r_t):** Controls which parts of the previous hidden state should be forgotten or reset.
- **Candidate Activation (h~_t):** Represents the new candidate hidden state, which combines the previous hidden state and the current input.

Traffic data is preprocessed and organized into sequences, with each sequence containing historical traffic observations. The goal is to use this historical data to predict future traffic conditions. At each time step, the GRU model receives input features, which can include historical traffic data for that time step and contextual information such as time of day, day of the week, and weather conditions. The GRU model is trained using historical traffic data. During training, the model's parameters, including weights and biases, are adjusted to minimize a loss function, such as mean squared error. The model learns to capture temporal patterns and dependencies in the traffic data. Once trained, the GRU model can make predictions for future traffic conditions given a sequence of historical traffic data. These predictions can include traffic volume, speed, or congestion levels. The performance of the GRU-based traffic prediction model is evaluated using metrics like MAE or RMSE. These metrics assess how well the model's predictions align with the actual traffic data. If the GRU model demonstrates strong predictive performance during evaluation, it can be deployed in real-world traffic management systems. This enables traffic authorities to make informed decisions and respond effectively to changing traffic conditions. Traffic patterns can evolve over time due to various factors, so the GRU model may require periodic retraining with updated data to maintain its accuracy.

In summary, the GRU is a powerful neural network architecture for traffic prediction on roads. It excels at capturing temporal dependencies in sequential data, making it a valuable tool for traffic management and optimization. GRU-based models can help improve traffic flow and reduce congestion by providing insights into future traffic conditions.

1. **Real-Time Traffic Monitoring:** Machine learning algorithms process real-time data from sources like traffic cameras, GPS devices, and road sensors to monitor current traffic conditions. Techniques like computer vision and anomaly detection identify incidents, congestion, and accidents as they occur.
2. **Traffic Signal Optimization:** Reinforcement learning (RL) algorithms optimize traffic signal timings dynamically based on real-time traffic data. Adaptive traffic signal systems adjust signal cycles to minimize wait times, reduce congestion, and improve traffic flow during peak hours.
3. **Route Planning and Navigation:** Machine learning algorithms power navigation apps that suggest optimal routes for drivers based on current traffic conditions. These apps use RL and deep RL to update routes in real time as new data becomes available.
4. **Congestion Management:** Machine learning can identify congestion-prone areas and recommend strategies to alleviate traffic bottlenecks. Clustering and pattern recognition techniques help identify recurring congestion patterns. Congestion management on roads using machine learning techniques involves leveraging data and algorithms to monitor, predict, and

mitigate traffic congestion. Here's an overview of how machine learning can be applied to congestion management:

To manage congestion, first need to collect relevant data. This can include real-time traffic data from sources such as GPS devices, traffic cameras, road sensors, and mobile apps. Additionally, historical traffic data, weather information, and special events calendars can be valuable. Prepare and clean the collected data. This involves handling missing values, normalizing data, and ensuring data consistency and quality. Machine learning models, such as time series forecasting models, can predict future traffic conditions based on historical data and real-time information. Models like autoregressive integrated moving average (ARIMA), exponential smoothing, or more advanced techniques like LSTM and GRU can be used for this purpose. Machine learning can assist in finding the optimal routes for vehicles to minimize congestion. Algorithms like A* search, Dijkstra's algorithm, or RL can be used to optimize routing.

Adaptive traffic signal systems can be implemented using machine learning techniques to optimize signal timings based on real-time traffic data. This helps in reducing wait times and improving traffic flow. Machine learning models can monitor real-time traffic conditions and issue alerts to drivers, suggesting alternate routes or advising on the best times to travel to avoid congestion. Machine learning can be used to detect anomalies or unusual patterns in traffic data. When unusual congestion occurs, alerts can be sent to traffic management authorities for quick intervention. Machine learning can predict when road infrastructure, such as traffic lights or road signs, is likely to fail. This proactive maintenance approach helps in preventing congestion due to equipment breakdowns. Machine learning can optimize public transportation schedules and routes based on passenger demand and real-time traffic conditions, reducing congestion by encouraging the use of public transit. Machine learning models can predict areas with a high likelihood of traffic violations or accidents, allowing law enforcement agencies to focus their efforts on specific locations. Machine learning can facilitate data sharing and collaboration among various stakeholders, including traffic management authorities, transportation companies, and mobile app developers, to better manage congestion collectively. Machine learning models should continuously adapt and learn from new data to improve their accuracy and effectiveness in congestion management. By applying machine learning techniques to congestion management, traffic authorities can make data-driven decisions, reduce traffic congestion, improve traffic flow, and enhance the overall efficiency of transportation systems, ultimately leading to a better commuting experience for everyone on the road.

5. **Accident Detection and Response:** Computer vision and image recognition models can analyze traffic camera footage to detect accidents and incidents in real time. These models trigger alerts to emergency services and traffic management authorities for swift response.

6. **Public Transportation Optimization:** Machine learning models predict passenger demand, optimize bus and train schedules, and recommend route adjustments for public transportation systems. These models use regression analysis and neural networks to make data-driven decisions.
7. **Parking Management:** Machine learning predicts parking availability in real-time, guiding drivers to open parking spaces. RL can be used to optimize parking pricing structures and encourage efficient use of parking resources.
8. **Traffic Law Enforcement:** Automated traffic law enforcement systems use machine learning techniques like image recognition to detect violations such as speeding or running red lights. These systems generate citations without human intervention.
9. **Data-Driven Decision-Making:** Machine learning insights inform data-driven decisions about infrastructure upgrades, road maintenance, and traffic control measures. Decision trees and random forests help prioritize projects based on their impact.
10. **Environmental Impact Reduction:** Machine learning contributes to reducing environmental impact by optimizing traffic flow, reducing congestion, and promoting efficient transportation. This leads to decreased fuel consumption and greenhouse gas emissions.
11. **Emergency Response Planning:** Machine learning models predict traffic patterns during emergencies or disasters, enabling emergency services to plan for effective response and resource allocation.

These machine learning techniques collectively enhance traffic management, making roads safer, more efficient, and environmentally friendly. They empower traffic authorities to make data-driven decisions, respond to incidents swiftly, and optimize transportation systems to accommodate growing urban populations and evolving mobility needs.

8.4 OPTIMIZED ROUTING SCHEME

RL can be used to optimize routing by training agents to make routing decisions that maximize a specific objective or reward. Here's how RL can be applied to routing optimization:

1. **Define the Problem:**
   - Determine the objective or reward function you want to optimize. For example, you may want to minimize travel time, reduce fuel consumption, or balance traffic flow across different routes.
2. **State Space and Actions:**
   - Define the state space, which includes information about the current traffic conditions, road network, and any other relevant data. Specify the available actions that the routing agent can take, such as selecting a route or making specific navigation choices at intersections.

3. **Reward Function:**
   - Create a reward function that quantifies how well the agent is performing with respect to the defined objective. The reward function should provide positive or negative feedback to guide the agent's learning.
4. **Q-Learning or Policy Gradient Methods:**
   - Two common approaches are Q-learning and policy gradient methods like Proximal Policy Optimization (PPO) or Trust Region Policy Optimization (TRPO). TRPO is a RL algorithm that is significant for several reasons:
5. **Stability and Robustness:**
   TRPO is known for its stability and robustness in training RL agents. It uses a trust region approach to limit policy updates, ensuring that policy changes are incremental and do not lead to catastrophic performance degradation. This property is especially important when training agents for complex and high-dimensional environments. TRPO tends to be more sample-efficient compared to some other RL algorithms. It achieves good results with fewer samples, making it suitable for applications where data collection is costly or time-consuming. TRPO is effective in handling problems with large action spaces or continuous action spaces. It can be applied to a wide range of problems, including robotic control, autonomous navigation, and game playing. TRPO focuses on optimizing the policy directly, making it well-suited for tasks where the optimal policy is the primary objective. This is particularly important in applications such as autonomous driving, where safety and policy reliability are critical. TRPO employs a natural gradient method, which helps in finding more efficient policy updates compared to simple gradient descent. The natural gradient accounts for the underlying geometry of the policy space, leading to more stable convergence. TRPO's trust region constraint ensures that policy updates are conservative, avoiding large deviations from the current policy. This is advantageous when dealing with real-world applications where safety is a concern. TRPO can be used to evaluate the performance of different policies efficiently. Comparing policies within the trust region helps practitioners understand the trade-offs between different strategies and select the most suitable one. TRPO is a model-free RL algorithm, which means it does not require a model of the environment dynamics. This makes it applicable to a wide range of tasks without the need for prior knowledge about the environment. TRPO is built on solid theoretical foundations, which provide insights into its convergence properties and guarantee improved policy performance. TRPO has been successfully applied in various real-world applications, including robotics, autonomous vehicles, and control systems, demonstrating its practical significance in solving complex problems.

   Despite its advantages, it's important to note that TRPO has some limitations, including computational complexity and the need for careful hyperparameter tuning. Nonetheless, TRPO's significance lies in its ability to provide stable and efficient solutions to challenging RL problems, making it a valuable tool in the field of machine learning and robotics.

a. **Q-Learning:** Q-learning involves estimating the quality (Q-value) of taking a specific action in a given state. The Q-values are updated iteratively using the Bellman equation and a learning rate. The agent learns to select actions that maximize the expected cumulative reward.
b. **Policy Gradient Methods:** Policy gradient methods directly parameterize the agent's policy (the probability distribution over actions) and adjust the policy parameters to maximize expected rewards. These methods are well-suited for continuous action spaces.

6. **Training Data:** Gather training data that includes historical traffic data, route choices, and their outcomes. This data will be used to train the RL agent.
7. **Training Process:**
   - Train the RL agent using the collected data and the defined reward function. The agent explores different routing options and updates its policy to improve its performance over time.
8. **Exploration vs. Exploitation:** During training, balance exploration (trying new routes) and exploitation (choosing known good routes) to ensure that the agent learns the optimal routing policy.
9. **Simulation Environment:** Create a simulation environment that mimics real-world traffic conditions and routing scenarios. This environment is where the RL agent learns and tests its routing strategies.
10. **Testing and Evaluation:**
    - After training, evaluate the RL agent's performance in a realistic environment by simulating routing scenarios and measuring its ability to optimize routing based on the defined objective.
11. **Deployment:** Once the RL agent demonstrates satisfactory performance, it can be deployed in real-world routing applications. It can provide routing recommendations to drivers, traffic management systems, or autonomous vehicles.
12. **Continuous Learning:** To adapt to changing traffic conditions and road network updates, the RL agent can be continuously retrained with new data.

RL for routing optimization offers the advantage of adapting to dynamic traffic conditions and learning optimal routing strategies over time. It can be a valuable tool for managing traffic congestion, reducing travel times, and improving overall transportation efficiency.

8.5 CONCLUSION

The specialized accident detection system can be easily added to vehicles that weren't initially equipped with it during the manufacturing process. To reduce the chance of false alarms, users have the choice to turn the system on or off using a user input switch. Moreover, there's a secure server with login credentials for administrative staff, enabling the simultaneous monitoring of ambulance dispatch services for multiple accidents and efficient tracking of ambulance driver performance. The accompanying Android app greatly aids ambulance drivers in navigating through heavy traffic by automatically suggesting less congested routes. Implementing this comprehensive solution that covers both road traffic accident detection and ambulance management significantly cuts down the critical time needed for post-traumatic medical care, ultimately lowering mortality rates. This approach also promotes standardizing service delivery processes by reducing the need for human intervention. Such a fully automated system is immensely valuable, not only in everyday situations but also during natural disasters, where a quick and precise response is crucial.

REFERENCES

1. Kaur, G., & Kakkar, D. (2022). Hybrid optimization enabled trust-based secure routing with deep learning-based attack detection in VANET. Ad Hoc Networks, 136, 102961.
2. Sankar, S. H., Jayadev, K., Suraj, B., & Aparna, P. (2016, November). A comprehensive solution to road traffic accident detection and ambulance management. In *2016 International Conference on Advances in Electrical, Electronic and Systems Engineering (ICAEES)* (pp. 43–47). IEEE, Putrajaya, Malaysia.
3. Feng, H., Chen, D., & Lv, Z. (2022). Blockchain in digital twins-based vehicle management in VANETs. IEEE Transactions on Intelligent Transportation Systems, 23, 19613–19623.
4. Kamijo, S., Matsushita, Y., Ikeuchi, K., & Sakauchi, M. (2000). Traffic monitoring and accident detection at intersections. IEEE Transactions on Intelligent Transportation Systems, 1(2), 108–118.
5. Zhang, T., Xu, C., Zhang, B., Shen, J., Kuang, X., & Grieco, L. A. (2022). Toward attack-resistant route mutation for VANETs: An online and adaptive multiagent reinforcement learning approach. IEEE Transactions on Intelligent Transportation Systems. https://doi.org/10.1109/TITS.2022.3198507
6. Andersson, T., & Varbrand, P. (2007). Decision support tools for ambulance dispatch and relocation. Journal of the Operational Research Society, 58(2), 195–201.
7. Azhdari, M. S., Barati, A., & Barati, H. (2022). A cluster-based routing method with authentication capability in vehicular ad hoc networks (VANETs). Journal of Parallel and Distributed Computing, 169, 1–23.
8. Cárdenas, L. L., León, J. P. A., & Mezher, A. M. (2022). GraTree: A gradient boosting decision tree based multimetric routing protocol for vehicular ad hoc networks. Ad Hoc Networks, 137. https://doi.org/10.1016/j.adhoc.2022.102995
9. Nahar, A., & Das, D. (2023). MetaLearn: Optimizing routing heuristics with a hybrid meta-learning approach in vehicular ad-hoc networks. Ad Hoc Networks, 138. https://doi.org/10.1016/j.adhoc.2022.102996
10. Darabkh, K. A., Alkhader, B. Z., Ala'F, K., Jubair, F., & Abdel-Majeed, M. (2022). ICDRP-f-SDVN: An innovative cluster-based dual-phase routing protocol using fog computing and software-defined vehicular network. Vehicular Communications, 34, 100453.
11. Sun, G., Zhang, Y., Yu, H., Du, X., & Guizani, M. (2019). Intersection fog-based distributed routing for V2V communication in urban vehicular ad hoc networks. IEEE Transactions on Intelligent Transportation Systems, 21(6), 2409–2426.
12. Taherkhani, N., & Pierre, S. (2016). Centralized and localized data congestion control strategy for vehicular ad hoc networks using a machine learning clustering algorithm. IEEE Transactions on Intelligent Transportation Systems, 17(11), 3275–3285.
13. Yadav, V. K., Verma, S., & Venkatesan, S. (2020). Efficient and secure location-based services scheme in VANET. IEEE Transactions on Vehicular Technology, 69(11), 13567–13578.

14. Khatri, S., Vachhani, H., Shah, S., Bhatia, J., Chaturvedi, M., Tanwar, S., & Kumar, N. (2021). Machine learning models and techniques for VANET based traffic management: Implementation issues and challenges. Peer-to-Peer Networking and Applications, 14, 1778–1805.
15. Shrestha, R., Bajracharya, R., Shrestha, A. P., & Nam, S. Y. (2020). A new type of blockchain for secure message exchange in VANET. Digital Communications and Networks, 6(2), 177–186.
16. Hosmani, S., & Mathapati, B. (2021). R2SCDT: Robust and reliable secure clustering and data transmission in vehicular ad hoc network using weight evaluation. Journal of Ambient Intelligence and Humanized Computing, 14, 1–18.
17. Haghighi, M. S., & Aziminejad, Z. (2019). Highly anonymous mobility-tolerant location-based onion routing for VANETs. IEEE Internet of Things Journal, 7(4), 2582–2590.
18. Wang, X., Hu, J., Lin, H., Garg, S., Kaddoum, G., Jalilpiran, M., & Hossain, M. S. QoS and privacy-aware routing for 5G enabled industrial internet of things: A federated reinforcement learning approach. IEEE Transactions on Industrial Informatics, 18, 4189–4197.
19. Li, W., & Song, H. (2015). ART: An attack-resistant trust management scheme for securing vehicular ad hoc networks. IEEE Transactions on Intelligent Transportation Systems, 17(4), 960–969.
20. Guo, J., Li, X., Liu, Z., Ma, J., Yang, C., Zhang, J., & Wu, D. (2020). TROVE: A context-awareness trust model for VANETs using reinforcement learning. IEEE Internet of Things Journal, 7(7), 6647–6662.
21. Naresh, V. S., Allavarpu, V. D., & Reddi, S. (2022). Blockchain IOTA sharding based scalable secure group communication in large VANETs. IEEE Internet of Things Journal. https://doi.org/10.1109/JIOT.2022.3222382
22. Abbasi, F., Zarei, M., & Rahmani, A. M. (2022). FWDP: A fuzzy logic-based vehicle weighting model for data prioritization in vehicular ad hoc networks. Vehicular Communications, 33, 100413.
23. Zhang, C., Li, W., Luo, Y., & Hu, Y. (2020). AIT: An AI-enabled trust management system for vehicular networks using blockchain technology. IEEE Internet of Things Journal, 8(5), 3157–3169.
24. Mehra, A., Mandal, M., Narang, P., & Chamola, V. (2020). ReViewNet: A fast and resource-optimized network enabling safe autonomous driving in hazy weather conditions. IEEE Transactions on Intelligent Transportation Systems, 22(7), 4256–4266.
25. Kolandaisamy, R., Noor, R. M., Kolandaisamy, I., Ahmedy, I., Kiah, M. L. M., Tamil, M. E. M., & Nandy, T. (2021). A stream position performance analysis model based on DDoS attack detection for cluster-based routing in VANET. Journal of Ambient Intelligence and Humanized Computing, 12(6), 6599–6612.
26. Divya, N. S., Bobba, V., & Vatambeti, R. (2021). An adaptive cluster-based vehicular routing protocol for secure communication. Wireless Personal Communications, 127(5), 1–20.
27. Zhao, L., Bi, Z., Lin, M., Hawbani, A., Shi, J., & Guan, Y. (2021). An intelligent fuzzy-based routing scheme for software-defined vehicular networks. Computer Networks, 187, 107837.
28. Guo, C., Li, D., Chen, X., & Zhang, G. (2022). An adaptive V2R communication strategy based on data delivery delay estimation in VANETs. Vehicular Communications, 34, 100444.
29. Bao, X., Li, H., Zhao, G., Chang, L., Zhou, J., & Li, Y. (2020). Efficient clustering V2V routing based on PSO in VANETs. Measurement, 152, 107306.
30. Tang, Y., Cheng, N., Wu, W., Wang, M., Dai, Y., & Shen, X. (2019). Delay-minimization routing for heterogeneous VANETs with machine learning based mobility prediction. IEEE Transactions on Vehicular Technology, 68(4), 3967–3979.

31. Abhishek, N. V., Aman, M. N., Lim, T. J., & Sikdar, B. (2021). DRiVe: Detecting malicious roadside units in the internet of vehicles with low latency data integrity. IEEE Internet of Things Journal, 9(5), 3270–3281.
32. Bhabani, B., & Mahapatro, J. (2023). TRP: A TOPSIS-based RSU-enabled priority scheduling scheme to disseminate alert messages of WBAN sensors in hybrid VANETs. Peer-to-Peer Networking and Applications, 16, 1–19.
33. Bhoi, S. K., & Khilar, P. M. (2016). VehiHealth: An emergency routing protocol for vehicular ad hoc network to support healthcare system. Journal of Medical Systems, 40, 65. https://doi.org/10.1007/s10916-015-0420-2
34. Singh, P., Raw, R. S., Khan, A., Mohammed, A., Aly, A., & Le, D.-N. (2022). W-GeoR: Weighted geographical routing for VANET's health monitoring applications in urban traffic networks. IEEE Access, 10, 38850–38869. https://doi.org/10.1109/ACCESS.2021.3092426
35. Sundaravadivel, P., Kougianos, E., Mohanty, S. P., & Ganapathiraju, M. K. (Jan. 2018). Everything you wanted to know about smart health care: Evaluating the different technologies and components of the internet of things for better health. IEEE Consumer Electronics Magazine, 7(1), 18–28. https://doi.org/10.1109/MCE.2017.2755378
36. Behura, A., Srinivas, M., & Kabat, M. R. (2022). Giraffe kicking optimization algorithm provides efficient routing mechanism in the field of vehicular ad hoc networks. Journal of Ambient Intelligence and Humanized Computing, 13(8), 3989–4008.
37. Buvana, M., Loheswaran, K., Madhavi, K., Ponnusamy, S., Behura, A., & Jayavadivel, R. (2021). Improved resource management and utilization based on a fog-cloud computing system with IoT incorporated with classifier systems. Microprocessors and Microsystems, 103815. https://doi.org/10.1016/j.micpro.2020.103815
38. Behura, A., & Kabat, M. R. (2020). Energy-efficient optimization-based routing technique for wireless sensor network using machine learning. In Progress in Computing, Analytics and Networking: Proceedings of ICCAN 2019 (pp. 555–565). Springer, Singapore.
39. Behura, A. (2022). Optimized data transmission scheme based on proper channel coordination used in vehicular ad hoc networks. International Journal of Information Technology, 14(2), 1107–1116.
40. Behura, A., & Kabat, M. R. (2022). Optimization-Based Energy-Efficient Routing Scheme for Wireless Body Area Network. In: Mishra, S., Tripathy, H. K., Mallick, P. K., Sangaiah, A. K., & Chae, G.-S. (eds) Cognitive Big Data Intelligence with a Metaheuristic Approach (pp. 279–303). Academic Press.
41. Behura, A. (2021). A Deep Learning Application for Prediction of COVID-19. In: Mishra, S., Mallick, P. K., Tripathy, H. K., Chae, G.-S., & Mishra, B. S. P. (eds) Impact of AI and Data Science in Response to Coronavirus Pandemic (pp. 127–148). Springer.
42. Behura, A., & Panda, S. K. (2022). Role of Machine Learning in Big Data Peregrination. In: Kumar, V., Tiwari, P., Mishra, B. K., & Panda, S. K. (eds) Handbook of Research for Big Data (pp. 235–276). Apple Academic Press.
43. Behura, A. (2022). Intelligent Automotive Sector with IOT (Internet of Things) and Its Consequential Impact in Vehicular Ad Hoc Networks. In: Mohanty, S. N., Chatterjee, J. M., & Satpathy, S. (eds) Internet of Things and Its Applications (pp. 427–449). Springer.
44. Behura, A., Kabat, M. R., & Mohanty, S. N. (2022). The Fusion of IOT and Wireless Body Area Network. In: Mohanty, S. N., Chatterjee, J. M., & Satpathy, S. (eds) Internet of Things and Its Applications (pp. 195–220). Springer.
45. Behura, A., & Nandan Mohanty, S. (2022). Application of the Internet of Things (IoT) in Biomedical Engineering: Present Scenario and Challenges. In: Mohanty, S. N., Chatterjee, J. M., & Satpathy, S. (eds) Internet of Things and Its Applications (pp. 151–169). Springer.

46. Behura, A., Sahu, S., & Kabat, M. R. (2021). Advancement of Machine Learning and Cloud Computing in the Field of Smart Health Care. In: Mohanty, S. N., Chatterjee, J. M., Mangla, M., Satpathy, S., & Potluri, S. (eds) Machine Learning Approach for Cloud Data Analytics in IoT (pp. 273–306). Wiley.
47. Boualouache, A., Senouci, S. M., & Moussaoui, S. (2017). A survey on pseudonym changing strategies for vehicular ad-hoc networks. IEEE Communications Surveys Tutorials, 20(1), 770–790.
48. Zeng, K. (2006). Pseudonymous PKI for Ubiquitous Computing. In: Lopez, J., Samarati, P., & Ferrer, J. L. (eds) European Public Key Infrastructure Workshop (pp. 207–222). Springer.
49. Lu, R., Lin, X., Luan, T. H., Liang, X., & Shen, X. (2011). Pseudonym changing at social spots: An effective strategy for location privacy in VANETs. IEEE Transactions on Vehicular Technology, 61(1), 86–96.
50. Goyal, R., Mittal, N., Gupta, L., & Surana, A. (2023). Routing protocols in wireless body area networks: Architecture, challenges, and classification. *Wireless Communications and Mobile Computing*, 2023.
51. Fan, C. I., Hsu, R. H., Ho, P. H. (2011). Truly non-repudiation certificateless short signature scheme from bilinear pairings. Journal of Information Science and Engineering, 27, 969–982
52. Tsai, J. L. (2015). A new efficient certificateless short signature scheme using bilinear pairings. IEEE Systems Journal, 11(4), 2395–2402.
53. Nath, H. J., & Choudhury, H. (2022). A privacy-preserving mutual authentication scheme for group communication in VANET. Computer Communications, 192, 357–372.
54. Sedjelmaci, H., & Senouci, S. M. (2015). An accurate and efficient collaborative intrusion detection framework to secure vehicular networks. Computers Electrical Engineering, 43, 33–47.
55. Malina, L., Castella-Roca, J., Vives-Guasch, A., & Hajny, J. (2012, October). Short-Term Linkable Group Signatures With Categorized Batch Verification. In International Symposium on Foundations and Practice of Security (pp. 244–260). Springer, Berlin, Heidelberg.
56. Islam, S. H., Obaidat, M. S., Vijayakumar, P., Abdulhay, E., Li, F., & Reddy, M. K. C. (2018). A robust and efficient password-based conditional privacy preserving authentication and group-key agreement protocol for VANETs. Future Generation Computer Systems, 84, 216–227.

9 A Comparative Study of Machine Learning and Deep Learning Methods for Detecting Thyroid Disease

An Experimental Investigation

Jay Prakash Singh, Debolina Ghosh, Francis Palma, and Jagannath Singh

9.1 INTRODUCTION

Deep learning (DL) and machine learning (ML) have significantly impacted the field of disease detection and classification by enabling more accurate, efficient, and automated methods for analyzing complex medical data [1]. ML algorithms can process large volumes of medical data, such as images, patient records, and genomic data, to identify patterns and features that are difficult for human experts to discern. Convolutional Neural Networks (CNNs) excel at automatically learning relevant features from raw data, particularly in tasks like image analysis in medical domain [2]. DL models have shown remarkable success in tasks like early detection of diabetic retinopathy, cancer detection, and identifying neurological disorders from brain scans. Both ML and DL models have the capability to act as decision-support tools for medical professionals, offering treatment recommendations by analyzing patient data alongside established medical protocols. It's essential to recognize that despite the considerable potential exhibited by ML and DL in identifying and categorizing illnesses, their integration necessitates meticulous attention to ethical and confidentiality matters [3].

Thyroid-related ailments present a global health challenge impacting a substantial population. Central to various physiological functions, the thyroid gland orchestrates processes spanning metabolism, energy synthesis, and hormone equilibrium [4]. Instances like hypothyroidism and hyperthyroidism carry the potential for diverse symptoms and complexities, underscoring the significance of timely identification and management [5]. In this context, the adoption of emerging methodologies such

 DOI: 10.1201/9781032624891-9

as ML and DL acquires paramount importance due to their capacity to reshape diagnostics and ultimately enhance patient well-being [6].

9.1.1 Enhanced Diagnostic Precision

Conventional methodologies utilized for diagnosing thyroid diseases, such as blood tests and medical imaging, can be susceptible to subjective interpretation and human fallibility [7]. However, the application of ML and DL algorithms offers a distinct advantage. These algorithms can discern intricate patterns and associations within vast, diverse datasets, leading to diagnoses that are not only more precise but also consistently reliable. This ability to identify subtle patterns not readily apparent to human practitioners enhances the overall dependability of diagnoses.

9.1.2 Timely Detection and Proactive Measures

A notable strength of ML and DL lies in their capacity to detect subtle irregularities at an early stage [8]. Through comprehensive analysis of extensive patient information, these techniques can spot initial indications of thyroid irregularities, enabling timely intervention and treatment. Such timely detection has the potential to halt the advancement of thyroid conditions and alleviate the emergence of severe complications.

9.1.3 Personalized Treatment Approaches

ML and DL models are equipped to account for an individual's distinctive attributes, encompassing medical history, genetic composition, and lifestyle components [9]. This adaptability paves the way for tailored diagnostic and treatment strategies, tailored to the specific requirements of each patient. Personalized medical approaches heighten the efficacy of interventions, mitigate unfavorable effects, and amplify patient contentment.

9.1.4 Streamlined Data Analysis

In healthcare environments where prompt decisions hold paramount importance, ML and DL's capability to process and analyze copious medical data expeditiously is especially advantageous [10]. By mechanizing data analysis, these algorithms empower healthcare professionals to concentrate on patient care and the formulation of treatment strategies.

9.1.5 Navigating Complex Data Landscapes

Thyroid ailment diagnosis frequently necessitates the interpretation of diverse data categories, spanning medical images, laboratory findings, patient histories, and more. ML and DL models exhibit versatility, adept at handling heterogeneous data formats while gleaning valuable insights from each dimension. This comprehensive methodology for data analysis can result in more exhaustive and precise diagnoses [11].

9.1.6 Illuminating Research and Knowledge

Employing ML and DL methodologies for thyroid disease detection yields a profusion of data-derived insights. These insights bolster medical research, enriching our comprehension of disease mechanisms, predisposing factors, and responses to treatment regimens. This heightened knowledge advances the realm of medical science, guiding the creation of more efficacious therapeutic strategies [12].

9.1.7 Cost-Efficient Healthcare

The timely and precise diagnoses enabled by these advanced techniques can yield cost savings within healthcare systems [13]. Swift identification and effective intervention curtail complications, hospitalizations, and resource-intensive treatments. Consequently, this alleviates the financial burden borne by healthcare providers and patients alike.

The research is organized as follows: The second section presents an overview of pertinent preceding studies. The ensuing third section delves into our proposed methodologies, encapsulating dataset attributes, data refinement techniques, visualization approaches, specifics of our experimental design, and the proposed methodologies themselves. The fourth section critically evaluates and discusses the findings garnered from our experiments. In the fifth section, potential sources of challenges to validity are expounded upon. Lastly, the concluding section encapsulates the insights gleaned from the study and outlines potential avenues for future research ventures.

9.2 RELATED WORKS

In this section, we present some of the related existing works in the field of Thyroid disease detection using ML and DL. During the literature survey we found many research papers related to detection of thyroid based on available datasets consisting of clinical data from hospitals or images of thyroid gland. Here we present some of the most cited and important related work and their shortcomings.

Aversano et al. [14] have used the patients data set of hormonal parameters to predict whether the doses of Sodium Levothyroxine (LT4) should increase or decrease. The dataset consists of personal information, physical characteristics, and clinical data of 800 patients. The data set also contains clinical test reports and doctor's notes. Then SMOTE (Synthetic Minority Over-sampling TEchnique) is applied to mitigate class imbalance problems. Out of 135 actual attributes, 27 attributes are selected which represent the patient information and parameters of thyroid. The authors have developed 10 ML models for classification of final output in three classes. After discretization and balancing of the input data set, the Extra Tree Classifier performs best out of all 10 models used in this study with accuracy 84% and precision 85%.

In another work by Hamid et al. [15] ultrasound pictures were used for prediction of thyroid disease. In total, 7200 ultrasound images were cleaned and preprocessed and finally 2870 negative samples and 293 positive samples were found. As the data set was imbalanced, down-sampling was performed to make data set balanced; 25 attributes were fetched from the final images and a data set was prepared for prediction. The researchers employed four distinct ML algorithms: Decision Tree (DT), random forest, K-nearest neighbor (KNN), and naïve Bayes. To assess the effectiveness of these models, they employed performance metrics including sensitivity and specificity. The outcomes indicated that the random forest model yielded the highest prediction accuracy, boasting a sensitivity of 94.8% and specificity of 91%.

Another similar work was done by Poudel et al. [16], in which he used thyroid patients' images to classify the images into thyroid or non-thyroid images. In this work, first the ultrasound images of size 760 × 500 pixels are converted into texture patches of smaller size 20 × 20 pixels. Then, using CNN and other three traditional image processing techniques, the author tried to classify the input images. By employing CNN, the author measured a dice coefficient of 0.876 and a Harsdorf distance of 7.3. These metrics were instrumental in the categorization of thyroid tissues into either thyroid or non-thyroid tissues.

Abbad et al. [17] utilized a dataset gathered from three hospitals in Pakistan. In their study, they employed various ML algorithms such as KNN, Naïve Bayes, Support Vector Machine (SVM), DT, and logistic regression. These algorithms were tested both with and without feature selection techniques. The dataset encompassed clinical information from 309 patients, supplemented by 3 additional attributes: pulse rate, body mass, and blood pressure.

To enhance the efficiency of their ML models, the researchers applied L1- and L2-based feature selection methods. Their analysis led them to conclude that models employing L1-based feature selection exhibited superior accuracy in comparison to models employing L2-based feature selection. The output of experiment was found to be very good for Naive Bayes (100%), Logistic Regression (100%), and KNN (97.84%), but not so good for SVM and DT.

In a work by Pal et al. [18] they used the data set from UCI repository consisting of 3163 records and 24 thyroid features. The researchers employed three distinct ML models: DT, KNN, and Multi-Layer Perceptron. Their aim encompassed forecasting the probability of thyroid-related concerns in patients. To assess the proficiency of these models, they employed evaluative criteria such as accuracy and the area under the curve (AUC). They have found that out of three ML models, Multi-layer Perceptron performs better with accuracy 96% and area under curve 94.23. But, in this study the data set was imbalanced, with 2870 records not having thyroid and 293 records having thyroid.

Sultana and Islam [19] have used the dataset of 2800 patients from UCI repository. There were 28 attributes present in the dataset and binary classification was required. In the dataset there are 2723 records of non-thyroid patients and only 77 records of thyroid-positive patients. They had used the SMOTE technique for balancing the dataset. The experimentation phase encompassed the application of six distinct ML algorithms: SVM, AdaBoost, DT, Gradient Boosting, and Random Forest. The assessment of these models was carried out using a five-fold cross-validation technique. Notably, the Random Forest algorithm displayed the highest performance among the six models, with an accuracy of 99%.

Sankar et al. [20] have used the XGBoost algorithm for feature selection and studied the improvement in accuracy for different ML algorithms. The dataset from UCI knowledge discovery contained 215 instances. It is a multi-class dataset with three classes, i.e., normal, hyper-, and hypothyroid. The dataset had five features. They found that after applying the XGBoost algorithm the accuracy of KNN increased by 2%. Similarly, the accuracy of DT and logistic regression was enhanced by 12% and 17%, respectively.

Salman et al. [21] have used dataset of 1250 Iraqi people for predicting the types of thyroid disease, i.e., hypothyroidism, hyperthyroidism, and normal. They have used eight ML algorithms for prediction with and without feature selection. From the experiment they found that the accuracy of DT, Random Forest, and MLP is the best with 98.4%, 98.93%, and 97.6%, respectively, with feature selection.

Akhtar et al. [22] have tried to compare the effect of feature selection techniques on the performance of thyroid detection technique. They have applied three feature selection techniques, i.e., Recursive Feature Elimination (RFE), Select from Model (SFM), and Select k-Best (SKB). They have used Thyroid 0387 dataset downloaded from Knowledge Extraction based on Evolutionary Learning (KEEL) repository. For implementation, bagging and boosting-based classifiers such as KNN, Naïve Bayes, SVM, DT, and logistic regression were used. The author found that the performance of RFE with logistic regression was the best, with accuracy 99.27%, precision 97%, and recall 98%.

9.3 PROPOSED APPROACH

In this study, a comprehensive analysis was undertaken to assess the efficacy of various ML models in predicting thyroid disease. The employed classifiers encompass SVM, KNN, Logistic Regression, Random Forest, Gradient Boosting, AdaBoost, and DT Classifiers. As a culmination of this investigation, we advocate the integration of a CNN methodology to further elevate the precision and performance of thyroid disease detection.

9.3.1 Dataset Description

We have collected a primary dataset of 3772 patients from the Kaggle. This diagnosis dataset consists of a total number of 29 features (columns) and one target class. The dataset contains a variety of attributes, including demographic information like 'age' and 'sex,' as well as medical indicators such as 'on thyroxine,' 'query on thyroxine,' and 'on antithyroid medication.' Other factors like 'sick,' 'pregnant,' 'thyroid surgery,' 'I131 treatment,' 'query hypothyroid,' and 'query hyperthyroid' are also part of the dataset. Additional attributes encompass 'lithium,' 'goitre,' 'tumor,' 'hypopituitary,' 'psych,' 'TSH measured,' 'TSH,' 'T3 measured,' 'T3,' 'TT4 measured,' 'TT4,' 'T4U measured,' 'T4U,' 'FTI measured,' 'FTI,' 'TBG measured,' 'TBG,' 'referral source,' and finally, the 'binaryClass' attribute which signifies the target classification. The categorical presentation of the data can be observed in Figure 9.1.

9.3.1.1 Dataset Cleaning

Data cleaning plays an instrumental role in refining the dataset for analysis, ensuring that only pertinent features are considered, and mitigating the adverse effects of missing or erroneous data. This, in turn, cultivates a solid foundation for the subsequent application of ML algorithms, fostering accurate and reliable predictions.

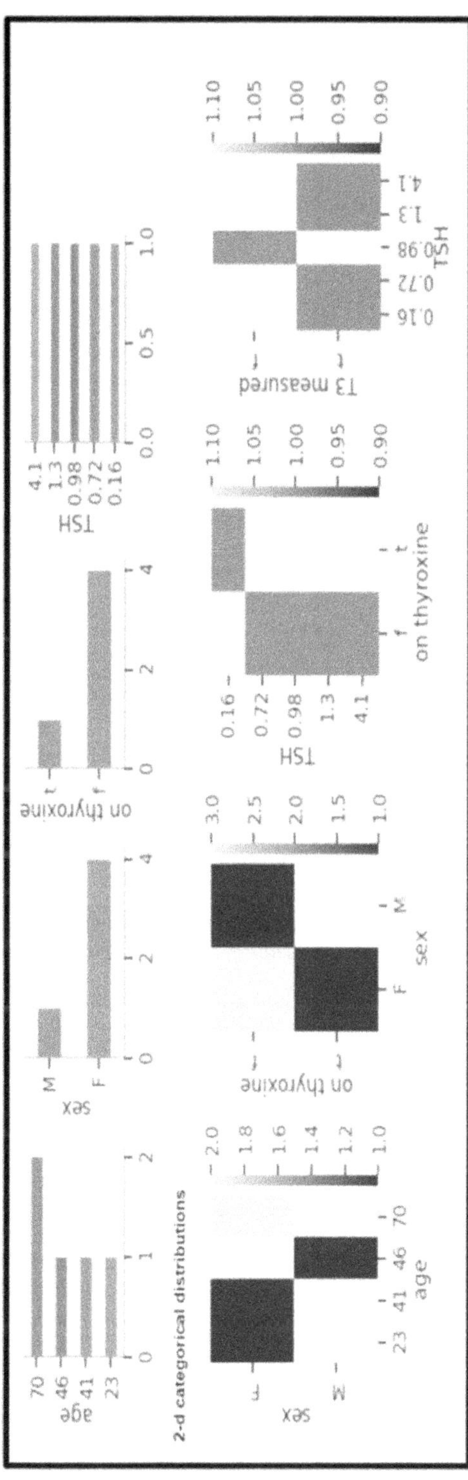

FIGURE 9.1 Categorical distribution of data.

```
 #   Column             Non-Null Count  Dtype
---  ------             --------------  -----
 0   age                3771 non-null   float64
 1   sex                3622 non-null   object
 2   sick               3772 non-null   object
 3   pregnant           3772 non-null   object
 4   thyroid surgery    3772 non-null   object
 5   I131 treatment     3772 non-null   object
 6   lithium            3772 non-null   object
 7   goitre             3772 non-null   object
 8   tumor              3772 non-null   object
 9   TSH                3403 non-null   float64
 10  T3                 3003 non-null   float64
 11  TT4                3541 non-null   float64
 12  T4U                3385 non-null   float64
 13  FTI                3387 non-null   float64
 14  Label              3772 non-null   object
dtypes: float64(6), object(9)
memory usage: 442.2+ KB
```

FIGURE 9.2 Data information.

Dataset which we obtained from Kaggle has many such features which need to be discarded as they were of no use in predicting thyroid disease. Consequently, the subsequent attributes were disregarded in the analysis: 'T3 measured,' 'TSH measured,' 'TT4 measured,' 'T4U measured,' 'FTI measured,' 'TBG measured,' 'TBG,' 'referral source,' 'on thyroxine,' 'query on thyroxine,' 'on antithyroid medication,' 'query hypothyroid,' 'query hyperthyroid,' 'hypopituitary,' and 'psych.' After removing these features, we now have an exact dataset with resultant features that is used for further research, as represented in Figure 9.2.

In the process of data cleaning, our next task was to deal with the missing data. Missing data details are presented in Figure 9.3.

We have replaced the missing data for features TSH, T3, TT4, T4U, and FTI with the mean of the total available data, and for age and sex we dropped the

```
age                  1
sex                150
sick                 0
pregnant             0
thyroid surgery      0
I131 treatment       0
lithium              0
goitre               0
tumor                0
TSH                369
T3                 769
TT4                231
T4U                387
FTI                385
Label                0
dtype: int64
```

FIGURE 9.3 Missing data report.

```
#    Column             Non-Null Count  Dtype
---  ------             --------------  -----
0    age                3620 non-null   int64
1    sex                3620 non-null   object
2    sick               3620 non-null   object
3    pregnant           3620 non-null   object
4    thyroid surgery    3620 non-null   object
5    I131 treatment     3620 non-null   object
6    lithium            3620 non-null   object
7    goitre             3620 non-null   object
8    tumor              3620 non-null   object
9    TSH                3620 non-null   float64
10   T3                 3620 non-null   float64
11   TT4                3620 non-null   int64
12   T4U                3620 non-null   float64
13   FTI                3620 non-null   int64
14   Label              3620 non-null   object
dtypes: float64(3), int64(3), object(9)
memory usage: 452.5+ KB
```

FIGURE 9.4 Final data description.

corresponding rows. After handling the NULL value issue, the description of final data is presented in Figure 9.4.

9.3.1.2 Dataset Visualization

Dataset visualization bridges the gap between raw data and meaningful insights, making it an indispensable tool in data analysis, research, and decision-making across various domains. For visualizing and better understanding the data distributions and relationships we have plotted a pair plot for Kernel Density Estimation (KDE). The corresponding plot is presented in Figure 9.5 and Figure 9.6 represents the regression (reg) plot. Regression plots (reg plots) are used to visualize the relationship between two continuous variables and to fit a regression model to the data. They provide insights into the strength, direction, and linearity of the relationship. From the KDE, presented in Figure 9.5, we can visualize that data points are well distributed, and also we can conclude that anomalies are not present in the data points. From the plotted regression plot for the variables (diagnostics items) we can say that all the variables are closely related and change in any variable impacts the other variable.

The correlation matrix plays a significant role in various stages of the ML workflow, from feature selection and engineering to model interpretation and validation. It helps in making informed decisions to improve the quality and performance of ML models, and hence correlation matrix is calculated for the features and presented in Figure 9.7. Heat maps are a powerful visualization tool in ML that facilitates the understanding of feature correlations, guides feature selection and engineering, aids in model interpretation, and assists in making informed decisions throughout the entire ML pipeline. Corresponding heat map is presented in Figure 9.8.

For better data visualization of the features, Box Plot of age, TSH, T3, TT4, and T4U are presented in Figure 9.9.

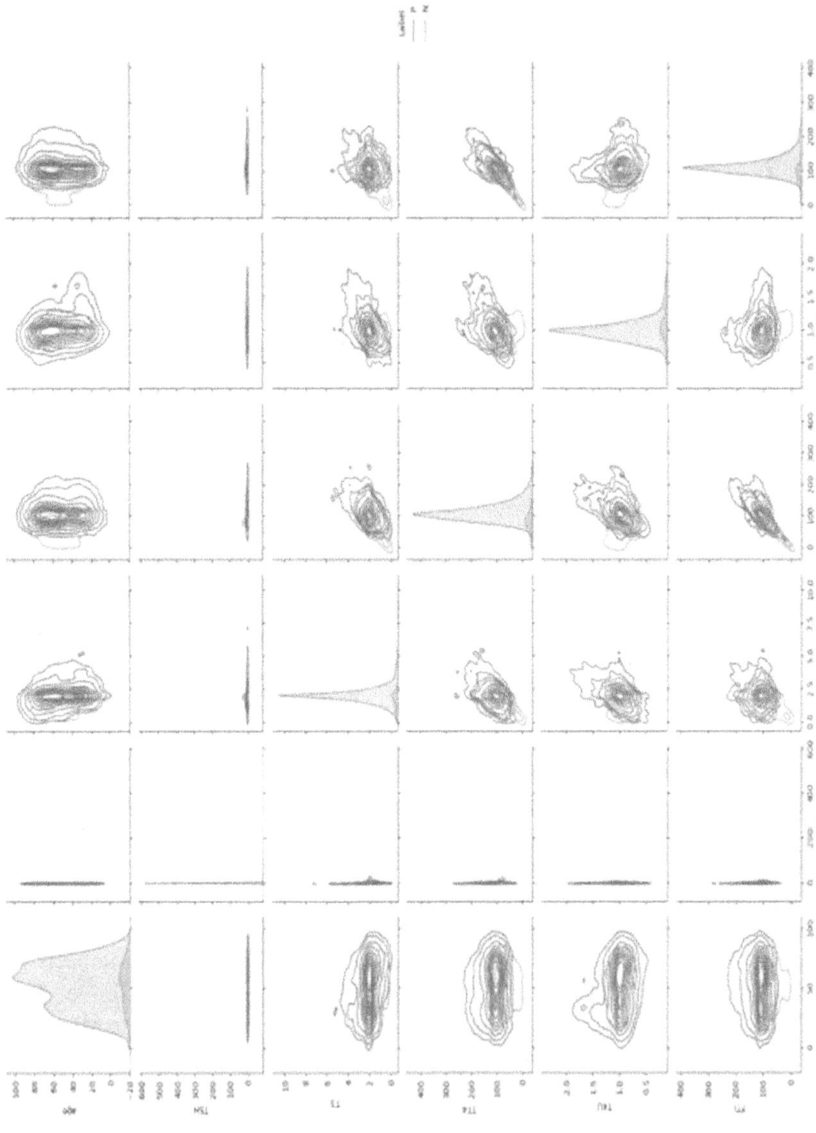

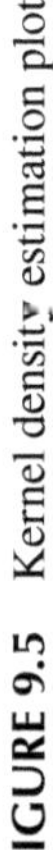

FIGURE 9.5 Kernel density estimation plot.

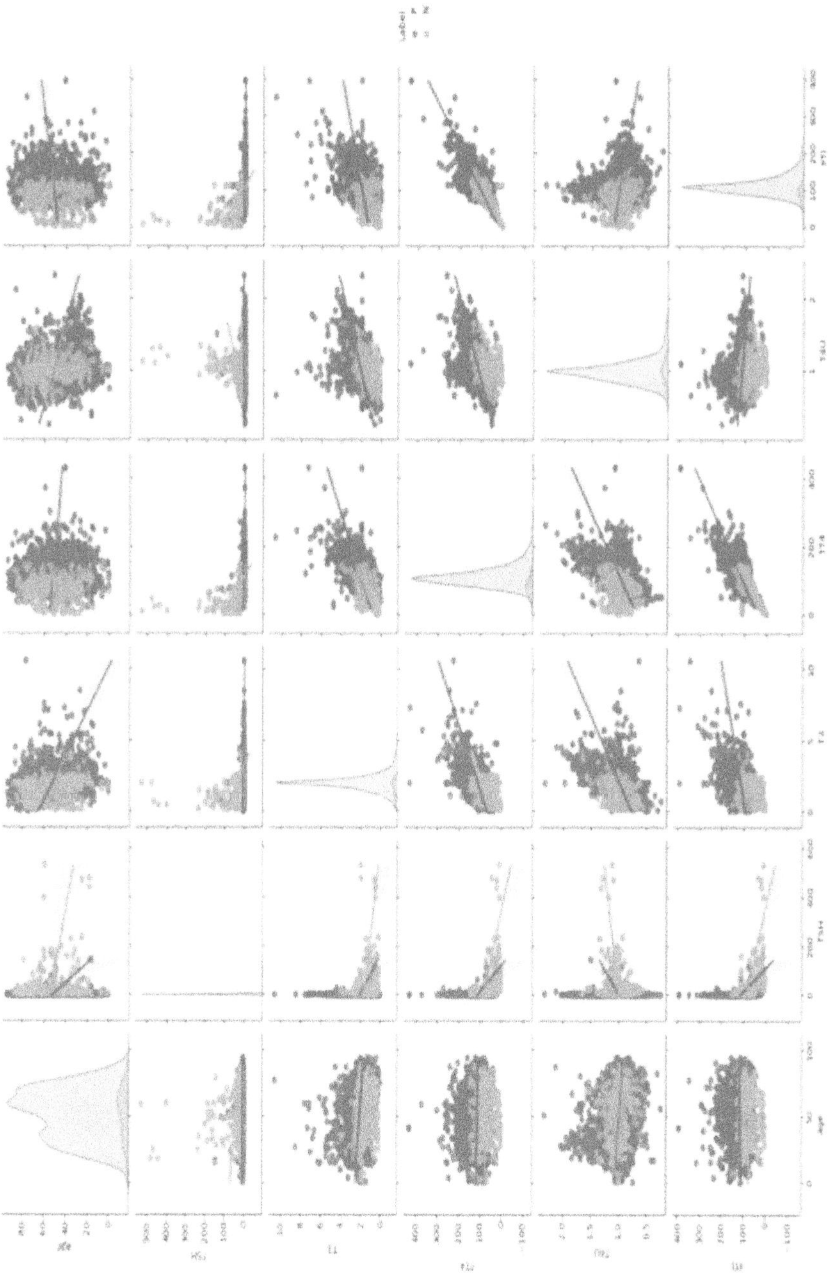

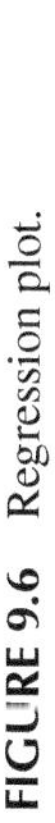

FIGURE 9.6 Regression plot.

	age	TSH	T3	TT4	T4U	FTI
age	1.000000	-0.046824	-0.233933	-0.041377	-0.171449	0.054944
TSH	-0.046824	1.000000	-0.156668	-0.268858	0.070878	-0.301982
T3	-0.233933	-0.156668	1.000000	0.511571	0.409039	0.311655
TT4	-0.041377	-0.268858	0.511571	1.000000	0.427210	0.780546
T4U	-0.171449	0.070878	0.409039	0.427210	1.000000	-0.171555
FTI	0.054944	-0.301982	0.311655	0.780546	-0.171555	1.000000

FIGURE 9.7 Correlation matrix.

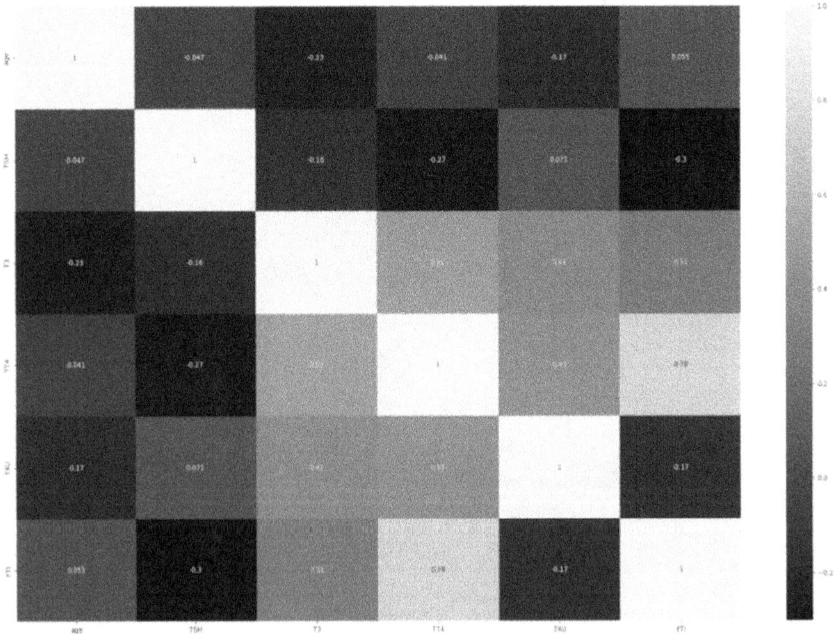

FIGURE 9.8 Heat map.

9.4 PROPOSED APPROACH

Proposed approach is presented in Figure 9.10. We have collected a dataset from Kaggle and then data cleaning is performed to remove the unwanted features and to deal with the not a number (NaN) and null data elements. We have trained various ML models by adopting hyperparameter tuning and testing is performed on the trained models. We executed training using a diverse set of ML algorithms, specifically including Logistic Regression, SVM, Random Forest, Gradient Boosting, KNN, AdaBoost Classifier, Multinomial Naive Bayes, and DT Classifier.

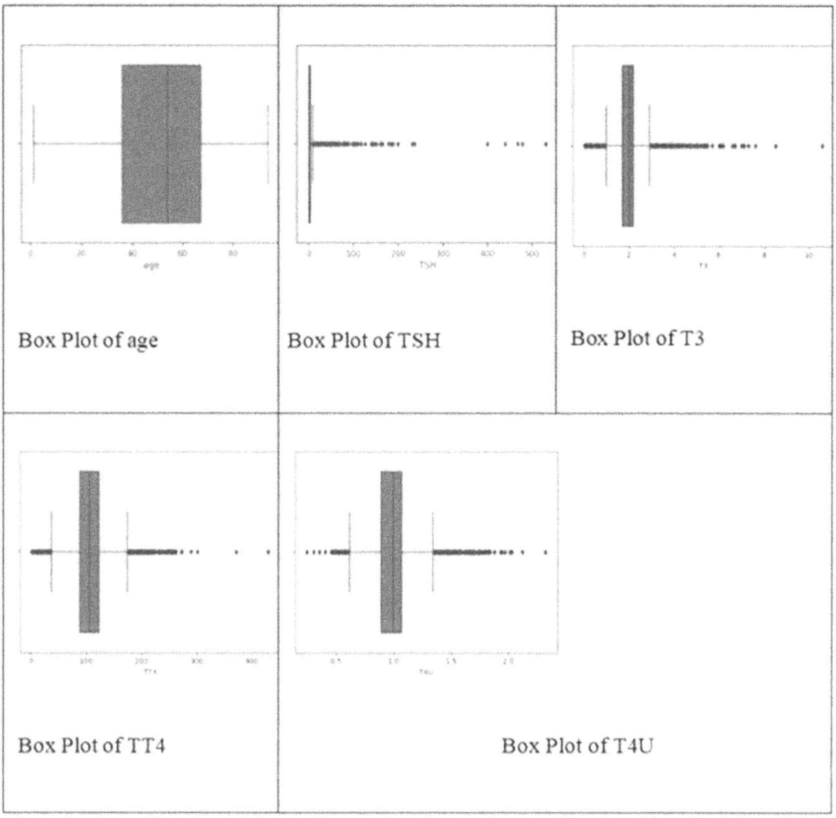

Box Plot of age

Box Plot of TSH

Box Plot of T3

Box Plot of TT4

Box Plot of T4U

FIGURE 9.9 Box plots of features.

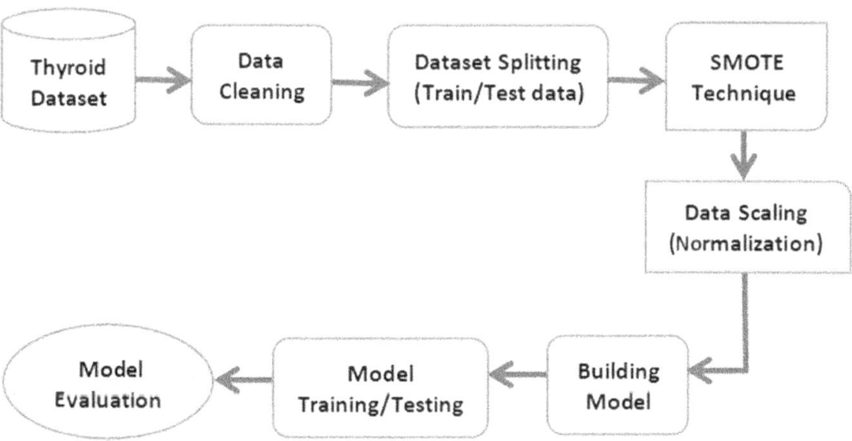

FIGURE 9.10 Flowchart of proposed approach.

For Logistic Regression we have considered hyperparameter as maximum iterations = 500, penalty as '12' and solver 'saga.' For the SVM, we have set the kernel as linear. For random forest we have tested accuracy for various n_estimators and found that for n_estimator 8, it performed far better as compared to other combinations. For Gradient Boosting Classifier we have tuned n_estimator to 15 and learning rate 0.2. For KNN, we have found promising results by tuning the hyperparameters as n_neighbors to 3, weights as uniform and the distance metric as Manhattan Distance. AdaBoost Classifier furnished promising results for n_estimators 6, learning rate 0.02, and random state 0. For Multinomial Naive Bayes, we have considered the smoothing parameter for Laplace smoothing alpha to be 0.1. For the DT Classifier we have considered 'gini' splitting criterion, set maximum depth of tree as 5, minimum number of samples required to split a node as 3, and minimum number of samples required in a leaf node as 1. Proposed modified CNN outperformed all the ML models. Under the same environment Modified CNN is trained by splitting the complete data in training-testing as 80:20. Sequential model is used with input layer and hidden layer activation function as ReLu and output layer activation function as Sigmoid. Model summary is presented in Figure 9.11. For the proposed modified CNN model we have used Adam optimizer, binary_crossentropy to capture loss, and to improve training stability and convergence we used 'ReduceLROnPlateau' callback. We have set validation accuracy as the monitored metric. If validation loss doesn't improve for 30 consecutive

```
_________________________________________________________________
 Layer (type)                Output Shape              Param #
=================================================================
 dense_30 (Dense)            (None, 256)               7424

 dropout_26 (Dropout)        (None, 256)               0

 dense_31 (Dense)            (None, 128)               32896

 dropout_27 (Dropout)        (None, 128)               0

 dense_32 (Dense)            (None, 64)                8256

 dropout_28 (Dropout)        (None, 64)                0

 dense_33 (Dense)            (None, 32)                2080

 dropout_29 (Dropout)        (None, 32)                0

 dense_34 (Dense)            (None, 1)                 33

=================================================================
Total params: 50,689
Trainable params: 50,689
Non-trainable params: 0
_________________________________________________________________
```

FIGURE 9.11 Modified CNN model summary.

iterations, the learning rate is to be reduced by a factor of 0.5 until it reaches the minimum threshold value of learning rate that is 1×10^{-5}. If validation loss doesn't improve for continuous 20 iterations then the training process will stop. Initially we considered 100 epochs but it stopped after 26 epochs based on criteria of early stopping.

9.5 RESULT AND DISCUSSION

In our research paper focused on thyroid disease detection, we have developed and evaluated various ML and DL models. The goal was to create effective tools for identifying thyroid diseases using a dataset of medical information. The ML models we used encompassed a wide spectrum of algorithms, including Logistic Regression, SVM, Random Forest, Gradient Boosting, KNN, AdaBoost Classifier, Multinomial Naive Bayes, and DT Classifier. Additionally, we employed a DL approach with a customized CNN architecture.

To train and assess the performance of these models, we employed a commonly used technique called data splitting. Specifically, we divided the available dataset into two parts: one containing 80% of the data for training and the other 20% for testing. This enabled us to simulate real-world scenarios where the models need to generalize well to new, unseen data. Positive for thyroid disease is represented by 1 and negative for thyroid disease is represented by 0. Furthermore, it's important to highlight that we ensured a consistent environment throughout our experiments. This means that we maintained uniform settings and configurations for all models, ensuring a fair and unbiased comparison.

To evaluate the models' effectiveness, we measured their performance using various performance measuring metrics. Evaluation metrics like precision, recall, F1 score, and accuracy provide different perspectives on a model's performance in classification tasks. Precision and recall balance false positives and false negatives, respectively. The F1 score combines both metrics for a balanced view. Accuracy represents the overall model performance, considering class distribution and class-specific performance. We have calculated all these evaluation metrics of the ML models, as shown in Table 9.1. It is observed that CNN is performing best with an accuracy of 99.4% and the Gradient Boosting model is the next with 98.9% accuracy.

TABLE 9.1
Performance Comparison of All Machine Learning Models

Model	F-1 Score	Recall	Precision	Accuracy
Logistic Regression	0.972	0.999	0.948	0.948
Support Vector Machine	0.972	0.999	0.946	0.946
Random Forest	0.993	0.991	0.994	0.986
Gradient Boosting	0.994	0.994	0.994	0.989
K-Nearest Neighbors	0.975	0.999	0.953	0.953
AdaBoost Classifier	0.992	0.987	0.998	0.986
Multinomial Naive Bayes	0.974	0.997	0.952	0.950
Decision Tree	0.992	0.991	0.993	0.985
CNN	0.934	0.881	0.987	0.994

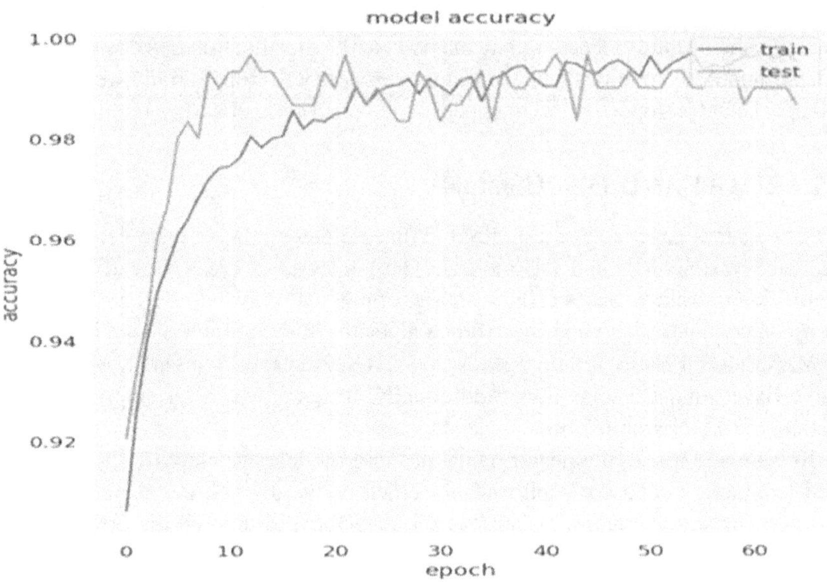

FIGURE 9.12 Modified CNN model accuracy graph.

For the modified CNN model, testing and training accuracy are presented in Figure 9.12. It is observed that CNN performs better during testing than training. The training and validation loss is presented in Figure 9.13. As expected, it is observed that loss during testing is less in comparison with training.

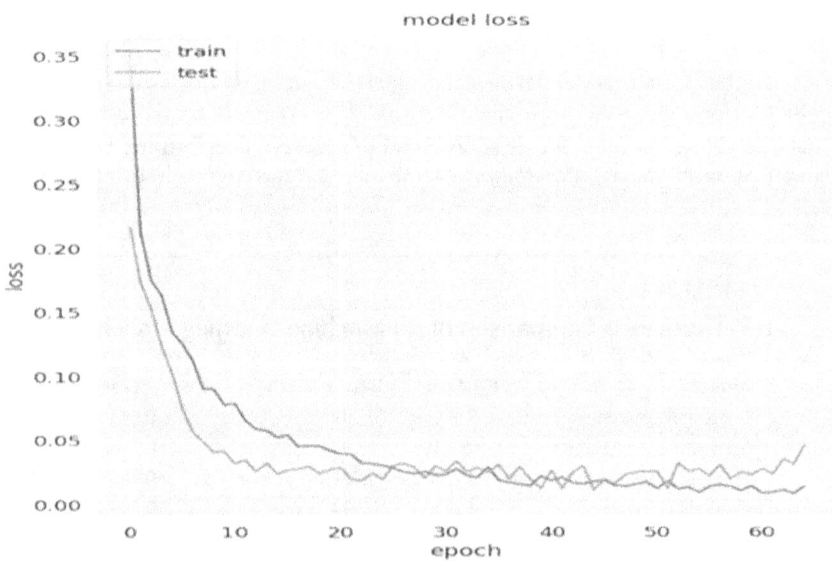

FIGURE 9.13 Modified CNN model loss graph.

When applying ML and DL techniques to thyroid disease detection, several threats to the validity of the results should be considered. These threats could impact the reliability, generalization, and applicability of the models. Some potential threats to validity include Data Bias, small dataset, domain shift, and validation approach.

Addressing these threats requires rigorous data preprocessing, careful model selection, extensive validation, domain expertise, and continuous monitoring of model performance. Awareness of these threats helps researchers and practitioners make informed decisions and develop reliable and effective thyroid disease detection systems.

9.6 CONCLUSION AND FUTURE WORK

In this chapter, we explored the effectiveness of various ML approaches and a modified CNN for the detection of thyroid disease. Our results demonstrate the significant potential of ML techniques in accurately classifying thyroid disease based on the provided dataset.

Among the ML approaches, Random Forest, Gradient Boosting, AdaBoost Classifier, and DT Classifier emerged as strong contenders, achieving accuracy rates of 98.6%, 98.9%, 98.6%, and 98.5% respectively. These results underscore the ability of ensemble methods and DT-based models to capture complex patterns within the data and make accurate predictions.

Interestingly, the modified CNN outperformed all the ML models, achieving an impressive accuracy of 99%. This highlights the power of DL in capturing intricate features from medical data. The superior performance of the modified CNN suggests its potential to provide highly accurate and reliable results, showcasing the synergy between DL and medical diagnostics.

While our study presents promising results, there are several avenues for future research and improvement. Investigating methods to enhance the interpretability of DL models, especially the modified CNN, is essential for gaining insights into the decision-making process and building trust with medical professionals. Exploring ensemble techniques that combine the strengths of multiple models could lead to further improvements in accuracy and robustness.

In conclusion, our study demonstrates the effectiveness of ML and DL techniques in thyroid disease detection. The exceptional accuracy achieved by the modified CNN indicates its potential for real-world medical applications. Future research should focus on refining these models, enhancing their interpretability, and seamlessly integrating them into clinical workflows to aid healthcare professionals in accurate and timely diagnosis.

REFERENCES

1. Allugunti, V. R. (2022). Breast cancer detection based on thermographic images using machine learning and deep learning algorithms. *International Journal of Engineering in Computer Science*, *4*(1), 49–56.

2. Budd, S., Robinson, E. C., & Kainz, B. (2021). A survey on active learning and human-in-the-loop deep learning for medical image analysis. *Medical Image Analysis, 71*, 102062.
3. Sungheetha, A. (2021). Design an early detection and classification for diabetic retinopathy by deep feature extraction based convolution neural network. *Journal of Trends in Computer Science and Smart Technology, 3*(2), 81–94.
4. Chaubey, G., Bisen, D., Arjaria, S., & Yadav, V. (2021). Thyroid disease prediction using machine learning approaches. *National Academy Science Letters, 44*(3), 233–238.
5. Chiovato, L., Magri, F., & Carlé, A. (2019). Hypothyroidism in context: Where we've been and where we're going. *Advances in Therapy, 36*, 47–58.
6. Zhou, C. M., Wang, Y., Xue, Q., Yang, J. J., & Zhu, Y. (2022). Predicting difficult airway intubation in thyroid surgery using multiple machine learning and deep learning algorithms. *Frontiers in Public Health, 10*, 937471.
7. Ma, X., Xi, B., Zhang, Y., Zhu, L., Sui, X., Tian, G., & Yang, J. (2020). A machine learning-based diagnosis of thyroid cancer using thyroid nodules ultrasound images. *Current Bioinformatics, 15*(4), 349–358.
8. Singh, V., Asari, V. K., & Rajasekaran, R. (2022). A deep neural network for early detection and prediction of chronic kidney disease. *Diagnostics, 12*(1), 116.
9. Parekh, V. S., & Jacobs, M. A. (2019). Deep learning and radiomics in precision medicine. *Expert Review of Precision Medicine and Drug Development, 4*(2), 59–72.
10. Ghosh, P., Azam, S., Jonkman, M., Karim, A., Shamrat, F. J. M., Ignatious, E., & De Boer, F. (2021). Efficient prediction of cardiovascular disease using machine learning algorithms with relief and LASSO feature selection techniques. *IEEE Access, 9*, 19304–19326.
11. Guleria, K., Sharma, S., Kumar, S., & Tiwari, S. (2022). Early prediction of hypothyroidism and multiclass classification using predictive machine learning and deep learning. *Measurement: Sensors, 24*, 100482.
12. Chai, X. (2020). Diagnosis method of thyroid disease combining knowledge graph and deep learning. *IEEE Access, 8*, 149787–149795.
13. Wurcel, V., Cicchetti, A., Garrison, L., Kip, M. M., Koffijberg, H., Kolbe, A., & Zamora, B. (2019). The value of diagnostic information in personalised healthcare: A comprehensive concept to facilitate bringing this technology into healthcare systems. *Public Health Genomics, 22*(1–2), 8–15.
14. Aversano, L., Bernardi, M. L., Cimitile, M., Iammarino, M., Macchia, P. E., Nettore, I. C., & Verdone, C. (2021). Thyroid disease treatment prediction with machine learning approaches. *Procedia Computer Science, 192*, 1031–1040.
15. Alyas, T., Hamid, M., Alissa, K., Faiz, T., Tabassum, N., & Ahmad, A. (2022). Empirical method for thyroid disease classification using a machine learning approach. *BioMed Research International, 2022*, 1–10.
16. Poudel, P., Illanes, A., Sadeghi, M., & Friebe, M. (2019, July). Patch based texture classification of thyroid ultrasound images using convolutional neural networks. In 2019 41st Annual International Conference of the IEEE Engineering in Medicine and Biology Society (EMBC) (pp. 5828–5831). IEEE, Berlin.
17. Abbad Ur Rehman, H., Lin, C. Y., Mushtaq, Z., & Su, S. F. (2021). Performance analysis of machine learning algorithms for thyroid disease. *Arabian Journal for Science and Engineering, 46*, 1–13.
18. Pal, M., Parija, S., & Panda, G. (2022). Enhanced prediction of thyroid disease using machine learning method. In 2022 IEEE VLSI Device Circuit and System (VLSI DCS) (pp. 199–204). IEEE, Kolkata.
19. Sultana, A., & Islam, R. (2023). Machine learning framework with feature selection approaches for thyroid disease classification and associated risk factors identification. *Journal of Electrical Systems and Information Technology, 10*(1), 1–23.

20. Sankar, S., Potti, A., Chandrika, G. N., & Ramasubbareddy, S. (2022). Thyroid disease prediction using XGBoost algorithms. *Journal of Mobile Multimedia*, *18*(3), 1–18.
21. Salman, M. T., AlGhazzawi, M. S., Al-Kamil, E. A., Al-Salmi, S., Yousuf, M. S., & Abdulla, T. S. (2023). Accuracy of ultrasound scans as compared to fine needle aspiration cytology in the diagnosis of thyroid nodules. *Cureus*, *15*(2), e35108. doi: 10.7759/cureus.35108
22. Akhtar, M. A., Agrawal, R., Brown, J., Sajjad, Y., & Craciunas, L. (2019, Jun 25). Thyroxine replacement for subfertile women with euthyroid autoimmune thyroid disease or subclinical hypothyroidism. *Cochrane Database Systematic Reviews*, *6*(6):CD011009. doi: 10.1002/14651858.CD011009.pub2

10 Sensory Smart Pills for Precision Drug Delivery

Shubham Suman, Priyanka Malakar, and Aadarsh Choudhary

10.1 INTRODUCTION

Modern technology helps people to make modern lifestyle smooth day by day with its up gradation in various ways, still there are some issues with the medical consumption system, it is more with the elder patients and also even with children. Non-adherence and negligence are the main issues behind this, which causes even death. Because of the various serious diseases, the sudden increases in the cost of hospitalization make the burden of medication become tough [1]. People with very serious diseases need to take a lot of medicines every day, but because of the lack of guidance or just simply the habit to forget things can make it very difficult. It is very crucial to take medicine at a proper time with a proper dose [2]. As per the need and required timing of the patient, a reminder system may use. It is also connected with keypad to change or set the timing and an alarm system also which will turn on at the present time. When the number of pills will get low, it will automatically send an order to the medical store [3]. An AI-IOT-based Smart Pill Expert System (SPES) which will be helpful to hospitals and even every single individual. With various sensors, this will work as a multitasking system. Which will confirm the right patient took the medicine at the right time [4].

10.2 RELATED WORKS

1. MCS-51 micro controller using a stepper motor can take the pill out from the box there is no such option where it can capture the taking time also the pills need to be filled up manually.
2. Another system called intelligent pill box (IPB) system can send the medical bag out on proper time also it can inform the family members/care persons via Skype if the bag is not taken. So the first thing which is required here is strong internet [5].
3. Medtracker system also can capture the time when the lid of the box is opened still it does not provide reminders [6].
4. In the traditional devices, those are becoming more reliable due to the usage of digital technology, which notifies the patients with various interfaces, text messages, etc. It can also help to not take the wrong pills with the help of low end security system. Still, various devices have some errors [7].
5. This pillbox system provides timing reminders for older patients for medication.

 DOI: 10.1201/9781032624891-10

6. In the paper "SMART MEDICINE DISPENSER" required android system to operate and also it store data on cloud and will sync as per different login. Using Bluetooth the system can be operated by Android and indicate which container is required now. The application with a home page can contain history, overview, and alarm system. It is difficult for the elders to operate because of technology but easy for others to track [8].
7. In "A SMART PILLBOX WITH REMIND AND CONSUMPTION CONFIRMATION FUNCTIONS," use matrix bar-code printed medicine bag instead of the internet. Which contains every detail of the patient. With the help of a camera patient can scan the bar-code and the UI will do the reminder and alarm function. Alarm will work with light, sound, and vibration. But there will be no interaction between patient and doctor [9].

The Internet of Things (IoT) is the network connecting the devices, which contain electronics, software, sensors, actuators, and connectivity which allow them to interact and exchange data without any human interaction. IoT with its growing interdisciplinary applications has transformed our living. The impact of IoT will be the most important and personal impact. The convergence of medicine and information technologies, such as the medical informatics, will be having transformation in healthcare as we know it, curbing costs, reducing inefficiencies, and saving lives [10]. Most patients with chronic diseases need to take medications over a prolonged period of time in order to stabilize their conditions. Ensuring that the patients consume the right medication at the appropriate time becomes crucial [11]. This study deals with the time, in particular, the Patient needs to take pills. The timing is set to the system initially reminding and it can be changed by the patient according to his requirement. The system will start an alarm at that particular time. To make the user-friendly system. This helps to change pills' time. After having pills, the user must have to put the no. of pills he removed from the box. As the no. of pills remains very few, the order for the particular pill is sent by the system automatically to medical shop. So, it is helpful to user to get the pill at particular time and avoid confusion among pills [12].

10.3 CASE STUDY

This chapter contains the proposal for alert-based reminder technology to take medical pills. To solve these issues, which happen to most of the older family members, it will work from time to time and also will send orders to medical shops when refill is required. In today's hectic and busy life, it is important to take pills properly for normal people including people with various diseases. Timing is very crucial for pills, for this, the system will alert on time and to keep record the person should update the status of taking pills [13]. In the case of related work, an MCS-51 micro controller using a stepper motor can take the pill out from the box there is no such option where it can capture the taking time also the pills need to be filled up manually. Another system called intelligent pill box (IPB) system can send the medical bag out on proper time also it can inform the family members/care persons via Skype if the bag is not taken. So the first thing which is required here is strong internet.

MedTracker system can also capture the time when the lid of the box is opened still it does not provide reminders. In the final proposed system, time setting for pills and also box number setting for different pills at the same time. The buzzer system will ring continuously until anyone is turning it off. After that the pills will come out. But also in here it is required to update the number of pills so when the pills are about to end the system can send the online purchase order also. All of this will work under ID3 algorithm [14]. As a result, the proposed smart pillbox system is a good alternative system to remind and confirm the consumption of medicine [15].

10.4 AREA OF APPLICATIONS

An AI-IOT-based SPES which is automatic. It can be used in old-age homes, hospitals, and healthcare centers where medical non-adherence can be seen. The failure rate of SPES is less than 5% and this system is a benefit for caregivers to track and monitor. In the modern and better lifestyle, technology gives us benefits. Still, medication error is a huge issue where 70% of adults do not follow due to negligence or non-adherence. World Health Organization (WHO) also mentioned various reasons for this error. This AI-IOT-based system will help to reduce the over increasing cost of hospitalization and will support every individual and patient also [16]. Nowadays, the market for automatic pill dispenser is increasing so the medical system can provide hassle free services. Healthcare and hospitals are using this technology combined with hardware and software to monitoring and generating information for patient medication. In the traditional devices, those are becoming more reliable due to the usage of digital technology that notifies the patients with various interfaces, text messages, etc. It can also help to not take the wrong pills with the help of low-end security system [17]. There are some pillboxes available in market, such as glow-cap and Glow Pack from Vitality: Vitality's glow-caps are adjustable and cellular connected which can fit anywhere. The cap and base station both use light and music to notify and also have calling system. This cap can automatically send a request for refill [18]. AdhereTech smart pill bottle: AdhereTech has a smart pill bottle which can sense the number of medicines to prevent overdose and the cellular connectivity is built directly into the bottle. The company does not have any plan to launch this product for normal consumer directly. Abiogenix's uBox: The Ubox connected with a Smartphone app can lock and unlock as per the scheduled time. It can inform family members for missing doses also. MedMinder's Maya & John: MedMinder comes with 28 compartments and 7-day pill dispenser system. While plugged in, it can send call, SMS, and email also. E-pill's Monitored MedSmart PLUS: E-pill is mainly using the market of elder and old age people to provide pill containers, wrist watches, and alarms. Simply, it stores and dispenses medicine, sends alerts to multiple people, and also can call and inform the caretaker for refill. Philips Medication Dispensing Service: Philips also comes with a non-portable large sized medication system, which anyone can use. For various events, it can call the caretaker to get a backup battery.

Nowadays, assistive technology (AT) has become a very important part of Telehealth. The remote connection between the care provider and the patient is called or known as Telehealth. Ethical concerns are a big matter while providing Telehealth in combination with AT, which caregivers need to follow as per the disciplines. it is a combined advanced technology where future research will try to work on good results and quality, where usage evidence can help to conduct. Prevalent use of technology has altered the way in which individuals communicate with others, delivering services to an individual through the use of electronic communication and remote Telehealth has become a promising service delivery alternative for some of the services provided under Telehealth in various disciplines include some individuals who receive services through Telehealth also rely on necessary tools. This population may also include individuals who advocate for AT devices, including the community connected to this topic includes individuals, whether they need these devices to navigate through their communities and communicate among peers and devices, as well as opportunities in the community for individuals to be able to successfully devices can be made low-cost, but many are very expensive due to advancements in technology, thus creating financial barriers for many individuals and families who truly need these devices to For some, an AT device is what can permit individuals to keep a Examples of low-tech AT devices may include cardboard communication.

10.5 WORKFLOW MODEL

This section addresses the workflow of smart pill dispensing box as shown in Figure 10.1. Telehealth & Assistive Technology many individuals depend on, thus making it an essential aspect of Telehealthcare for those who Similar to Telehealth, AT is considered an umbrella term, as AT E-servant is a system that can be programmed

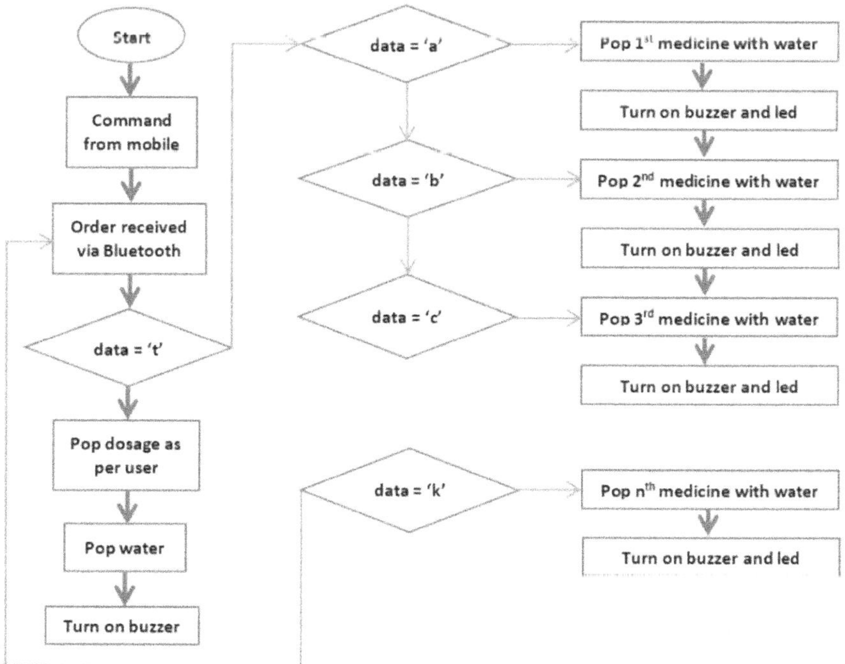

FIGURE 10.1 Workflow of smart pill dispensing box.

to assist individuals with their AT devices and home to ensure safety. Emergency management in the home for elderly individuals to ensure safety and adequate care. AT devices do not serve just one sole purpose, as they provide a vast range of devices that can serve multiple functions such as communication and motor assistance, they can also other AT devices focus mainly on the caretaker's role in providing support for caretakers of individuals with dementia.

Designed for the caretakers of individuals with dementia, and how they can improve the overall person with dementia, Bossen et al. Caretaker's use of technology to support the person with dementia. AT devices are also a useful part of speech and language therapy, which are used for children and adults to share their needs. This device is used to aid individuals with complex communication needs (CNN) and is referred to as augmentative alternative communication (ACC). Speech generating device (SGD) is one of the models of AAC devices. Most of the non-verbal or minimally verbal individuals used AAC devices as an alternative option for speech. The main challenge of tele-AAC is the lack of trained people who can provide the service [19]. As per the code of ethics, all healthcare fields are bound to follow a code to ensure professional patient care. They also need to provide the service with which they are trained with or it could negatively affect client services also raised ethical concerns. And there is a shortage of SLPs trained in AAC use, where individuals or parents expect treatment from a trained person. One more concern includes the validity of assessments, which needs attention including the analysis and implementation. It is very much required to conduct the test properly so the lack can be identified. So it could be decided what kind of therapy is required, either face to face or remote. Telehealth is not a new product and it exists in various forms to support individuals for daily purposes and also to monitor their activities. But still, there is not enough research to brief the benefits and disadvantages of this service. Many people use AT, but it is highly recommended for clinicians to become familiar with the AT so they can give their best to their field.

Also, it is very important to follow the code of ethics so the treatment can be useful and individuals get the most accurate treatment as per their needs and situation. AT and telecare are kind of a device which allows anyone especially dementia people to do any task which they normally can't do. It helps them to live freely and safely. This paper presents the scene where people with dementia or their caregivers using this technology in daily life. The trial is investigating the effectiveness of telecare and how helpful it is for people with chronic diseases, where we got mixed results. Like its expensive, it does not reduce the number of hospital-going people but it gives positive hope to the patients. Previous studies have mentioned how this AT will improve everyday usage and requirements for the patients, but this research did not mention people with dementia as a participating group. One study with caregivers and therapists shows various types of technologies to help dementia people, which are identified by effectiveness, low cost, and usefulness. Also, it informed us about the problems like burden, installation issues, and lack of safety.

But this study highlighted upon caregivers which raises questions that how people with dementia will get 100% benefit from this where the caregivers have very limited ability to know what they want. Where direct involvement in the research can improve their experience. Other research showed how this kind of technology affects the life of dementia people. They dislike the fact that always they are under the surveillance of caregivers. Also, caregivers said that AT should justify intruding in the life of dementia people. This explains the tension and lack of balance in daily life. Recent research showed the difficult issues with this technology, where people with dementia or caregivers may face problems getting the information of available services. The lack of details of the service providers may create a problem for dementia people to acquire and receive instruction. When they get the technology they were unable to install it as per the DIY instructions. Practice is a connection between human action and social structures, as per social science. Also, as Practice theorist Pierre Bourdieu said, habitus framed how society provided humans with certain dispositions. This structured how humans could act in various situations. But such theory dominates the central tensions of social science. Other scholars explained practices as unintentional or intentional political implications. To find the effectiveness of this technology, the team worked on human practices and activities. This study used a design to investigate how dementia people using or not using the ATT which is offered to them. The ethnographic approach used in this study focuses on recent research and observation on practices on dementia people and caregivers.

To provide proper results and findings, the scholars formulated a credible, dependable, and confirmable process for data collection. A purposive sampling strategy was used to select participants with experience of various characteristics from the wide community. Participants and researchers working on various authorities were recruited by the team. The study included nine case observations of six months visits, each contains at least one dementia person and their caregiver. A total of 208 hours of observation took place by the fieldworker. The conversation between the participants and researchers shows the contextual details. Fieldworkers also took notes, which served as an aide-memoire. The study team analyzed each case through computer-assisted analysis software called Nvivo, the main highlighted point is how dementia people and caregivers try to fit ATT in their daily life. To compare the results-focused coding was also used. In the result and case study we can see that in the draper's case, the mother and son tried to fit the fall detector into their lives. Their case teaches the importance of social connections and the importance of a technology-enabled care system. This raised the issue of passive devices where the trigger will be automatically charged in situations where the person does not need to perform it because dementia patients have memory difficulties.

It is also important for the patient or caregivers to trust the technology as per the user requirement. In Stewart's case, we can see the importance of using established material to achieve the appropriate outcome. Because the familiar location may support their orientation, which is relied on in the older memories. Brown's case demonstrated how devices may be adapted to local circumstances suitable to the person. Although the person switched off the device, its co-location provided the need to remember. The intro of ATT shows us how the care practices could update from face-to-face interaction to technological devices. The result shows how people adopt and use these technologies for care giving also how they fit into everyday life. This helps dementia people to live independently without the presence of caregivers. ATT can give caregivers peace of mind, but also some challenges like the need to attend and understand the configuration. Previous research has drawn the concept of bricolage, where people adopt the habit of using materials.

The effectiveness of the technology will work with the participants' social condition and with the interpreting power on how to use the device. Also, it requires people to make choices as to how it can fit on bodies or around spaces. Individual caregivers and available ATT can make the care giving process more easy and do daily activities. The capacity of caregivers may change but the effectiveness of the technology remains the same. These findings highlighted the consequences of ATT usage in the real world. It showed the need for technology with the changing times and lifestyles. This study informed that dementia care only through a good and proper amount of practices can create and provide the proper implementation of the technology.

10.6 CONCLUSION

The entire globe has witnessed a pandemic which created a demand to put emphasis on health. Many researches have been carried out to make healthcare at ease and fingertips. The authors in this chapter have visualized the need of healthcare and how the use of IoT can make self-care at the fingertips. This methodology will decline the hospitalization rate and also decrease the load of the health workers. Smart pills box is a booming instrument to solve problems like irregular medication and selection of wrong pills. It also makes monitoring the medication intake procedure of any elderly person resulting in quick action to safeguard them. This pill box has a mechanism of popping medication by the command given from its mobile application.

REFERENCES

1. Pedi Reddy, J. E., & Chavan, A., "AI-IoT Based Smart Pill Expert System," 2020 4th International Conference on Trends in Electronics and Informatics (ICOEI) (48184), 2020, pp. 407–414. doi: 10.1109/ICOEI48184.2020.9142946.
2. Dutta, P., & Mishra, S. (2022). A comprehensive review analysis of Alzheimer's disorder using machine learning approach. Augmented Intelligence in Healthcare: A Pragmatic and Integrated Analysis, 1, 63–76.
3. Moirangthem, B., Tambe, P., Panat, L., Chitra, P., & Singh, B. P. (2019, Feb). Technology survey of pillbox and design using IOT. International Research Journal of Engineering and Technology (IRJET), 6.
4. Sahoo, P. K., Mishra, S., Panigrahi, R., Bhoi, A. K., & Barsocchi, P. (2022). An improvised deep-learning-based mask r-CNN model for laryngeal cancer detection using CT images. Sensors, 22(22), 8834.
5. Shinde, S., Kadeskar, T., Patil, P., & Barathe, R. (2017, Dec). A smart pill box with remind and consumption using IOT. International Research Journal of Engineering and Technology (IRJET), p–ISSN: 2395-0072.
6. Mohapatra, S. K., Mishra, S., Tripathy, H. K., & Alkhayyat, A. (2022). A sustainable data-driven energy consumption assessment model for building infrastructures in resource constraint environment. Sustainable Energy Technologies and Assessments, 53, 102697.
7. Mishra, S., Thakkar, H. K., Singh, P., & Sharma, G. (2022). A decisive metaheuristic attribute selector enabled combined unsupervised-supervised model for chronic disease risk assessment. Computational Intelligence and Neuroscience, 2022, 1–17.
8. Antoun, W., Abdo, A., & Yaman, S. A. "Smart Medicine Dispenser (SMD)," 2018 IEEE 4th Middle East Conference on Biomedical Engineering(MECBME), Tunis, Tunisia.

9. Wu, H.-K., Wong, C.-M., Liu, P.-H., Peng, S.-P., Wang, X.-C., Lin, C.-H., & Tu, K.-H. (2015). "A Smart Pill Box with Remind and Consumption Confirmation Functions," IEEE 4th Global Conference on Consumer Electronics (GCCE), October 10-13, 2023, Nara, Japan.
10. Chakraborty, S., Sahoo, K. S., Mishra, S., & Islam, S. M. (2022, April). "AI Driven Cough Voice-Based COVID Detection Framework Using Spectrographic Imaging: An Improved Technology," 2022 IEEE 7th International Conference for Convergence in Technology (I2CT), pp. 1–7. IEEE, Pune, India.
11. Suman, S., Mishra, S., Sahoo, K. S., & Nayyar, A. (2022). Vision navigator: A smart and intelligent obstacle recognition model for visually impaired users. Mobile Information Systems, 2022, 1–15.
12. Huang, S., Chang, H., Jhu, Y., & Chen, G. (2014). "The intelligent pillbox design and implementation," 2014 IEEE International Conference on Consumer Electronics, pp. 235–236. IEEE, Taiwan.
13. Schmeler, M. R., Schein, R. M., McCue, M., Betz, K. (2009). Telerehabilitation clinical and vocational applications for assistive technology: research, opportunities, and challenges. Int J Telerehabil, 1(1), 59–72. https://doi.org/10.5195/ijt.2009.6014
14. Lariviere, M., Poland, F., & Woolham, J. et al. (2021). Placing assistive technology and telecare in everyday practices of people with dementia and their caregivers: Findings from an embedded ethnography of a national dementia trial. BMC Geriatrics, 21, 121. https://doi.org/10.1186/s12877-020-01896-y. Published 15 February 2021.
15. Raghuwanshi, S., Singh, M., Rath, S., & Mishra, S. (2022). Prominent Cancer Risk Detection Using Ensemble Learning. In: Mallick, P. K., Balas, V. E., Bhoi, A. K., Zobaa, A. F. (eds) Cognitive Informatics and Soft Computing (pp. 677–689). Springer, Singapore.
16. Patnaik, M., & Mishra, S. (2022). Indoor Positioning System Assisted Big Data Analytics in Smart Healthcare. In: Mishra, S., González-Briones, A., Bhoi, A. K., Mallick, P. K., Corchado, J. M. (eds) Connected e-Health (pp. 393–415). Springer, Cham.
17. Chandrayan, S. S., Suman, S., & Mazumder, T. (2021). IoT for COVID-19: A Descriptive Viewpoint. In: Mishra, S., Mallick, P. K., Tripathy, H. K., Chae, G. S., Mishra, B. S. P. (eds) Impact of AI and Data Science in Response to Coronavirus Pandemic. Algorithms for Intelligent Systems. Springer, Singapore. https://doi.org/10.1007/978-981-16-2786-6_10
18. Sivani, T., & Mishra, S. (2022). Wearable Devices: Evolution and Usage in Remote Patient Monitoring System. In: Mishra, S., González-Briones, A., Bhoi, A. K., Mallick, P. K., Corchado, J. M. (eds) Connected e-Health (pp. 311–332). Springer, Cham.
19. Sinha, K., Miranda, A. O., & Mishra, S. (2022). Real-Time Sign Language Translator. In: Mallick, P. K., Balas, V. E., Bhoi, A. K., Zobaa, A. F. (eds) Cognitive Informatics and Soft Computing (pp. 477–489). Springer, Singapore.

11 Smart and Assertable Approach for Brain Tumor Detection

Rishika Singh, Kashish Kaur, and Aditi Yadav

11.1 INTRODUCTION

In the present age information technology is broadly used. Because of science and technology advancements, traditional medicine centered around biotechnology is gradually embracing digitization and the integration of information. This evolution can even be observed in the implementation of groundbreaking information technology in smart healthcare. Smart healthcare represents a comprehensive transformation which goes much beyond being just a technological advancement [1].

The term smart healthcare is used to describe a healthcare system that can actively manage and smartly address the medical ecosystem demands (as depicted in Figure 11.1). By leveraging technologies like smart body-worn equipment, the Internet of Things (IoT), and smartphone-based online service, smart healthcare provides real-time retrieval of information and promotes connectivity between individuals, resources, and healthcare organizations. It encourages good communication among all entities of clinical domain, and also makes sure that users get essential support, aids in decisive facilitating processes, and optimizes the reliable utilization of resources. If simply stated, sensor-based healthcare represents a higher degree of knowledge generation within the Medicare field.

One of the primary goals of smart healthcare is to support consumers by keeping them informed about their medical condition and promoting awareness about health conditions. With the help of smart healthcare, individuals can handle certain emergency situations on their own. The main goal is to enhance the quality of user experience and well-being. Smart healthcare maximizes the utilization of existing resources, helps in remote patient monitoring, and even lowers treatment costs for users. Additionally, it enables healthcare practitioners to extend their services globally. A well-functioning smart healthcare system plays an important role in encouraging a healthy lifestyle for residents, particularly in the context of the growing trend toward smart cities.

From the beginning of the 21st century, prolonged risks have increasingly dominated the landscape of human illnesses and have become an emerging epidemic in the world that we live in today. These diseases have a prolonged duration, incur significant costs, and currently have no cure. Consequently, it is crucial to manage these diseases effectively. The conventional approach to healthcare, centered around hospitals and physicians, seems inadequate to handle the growing patient count and health risks. Contrary to the recent medical control paradigm within modern clinical

DOI: 10.1201/9781032624891-11

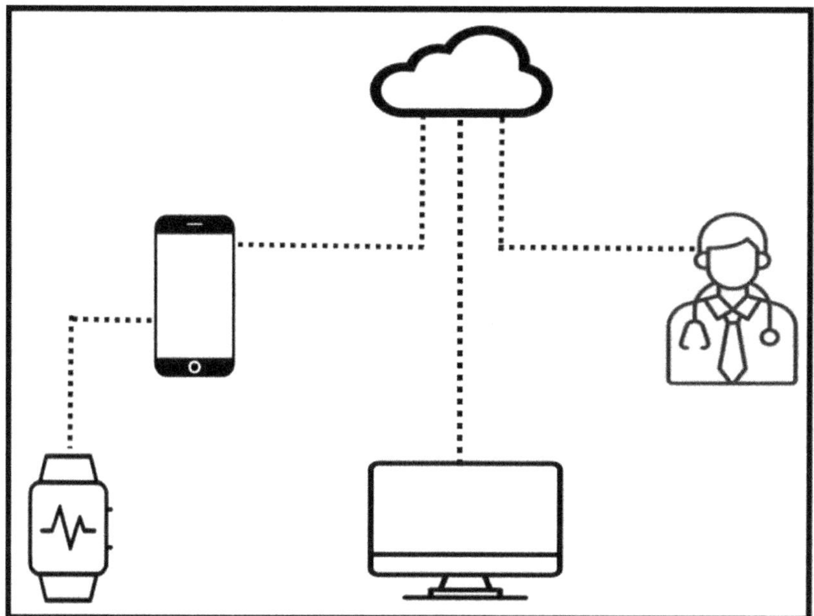

FIGURE 11.1 Smart healthcare using IoT.

service, it prioritizes self-regulation of patients. It gives importance to robust patient tracking, uninterrupted notification on medical status, and decision-making when it comes to health discrepancies. To address this challenge, the development of body-worn sensory equipment, IoT-based surrounding, and sensory-based medical data interface interconnected through sensors present an alternative. The current community Wearables enhance modern sensory units with energy-constrained devices intelligently and periodically, tracing several metrics parameters from users. These devices consume less power, provide enhanced comfort, and allow data integration along with clinical data from diverse domains. By shifting from episodic assessing to regular awareness and embedded Medicare, this strategy aims to manage the disease's progression better. It also simplifies disease prognosis tracking for medical organizations by minimizing associated risks. The emergence of smartphones, smartwatches, and similar devices has provided a new platform for such tracking. Attempts have been made to incorporate biosensors into cell phones, enabling users to closely monitor their surroundings and physical condition while increasing portability and utilizing high-performance smartphones.

In traditional disease risk prediction, health officials collect patient data, compare it with guidelines from authoritative organizations, and establish the prediction findings. However, this approach has delays and does not provide precise guidance to individuals. With reference to modern Medicare, health disorders projection takes on an adaptive and customized approach. It enables both patients and physicians to actively monitor their individual disease risks and take targeted preventive measures related to their respective assessment outcome. The latest health status detection framework gathers information from wearables and IoT applications, submits them at cloud storage through an internet work, and utilizes big data algorithms to evaluate the data. The predicted results are then delivered to customers within a short time span through information services. These methods are found to be efficient when it comes to supporting medical staff to design local medical procedures aimed at reducing disease risk. They also assist doctors and users to make proper variations in their lifestyles for the sake of their health.

11.1.1 Brain Tumor and IoT

The importance of IoT devices has increased in our daily lives, in the past few years. It is a platform that associates day-to-day entities integrated with firmware or sensory units online, allowing data collection and exchange between these devices. The healthcare sector is also adopting IoT technology to provide better services to patients.

As the tenth-leading cause of mortality, brain tumors (shown in Figure 11.2) have grown to be a serious issue in the healthcare society. At abroad zones, around 700,000 people have been detected with a brain tumor, with 80% being benign and 20% malignant. Recent statistics indicate that 78,980 adults have been identified with a brain tumor, of which 55,150 are benign and 23,830 are malignant, thereby supporting the statistics of recent studies. Additionally, it is forecast that almost 16,700 mortality in adults will be attributed to brain tumors, with 9,620 men and 7,080 women succumbing to this condition. Moreover, 4,830 children aged 0 to 19 are likely to get detected with brain tumors. The survival rates for brain tumors are

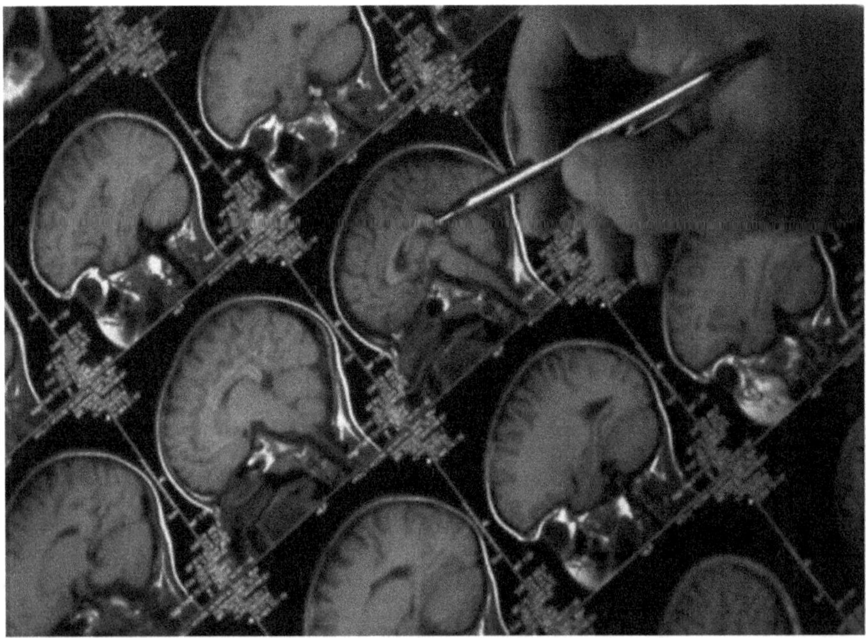

FIGURE 11.2 Brain tumor detection.

relatively low, with 34% of men and 36% of women surviving for at least five years. Given the challenges in treating brain tumors, modern technology is necessary for accurate and timely detection and classification.

The feasible diagnosis prior to a brain tumor is crucial in order to implement the proper treatment [2]. Although there is a diverse amount of brain tumors, they can mostly be divided into the following groups: Benign tumors, pre-malignant tumors, and malignant tumors are the three main categories.

This study proposes a smart automated brain tumor recognition model that categorizes different tumor symptoms based on their intrinsic properties, measured through sensors. Typically, the treatment of a brain risk is accomplished through magnetic resonance imaging (MRI). The conventional approach to identifying and classifying brain tumors from MRI scans heavily depends on human observation and the expertise of radiologists, which often leads to imprecise diagnoses. The proposed model addresses these challenges by employing computer-aided diagnostic methods, which offer significant advantages in accurately identifying and categorizing brain tumors from MRI scans [3].

This chapter is segmented into various sections which are as follows: Section 2 discusses the scope and need for the model, presenting an overview of the presented brain disorder assessment, diagnosis, and monitoring system. Section 3 further explores corresponding studies related to brain cancer prediction and diagnosis. Section 4, on the other hand, outlines the proposed IoT-based model for brain tumor detection. Section 5 shows the pros and cons of the model and Section 6 provides the conclusion and highlights the future work. Lastly, Section 7 provides the references used for this chapter.

11.2 SCOPE AND MOTIVATION

In the modern healthcare industry, advancements in informative and data sharing approaches have caused the growth of smart sensory computing. According to recent research brain cancer ranks as the tenth factor for losing life and has become a significant health issue. It has a severe impact on people's lives, with potentially fatal consequences if malignant cells are not detected timely. The need for precise image segmentation in conventional MRI-based methods makes detecting brain tumors challenging. The algorithms for MRI image classification are computationally complex and resource-intensive. This article proposes a time-saving and cost-effective alternative method for brain disorder assessment.

Considering the escalating number of brain tumor patients each year, the demand for a continuous and 24/7 monitoring system has become crucial. An IoT-based cancer patient monitoring system which is capable of timely identifying tumor-related symptoms at an early stage, continuously monitors diagnosed patients, and tracks the progress of the people who have undergone treatment. Our proposed model utilizes a wrist wearable device, the Mi Band 2, which integrates temperature and blood pressure sensors with an Arduino Uno for monitoring daily brain activities. By analyzing symptoms such as reduced deep sleep and elevated heart rate, the system is able to detect the likelihood of brain tumors and alert the individual accordingly. It even provides a list of hospitals and doctors for further confirmation and treatment, offering the convenience of booking appointments. In the second phase, an IoT-based framework is introduced, which is capable of employing cloud-based image analysis for early detection and precise classification of brain cancers. It ensures that the system can be accessed at any place and time. In the post-detection phase (phase 3), the Mi Band can be utilized for continuous body monitoring and promptly seeking assistance from a hospital in case of any emergencies. Implementing this proposed system would not only reduce the burden of tiring and costly hospital visits but would also enable people to receive high-quality medical care while residing at home.

11.3 RELATED WORKS

Srikanth et al. [4] proposed that the brain is composed of white masses of cells that form the central nervous system (CNS) in the human body. A brain tumor is an abnormal growth of cells that occurs when cells rapidly multiply and can be life-threatening if not detected early.

The precise and timely detection of the stage of a brain tumor has a significant impact on diagnosing it at an early stage, as well as on patient treatment decisions and evaluating tumor growth. With this information, the most suitable treatment approach, whether it be radiation therapy, surgery, or chemotherapy, can be determined. Consequently, if a tumor is accurately detected at an early stage, the chances of survival for a patient with a tumor can be significantly improved. Numerous studies analyzed several approaches to detect brain disorder regions in MRI images using conventional machine learning (ML) and deep learning (DL) approaches. Raheleh Hashemzehi et al. [5] introduced a hybrid approach that combines a convolutional neural network (CNN) with a Neural Autoregressive Distribution Estimation (NADE) to classify brain cancer based on MRI images. They automatically extracted features and calculated the data distribution. In a similar vein, authors in Ref. [6] presented a groundbreaking technique for fully automated sensor–driven brain risk analysis. This method incorporates carefully curated features, including specific mean force, Histogram of Oriented Gradients (HOG), and Local Binary Pattern (LBP). The authors then employed support vector machine (SVM) for pixel grouping using confidence surface modality (CSM). The CSM utilized a unique three-path CNN architecture, leveraging the provided MRI data.

Zacharaki et al. [7] highlighted a system for detecting many levels of gliomas using SVMs and K-nearest neighbors (KNNs), including binary classification of high and low grades. The multi-categorization gave an efficiency of 85%, while the binary classification noted an accuracy of 88%. Study in Ref. [8] developed a technique to improve the efficiency of brain tumor detection by enlarging the tumor region through image dilation and dividing it into sub-regions. By incorporating ring shape segmentation and tumor region expansion, they generated an optimum efficiency of around 91%. In Ref. [9], a hybrid approach combining SVM and fuzzy set categorization was discussed for brain tumor classification. The experiment utilized brain tumor MR images obtained from the Internet Brain Segmentation Repository and Diagnostic Centers, and significant results were obtained in the classification of brain MRI images using the SVM classifier. In publication Ref. [10], an IoT system based on radio frequency identification (RFID) technology for healthcare systems was proposed, with support from the National Natural Science Foundation (NSF) of the People's Republic of China and the Higher Education Doctoral Fund of the Ministry of Education. The authors of Ref. [11] introduced an IoT-based system for malignancy prediction, focusing on three physical symptoms, although the accuracy of their approach was not satisfactory [12]. Study in [12] discussed a brain risk prediction model based on image segmentation and an SVM algorithm. K-means clustering was utilized for segmentation, and tumor images were categorized as malignant or benign. The identified images and their features were added to the SVM database to enhance the system's accuracy [13]. Study in [13] discussed IoT-based healthcare systems, specifically addressing online healthcare and highlighting the foundational role of the IoT.

11.4 PROPOSED MODEL

This section describes a three-phase model proposed to detect brain disorders prior to using IoT. The first phase (Figure 11.3) is the detection stage, where patients can monitor early symptoms of brain tumors with the help of a mi band or similar device. In the second phase (Figure 11.4), the data collected from the mi band is analyzed to detect brain tumors. This phase is essential and includes sending data to specialists for enhancing the patient's experience. The third and final phase of the model (Figure 11.5) is known as the fallback stage. It focuses mainly on addressing the

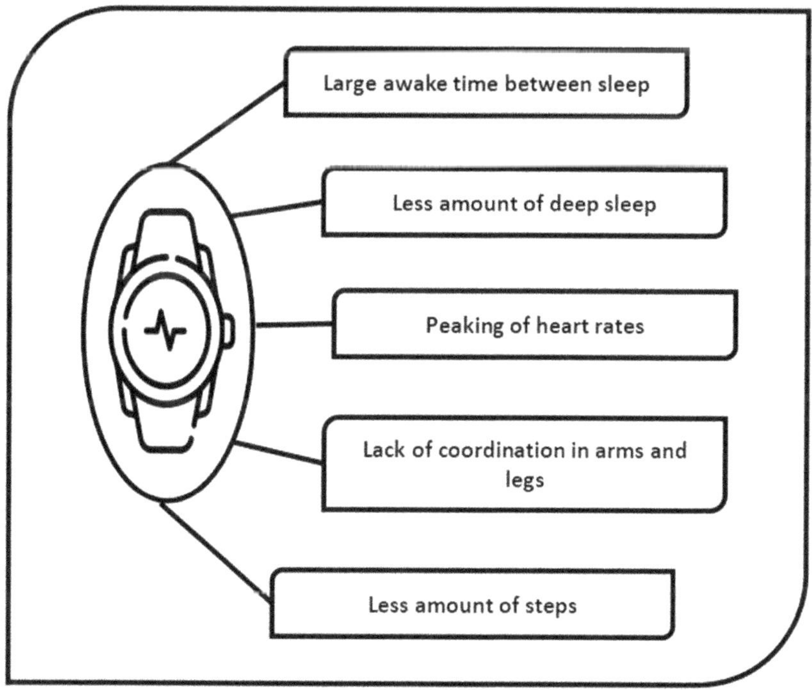

FIGURE 11.3 Using Mi band for the early detection of brain tumor

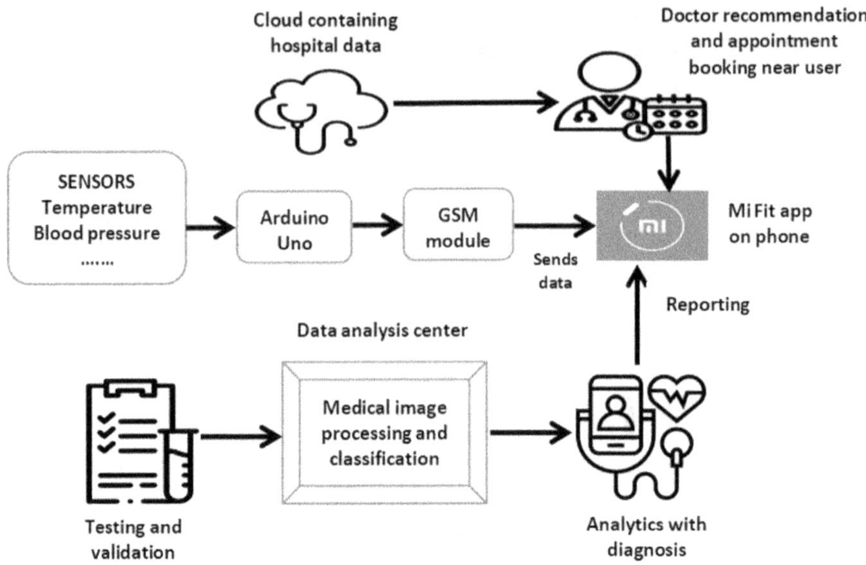

FIGURE 11.4 Analysis and reporting of the patient's health conditions.

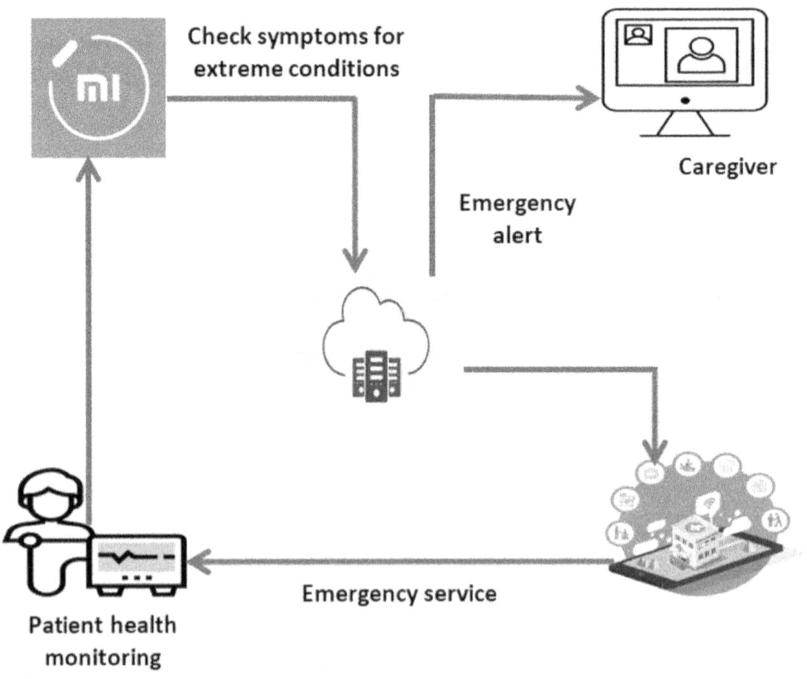

FIGURE 11.5 Emergency alert system by continuous monitoring of the patient's health conditions.

patient's critical health situations and acts as a reliable backup. It provides necessary support in emergencies, which is why it is referred to as the fallback stage.

Phase 1: Detection of Symptoms Using Mi Band Sensors

In this phase, the experiment uses the Xiaomi "Mi Band" wristband [14], which incorporates various sensors such as an optical heart rate monitor, accelerometer, vibration engine, ambient light, gyroscope, and altimeter. The pedometer on the Mi Band employs an improved algorithm for more accurate step counting. The accelerometer provides precise step counts and tracks overall activity duration. With the help of an optical heart rate monitor sensor, the device measures heart rate and records deep sleep patterns. By utilizing a heart rate sleep assistant that detects heart rate during sleep, this device captures sleep patterns, including deep sleep, periods of wakefulness between sleep cycles, and light sleep. The experimental data (shown in Figure 11.3) from the paper [14] were used for detection of symptoms in our proposed model. Table 11.1 highlights the classification of brain tumor risks symptoms.

TABLE 11.1
Classification of Brain Tumor Symptoms

Symptoms	Classification Symptoms	Time
Headache	1. High blood pressure 2. Increase body temperature 3. Accompanied by vomiting	1. Usually, steady pain after walking in the morning 2. Get better within a few hours
Seizures	1. Nausea and vomiting 2. Increasing heart rate 3. Increasing blood pressure	1. Any time 2. Blood pressure and heart rate get normal after 30 min of seizures
Vomiting or nausea	1. Increased body temperature 2. High heart rate 3. High blood pressure	1. May occur in the morning 2. When changing position
Walking problem	1. Less no. of steps as compared to normal 2. Lack of coordination in the arms or legs	1. Any time of the day, face difficulties to walk
Drowsiness or sleeping problem	1. Insomnia 2. Less amount of deep sleep	1. Falling asleep during the day 2. Not sleeping until 5/6 AM on some days
Vision changes	1. Low heart rate 2. High blood pressure 3. Headache	1. After waking up from sleep 2. Double or triple vision in one eye 3. Suddenly change posture
Fatigue	1. Difficult in sleeping 2. Headache 3. A large amount of awake time in between sleep 4. Vision changes	1. Whole day patient experiences this symptom

TABLE 11.2
Blood Pressure Chart

Blood Pressure	Systolic	Diastolic
High	Systolic > 140	Diastolic > 140
Low	Systolic < 90	Diastolic < 60
Normal	90 < Systolic < 140	60 < Systolic <90

Table 11.2 summarizes the blood pressure chart and Table 11.3 denotes the body normal temperature analysis.

For the detection of brain tumors, seven common symptoms are taken into consideration: fatigue, vomiting or nausea, vision changes, headache, seizures, drowsiness or sleeping issues, and walking problems (compared to individuals without any walking difficulties). The first step involves categorizing these symptoms and associated information. And then the sensors are used to capture the relevant information.

The wearable wristband shown in Figure 11.3 can measure most of these symptoms. Additionally, in order to measure body temperature and blood pressure individual sensors are employed. All of these sensors, along with the wristband, are connected to an Arduino Uno. Using the global system, the Arduino Uno transmits the sensor data to Android smartphones for mobile communication (GSM) module.

The wristband is linked to the Android smartphone through the Mi Fit app to gather data from the devices. The collected data is sent to the app's database, where it is analyzed on the basis of the symptoms observed in previous patients. The Mi Fit app interface is designed for providing expert recommendations, simplifying the process of booking appointments, and enhancing its usability for patients.

Phase 2: Diagnosis and Analysis

The second phase of this model is the most critical one among all the remaining phases and relies on an IoT system, as depicted in Figure 11.4 [15]. The architecture mentioned above is known as a multi-user access system since it enables multiple users to connect to the cloud simultaneously [16, 17]. There is a shared receiver

TABLE 11.3
Body Normal Temperature

Age	Heart	Average Sleep Hours
0 to 2 months	120 to 160	12 to 18
3 months to 1 year	80 to 140	14 to 15
1 to 3 years	80 to 130	12 to 14
3 to 5 years	80 to 120	11 to 13
6 to 12 years	70 to 110	10 to 11
Age > 13 years	60 to 110	8.5 to 10

among all the users of the device. The development of an IoT system with cloud administration is used for the classification of brain tumors. Utilizing the cloud as a distributed environment offers the most efficient solution for a medical system, facilitating easier access to data by doctors.

The proposed IoT framework comprises four primary phases:

1. Data gathering
2. Classification and image processing
3. Diagnosis
4. User interface

In the first phase, data from the mi band is collected and sent to the Mi Fit app on the user's mobile application. From there, it is stored in the cloud and forwarded to the relevant authorities for further processing and analysis to make informed decisions about the patient's current health conditions [18]. The patient can view their report through the mi fit app, and the app also provides doctor recommendations to facilitate more efficient appointment scheduling, resulting in reduction of the patient's workload.

The primary objective of this framework is to decrease mortality rates by early detection of malignant tumors. During the analytics phase, the patient can access their database to review the classification results. By uploading an MRI scan, we receive a near-instantaneous classification result, based on which a radiologist can detect the presence as well as the type of a tumor. The resulting report is then forwarded to the patient's doctor, who will make the most appropriate decisions in favor of the patient's health [19].

In the system implemented in this research paper, each user has a transmitter and a receiver. The transmitter is responsible for preparing the scanned image of the patient for transmission, while the receiver decodes the received image and extracts its features to enable early detection of brain tumors.

Phase 3: SOS

The third and final stage of the proposed model comes under the emergency phase, which adds an extra layer of reliability to the implemented model. As shown in Figure 11.3, this phase involves continuous monitoring of the patient's body conditions post diagnosis. The data collected is sent to the cloud through the Mi Fit app to ensure that the body levels remain normal without any abnormalities. In the event of any abnormality, an emergency alert is sent to both the patient's designated local guardian and the nearest healthcare facility [20].

All the phases combined make the model highly efficient, reducing expenses and minimizing exhaustive procedures for the patient while optimizing the utilization of resources by medical authorities. This model proves to be a boon to the current healthcare system, enhancing the patient's overall experience while conserving healthcare resources. For instance, consider an individual experiencing early symptoms of a brain tumor who happens to be a mi band user. The entire process of detection and diagnosis becomes significantly less burdensome with the implementation of this model. As a result, resources are saved, and the overall process of detection, analysis, and diagnosis becomes more streamlined [21].

11.5 BENEFITS OF THE PROPOSED MODEL

- **Early Detection:** The foremost thing when it comes to diseases is early detection. The entire idea behind this model is to help people get a diagnosis as early as possible to avoid a situation wherein the patient loses their life just because of late detection [22]. The sensors installed within the band help the user go on with everyday activities while subtly monitoring any or all health risks involved.
- **Accessible:** Accessible electronic information technology is a technology that can be used by people with different abilities and disabilities. It complies with universal design principles. Each user can use technology according to their needs. Diagnosis at the hands of the user, just a click away is one of the major goals of the use of IoT devices to detect diseases. In spite of the industrialization and enhanced importance of healthcare facilities, especially in the post pandemic world, not many people in the world have easy access to healthcare facilities [23]. However, wearing a Mi Band on your hand and having a constant healthcare system backing you up makes it pretty accessible and efficient for the patient. So this project reduces the cost, time, and effort spent in visiting the hospital in person unless the risks are high.
- **User-Friendly Interface:** The interface is an intermediary between the user and the system. The user will be able to communicate their needs to the system through the interface, and the system will fulfill them. An interface is said to be "user-friendly" if it is not built with a specific target audience in mind or without one in particular but with the goal of maximizing user convenience [24]. This model keeps in mind the user's convenience as a priority so that it is easy for the patient to access. Whether it is the early detection of symptoms, the doctor's recommendations, or the emergency services, all of these features make the system pretty user-friendly.
- **Time-Saving:** This system is also efficient in terms of accessibility and resource-saving along with saving the time of the user. The time that is wasted in unnecessary hospital visits, for testing as well as the report is saved through this entire system [25].
- **Emergency Situations:** The last stage of the proposed model has the feature of not just sending a notification to the local guardian of the patient but also the closest healthcare facilities will be informed to take the necessary steps with reference to the patient's safety.

11.6 ISSUES WITH THE PROPOSED MODEL

Table 11.4 highlights a comparison analysis between the proposed model and the traditional approach.

- **Faulty Sensors:** Sensing devices present on the Mi Band are the base of this project. Whether it is the first phase of early detection or the constant monitoring to sense an emergency situation beforehand, the sensors play an important role [26]. If there is a situation where the sensors are not working properly, the entire system will collapse and it would be a waste of resources, time, and effort.

TABLE 11.4
Traditional Approach vs. the Proposed Model

Traditional Method	Proposed Method
Mostly tumors are detected at a very late stage because of little to no noticeable changes	Early diagnosis is possible
Accessing hospital facilities is difficult for a lot of people due to many reasons like transportation, geographical location, etc.	It is easily accessible
A lot of time is wasted in unnecessary hospital visits, for testing as well as the report	Saves a lot of time as everything is accessible through the cloud
It is not cost efficient	It is cost efficient
Lack of prompt medical attention causes death of many emergency patients	It can contact the hospital right away in the event of an emergency

- **Overlapping Symptoms:** Some diseases have similar symptoms; this similarity sometimes might lead to inaccurate detection. Brain tumor misdiagnosis can commonly be diagnosed as the following diseases: Alzheimer's disease, Encephalitis, or something as common as headaches or mere migraines for that matter [27]. This makes the system a little misleading because even though it increases the odds of early detection, at the same time it might lead to a wrong prediction and unnecessary damage can be caused as a result.
- **False Alarm:** The third stage of the model is the most important in case of an emergency situation but there is a chance that sometimes a small miscalculation can lead to a false alarm which can be dangerous [28].

11.7 CONCLUSION AND FUTURE WORKS

Rising cancer incidence rates have become a major issue in the world that we live in today. This is mostly caused due to the dearth of proper medical facilities and the high cost of care [29].

Complex cancer patients are in an even worse situation because they need to be monitored constantly in order to make accurate diagnoses and treatment choices. Moreover, early cancer detection and therapy can resolve a lot of disease-related problems. An expert automated system is required to detect brain tumors at an early stage, allowing improved pharmaceutical treatment and maybe even sparing the patient from an invasive surgery. The development of wireless connectivity, embedded technologies, and remote data collection can significantly aid when it comes down to the early detection and treatment of cancer.

In conclusion, throughout this research an IoT-based technique for the automatic detection of brain cancers has been stated. The daily activities of both people with brain tumors and healthy people are monitored using a wearable wristband gadget through temperature sensors and blood pressure sensors. It examines numerous brain tumor symptoms and categorizes them as chosen common symptoms. Experimental datasets from both brain tumor patients and normal populations demonstrate the accuracy of the proposed method for the automatic detection of brain tumors using IoT. It also aids in the subsequent processes of analysis and ongoing monitoring post-detection. The suggested portable system is less time-consuming, more economical, and simpler to use.

A further direction of this work would be to further evaluate the performance of the proposed prototype.

REFERENCES

1. Quick Brain Tumor Facts-National Brain Tumor Society. (2021). http://braintumor.org/brain-tumor-information/brain-tumor-facts (Last accessed: 23 January, 2021).
2. Abhishek, Tripathy, H.K., & Mishra, S. (2022). A Succinct Analytical Study of the Usability of Encryption Methods in Healthcare Data Security. In: Tripathy, B.K., Lingras, P., Kar, A.K., Chowdhary, C.L. (eds) Next Generation Healthcare Informatics. Studies in Computational Intelligence, vol 1039. Springer, Singapore. https://doi.org/10.1007/978-981-19-2416-3_7
3. Sivani, T., & Mishra, S. (2022). Wearable Devices: Evolution and Usage in Remote Patient Monitoring System. In: Mishra, S., González-Briones, A., Bhoi, A. K., Mallick, P. K., Corchado, J. M. (eds) Connected e-Health (pp. 311–332). Springer, Cham.
4. Srikanth, B., & Suryanaraana, S.V. (2021). Multi-class classification of brain tumor images using data augmentation with deep neural network. Materials Today: Proceedings, 1–20.
5. Hashemzehi, R., Mahdavi, S.J.S., Kheirabadi, M., & Kamel, S.R. (2020). Detection of brain tumors from MRI images base on deep learning using hybrid model CNN and NADE. Biocybern Biomed Eng 40(3):1225–1232.
6. Khan, H., Shah, P.M., Shah, M.A., Islam, S., & Rodrigues, J.J.P.C. (2020). Cascading handcrafted features and convolutional neural network for IoT-enabled brain tumor segmentation. Comput Commun 153:196–207.
7. Zacharaki, E., Wang, S., Chawla, S., Soo Yoo, D., Wolf, R., Melhem, E., & Davatzikos, C. (2009). Classification of brain tumor type and grade using MRI texture and shape in a machine learning scheme. Magn Reson Med 62(6):1609–1618. https://doi.org/10.1002/mrm.22147
8. Cheng, J., Huang, W., Cao, S., Yang, R., Yang, W., Yun, Z., Wang, Z., & Feng, Q. (2015). Correction: Enhanced performance of brain tumor classification via tumor region augmentation and partition. PLoS ONE 10(12):e0144479. https://doi.org/10.1371/journal.pone.0140381
9. Birnale, D.B., & Patil, S.N. (2016). Brain tumor MRI image segmentation using FCM and SVM techniques. Int J Eng Sci Comput 6(12):479–486.
10. Talpur, S.H. (2013). The appliance pervasive of internet of things in healthcare systems. Int J Comput Sci Issues 10(1):No. 1.
11. Rahman, M.L., Shehab, S.H., Chowdhury, Z.H., & Datta, A.K. (2020). "Predicting the Possibility of Being Malignant Tumor Based on Physical Symptoms using IoT," *2020 IEEE Region 10 Symposium (TENSYMP)*, pp. 26–30. doi: 10.1109/TENSYMP50017.2020.9230941
12. Telrandhe, S.R., Pimpalkar, A., & Kendhe, A. (2016). Implementation of brain tumor detection using segmentation algorithm & SVM. Int J Comput Sci Eng 8(7). https://doi.org/10.1109/STARTUP.2016.7583949
13. Shinde Sayali, P., & Phalle Vaibhavi, N. (2017). A survey paper on internet of things based healthcare system. Int Adv Res J Sci Eng Technol 4(Special Issue 4):131–133.
14. Sahoo, P.K., Mishra, S., Panigrahi, R., Bhoi, A.K., & Barsocchi, P. (2022). An improvised deep-learning-based mask r-CNN model for laryngeal cancer detection using CT images. Sensors 22(22):8834.

15. Mishra, S., Jena, L., Tripathy, H.K., & Gaber, T. (2022). Prioritized and predictive intelligence of things enabled waste management model in smart and sustainable environment. PloS One 17(8):e0272383.
16. Khan, M.A., Lali, I.U., Rehman, A., Ishaq, M., Sharif, M., & Saba, T. et al. (2019). Brain tumor detection and classification: A framework of marker-based watershed algorithm and multilevel priority features selection. Microsc Res Tech 82:909–922.
17. Koziol, L.F., Budding, D.E., & Chidekel, D. (2012). From movement to thought: Executive function, embodied cognition, and the cerebellum. Cerebellum 11:505–525.
18. Mishra, S., Thakkar, H.K., Singh, P., & Sharma, G. (2022). A decisive metaheuristic attribute selector enabled combined unsupervised-supervised model for chronic disease risk assessment. Comput Intell Neurosci 2022:1–22.
19. Sajjad, S., Hanan Abdullah, A., Sharif, M., & Mohsin, S. (2014). Psychotherapy through video game to target illness related problematic behaviors of children with brain tumor. Curr Med Imaging 10:62–72.
20. Chakraborty, S., Sahoo, K.S., Mishra, S., & Islam, S.M. (2022, April). "AI Driven Cough Voice-Based COVID Detection Framework Using Spectrographic Imaging: An Improved Technology," *2022 IEEE 7th International Conference for Convergence in Technology (I2CT)*, pp. 1–7. IEEE.
21. Saba, T., Mohamed, A.S., El-Affendi, M., Amin, J., & Sharif, M. (2020). Brain tumor detection using fusion of hand crafted and deep learning features. Cogn Syst Res 59:221–230.
22. Tripathy, H.K., Mishra, S., Suman, S., Nayyar, A., & Sahoo, K.S. (2022). Smart COVID-shield: An IoT driven reliable and automated prototype model for COVID-19 symptoms tracking. Computing 104:1–22.
23. Raghuwanshi, S., Singh, M., Rath, S., & Mishra, S. (2022). Prominent Cancer Risk Detection Using Ensemble Learning. In: Mallick, P. K., Balas, V. E., Bhoi, A. K., Zobaa, A. F. (eds) Cognitive Informatics and Soft Computing (pp. 677–689). Springer, Singapore.
24. Ohgaki, H., & Kleihues, P. (2013). The definition of primary and secondary glioblastoma. Clin Cancer Res 19:764–772.
25. Chakraborty, S., & Mishra, S. (2022). A Smart Farming-Based Recommendation System Using Collaborative Machine Learning and Image Processing. In: Mallick, P. K., Balas, V. E., Bhoi, A. K., Zobaa, A. F. (eds) Cognitive Informatics and Soft Computing (pp. 703–716). Springer, Singapore.
26. Amin, J., Sharif, M., Anjum, M.A., Raza, M., & Bukhari, S.A.C. (2020). Convolutional neural network with batch normalization for glioma and stroke lesion detection using MRI. Cogn Syst Res 59:304–311.
27. Mishra, Y., Mishra, S., & Mallick, P.K. (2022). A Regression Approach Towards Climate Forecasting Analysis in India. In: Mallick, P. K., Balas, V. E., Bhoi, A. K., Zobaa, A. F. (eds) Cognitive Informatics and Soft Computing (pp. 457–465). Springer, Singapore.
28. De, A., & Mishra, S. (2022). Augmented Intelligence in Mental Health Care: Sentiment Analysis and Emotion Detection with Health Care Perspective. In: Mishra, S., Tripathy, H. K., Mallick. P., Shaalan, K. (eds) Augmented Intelligence in Healthcare: A Pragmatic and Integrated Analysis (pp. 205–235). Springer.
29. Mohapatra, S.K., Mishra, S., Tripathy, H.K., Bhoi, A.K., & Barsocchi, P. (2021). A pragmatic investigation of energy consumption and utilization models in the urban sector using predictive intelligence approaches. Energies 14(13):3900.

12 Cardiac Disease Risks Pattern Recognition Using Advanced Predictive Analytics

Sayan Garai, Prachi Kashyap, Shayan Irfan, and Ananya Pareek

12.1 INTRODUCTION

In today's time, heart diseases and heart failure are becoming more prevalent globally. In spite of technological advancement in the medical field which includes both detection and course of surgery or treatment, cardiac disease is one of the biggest reasons for death, known for one-third of global deaths annually and even the main reason behind early deaths. The only way out of this cycle is early and precise diagnosis which is the best way out to improve this scenario. The imaging of the cardiovascular space has a prominent role in diagnostic decision making. The existing systems of image assessment are mainly dependent on observable understanding of qualitative and quantitative techniques of cardiac structure images. For optimizing this diagnostic space of cardiac imaging, there is a need for more prominent techniques that would produce breakthrough in the space of analysis of imaging techniques which would grant higher classification and provide better results. Over the decade, the development of advanced topics including big data, predictive analysis (machine learning, ML), and abundant resources of high computational power are the main driving factors behind the significant growth of artificial intelligence (AI) technologies in all arenas, even in the arena of imaging in the medical field. These predictive analysis (ML) techniques used for diagnosis based on image are dependent on models that are known to learn and adapt from previous available medical data through classification and identification of various disguised and complicated patterns based on the algorithms. The previous works have already demonstrated the additional assessment of image-based diagnosis of cardiovascular structures with predictive analysis (ML) for various units of essential and critical medical situation of significance such as ischemic heart disease and cardiac arrest, which can be prevented on early diagnosis. The advancement in the accomplishment of AI-driven assessment of images has now developed the capability to ease the extra load of serious cardiac ailment through the development of precise and fast-processing decision making in the diagnostic arena. Here, the main predictive analysis (ML) algorithms which have produced significant success in field of diagnosis have been studied and analyzed.

 DOI: 10.1201/9781032624891-12

The main objectives of the study are as follows:

- To identify the pattern of diseases based on the images collected.
- Collecting sources of cardiovascular imaging data.
- Identifying the predictive analysis (ML) algorithms useful in this medical space.

12.2 RELATED WORKS

In Ref. [1], the paper indicates that Decision Tree (DT) Classification works better than approaches based on Naive Bayes (NB), Logistic Regression (LR), Random Forest (RF), Support Vector Machine (SVM), and K-Nearest Neighbors (KNN). In Ref. [2], this paper demonstrates the stability of KNN with its N(8) neighbors for testing the caliber, susceptibility and preciseness, F1-score, and precision in comparison to other available effective methods, i.e., NB, SVM, DT Classifier with 4 or 18 features, and RF classifiers. In Ref. [3], the paper highlights the latest functioning of predictive analysis (ML) with medications based on cardiovascular diseases, giving importance to cardiological image production. In Ref. [4], the aim of this paper is to assume that some data mining tools can be used as a substitute for some complex, expensive, and sometimes dangerous medical examinations. In Ref. [5] various predictive analysis (ML) algos and deep learning (DL) are adapted to analyze the outcomes and run a summary of the University of California Irvine (UCI) predictive analysis (ML) cardiovascular disease datasets. In Ref. [6] this paper highlights the ability of learning models in the arena of cardiac ailments which proves to be promising because of its interesting outcomes, particularly SVM and boosting algorithm. In Ref. [7] this paper, the use of advanced amplified computation power in analytical space involving medicine and diagnostics has been under study since the 1960s. In Ref. [8] this paper, identification and prediction of cardiovascular ailments using various predictive analysis (ML) algorithms and used the prevailing datasets to calculate its outcome using various techniques for evaluation, such as susceptibility, selectivity, precision, F-measure, and grouping precision. In Ref. [9] this paper, the aim is to assess the behavior and type of risk because of bias in ML and non-ML studies for heart disease prediction of risk. Both AI and ML show promising results in risk prediction of crucial heart diseases. In Ref. [10], the paper highlights the accuracy of diagnosis and finding out of heart disease using ML algos and Python using various parameters from a significant and large range of datasets. In Ref. [11], the aim of this paper is to predict heart diseases precisely through heartbeats using different ML algorithms like RF and Gradient Boosting (GB) tree. In Ref. [12], the main aim of this paper is to predict cardiovascular disease based on predictive analysis (ML) that is highly precise. In Ref. [13], this paper describes the decrease in the number of deaths every year due to ischemic cardiovascular diseases by training the model to run an accurate detection of long-term (chronic) diseases using training and testing of different datasets. In Ref. [14], the paper talks about the utilization and usage of various methods such as Neural Networks (NN) and KNN for the evaluation of the diagnosis of heart disease. In Ref. [15], the paper provides a deep understanding and learning on the risk evaluation of cardiac ailment through the quantification and calculation of retinal vessels. In Ref. [16], this paper aims to present a literature analysis on the implementation of best predictive analysis (ML) classification algorithms on heart disease datasets. In Ref. [17], the paper proposes a new mixed approach for precise diagnosis of cardiac diseases using different predictive analysis (ML) techniques such as Logistic Regression Adaptive Boosting (LRAB), Multi-Objective Evolutionary Fuzzy Classifier (MOEFC), Fuzzy Unordered Rule Induction (FURIA), Genetic Fuzzy System-LogicBoost (GFSL), and Fuzzy Hybrid Genetic Based Machine Learning (FHGBML). In Ref. [18], the aim of the paper is to anticipate the risk of cardiovascular ailment by taking the help of supervised ML techniques by comparing the performance in terms of preciseness and susceptibility of supervised models. In Ref. [19], this paper aims to develop alternative ML-based Risk Prediction Models that might be better at predicting cardiovascular diseases using non-laboratory features. In Ref. [20], the paper proposes an approach for cardiovascular disease identification based on a set of features that can be obtained directly from cardiac sounds.

12.3 RELATED CASE STUDIES IN CARDIAC RISKS ANALYSIS

Here, these two things are employed—Rapid Application Development (RAD) and Prototype Design Specification (PDS). The RAD approach adapts to changes and accepts new inputs such as features and functionalities at every stage of the development process.

In Figure 12.1, the proposed model for the working of the aim has been shown in which data set based on many patients which is first split and then the model is trained based on this data set. After this, it is tested and then the model is deemed capable of making predictions regarding heart conditions. If the model is deemed fit, it is saved and then exported to Flask API. It is henceforth again verified by inputs given from users of the model, and then finally it starts to make predictions.

The functionality (system) here makes use of the heart data set, which can be found on kaggle.com. This data set includes 14 test-result characteristics from 1025 individuals. A set for training and a set for testing were created from the data set. Four predictive analysis techniques were used to train this data set: KNN, SVC, DT, and RF Classifier. The model which has the highest percentage of accuracy was utilized to

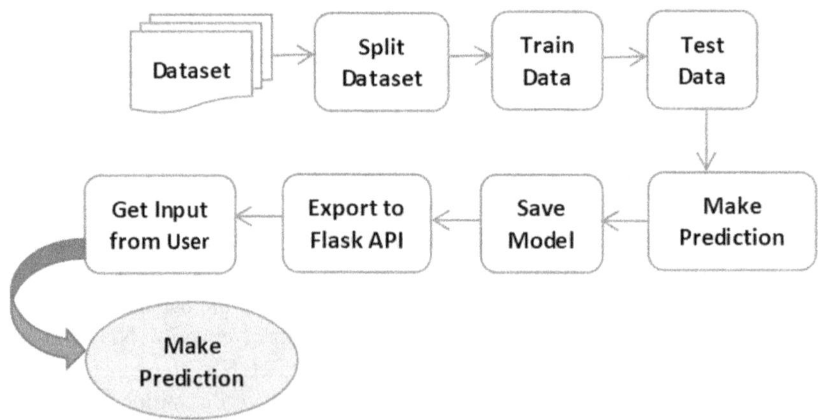

FIGURE 12.1 Proposed system model.

generate predictions after the four different training methods had been tested, trained, and checked for correctness. A site is loaded after saving and loading this trained model.

This trained model is loaded by Flask, an Application Programming Interface (AP1), which also collects user input to populate a form with results from the test. This data (inputs) is then sent to the model which has been trained, which will then analyze and assess whether the patient has a condition related to his/her heart or not.

In order to detect whether a patient has a cardiac condition or not, a predictive analysis (ML) model was trained for this study. This computer model makes use of a data set that includes 13 test results from various individuals. Make sure that there are no values containing zero, i.e., no Null values, by thoroughly cleaning and processing it. The x and y variables in this data set were separated, where the y variable has the output and the x variable holds the thirteen characteristics, which represent the various test outcomes. Standard Scale was being used to scale the x variable. Further subdivided into x-train, x-test, y-train, and y-test were the x and the y variables. These x-train and y-train were fitted or trained using the KNN, SVM, DT, and RF predictive analysis (ML) techniques. Using various n-values, the four algorithms were utilized to assess the accuracy rate of the findings. The highest precise result for K Neighbor is roughly 97.47% when $n = 1$; for SVM it is 98.83% when $n = 10$; for DT it is 98.83% when $n = 1$; and for RF it is 98.83% when $n = 10$ (the highest precise result for KNN is 97.47% when $n = 1$). Following accuracy testing, we employed DT Classifier, which has one of the most precise outcomes when producing predictions. Using the API Flask, the DT model was uploaded to the web. With the aid of Flask, we developed an HTML website with 13 inputs on which visitors could enter the results of several tests before passing the data to a model to determine whether or not they had heart disease. Additionally, the user may view the model's output online.

In Figure 12.2, an unfiltered data set is shown as it is collected and categorized under different columns, which will then be processed as given in Figure 12.3.

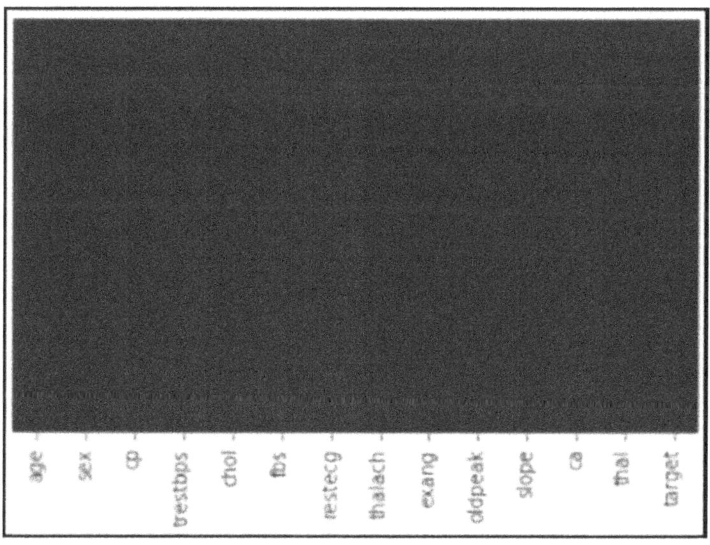

FIGURE 12.2 A raw unfiltered data set.

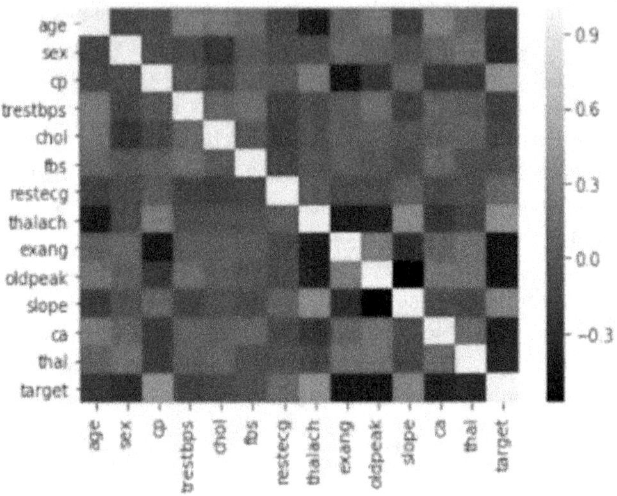

FIGURE 12.3 A correlation matrix of dataset.

Figure 12.3 shows correlation coefficients among distinct variables. Every box in the graph(table) depicts the relation between two variables. This is used to make the input of data into a more advanced and better form for better and advanced results and diagnosis.

	age	sex	cp	trestbps	chol	fbs	restecg	thalach	exang	oldpeak	slope	ca	thal
0	52	1	0	125	212	0	1	168	0	1.0	2	2	3
1	53	1	0	140	203	1	0	155	1	3.1	0	0	3
2	70	1	0	145	174	0	1	125	1	2.6	0	0	3
3	61	1	0	148	203	0	1	161	0	0.0	2	1	3
4	62	0	0	138	294	1	1	106	0	1.9	1	3	2
5	58	0	0	100	248	0	0	122	0	1.0	1	0	2
6	58	1	0	114	318	0	2	140	0	4.4	0	3	1
7	55	1	0	160	289	0	0	145	1	0.8	1	1	3
8	46	1	0	120	249	0	0	144	0	0.8	2	0	3
9	54	1	0	122	286	0	0	116	1	3.2	1	2	2
10	71	0	0	112	149	0	1	125	0	1.6	1	0	2
11	43	0	0	132	341	1	0	136	1	3.0	1	0	3
12	34	0	1	118	210	0	1	192	0	0.7	2	0	2
13	51	1	0	140	298	0	1	122	1	4.2	1	3	3
14	52	1	0	128	204	1	1	156	1	1.0	1	0	0
15	34	0	1	118	210	0	1	192	0	0.7	2	0	2
16	51	0	2	140	308	0	0	142	0	1.5	2	1	2

FIGURE 12.4 Training data for 1025 individuals.

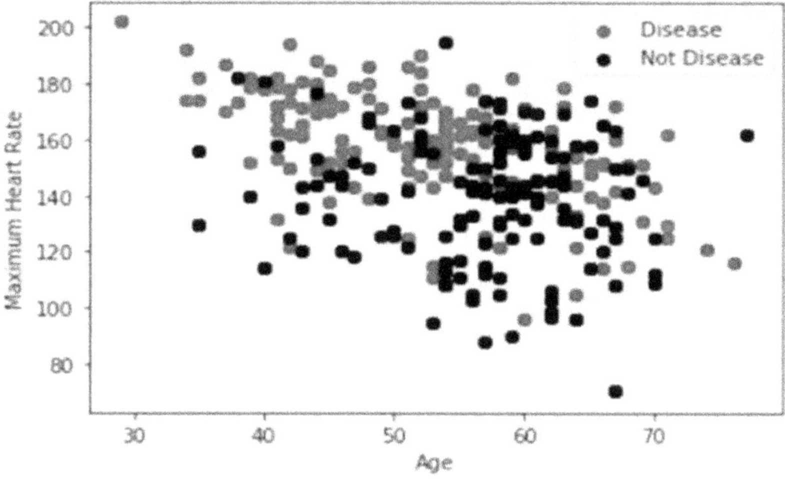

FIGURE 12.5 Scatter plot displaying the results of the test.

In Figure 12.4, a scatter plotting is demonstrated for the results of a test in which the ages and the maximum heart rate for people with heart disease and for people without a heart condition are specified.

In Figure 12.5, a scatter plotting is demonstrated for the results of a test in which the ages and the maximum heart rate for people with heart disease and for people without a heart condition are specified.

In Figure 12.6, another data plotting technique called histogram is displayed which simply shows the number of people against target 0 and 1.

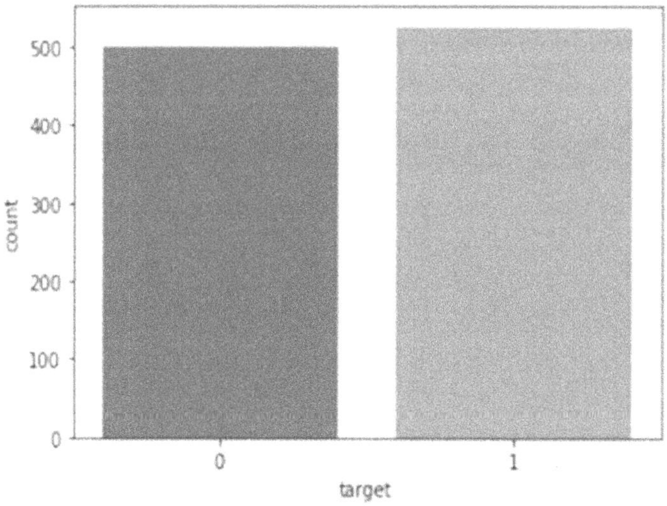

FIGURE 12.6 Histogram of the number of people.

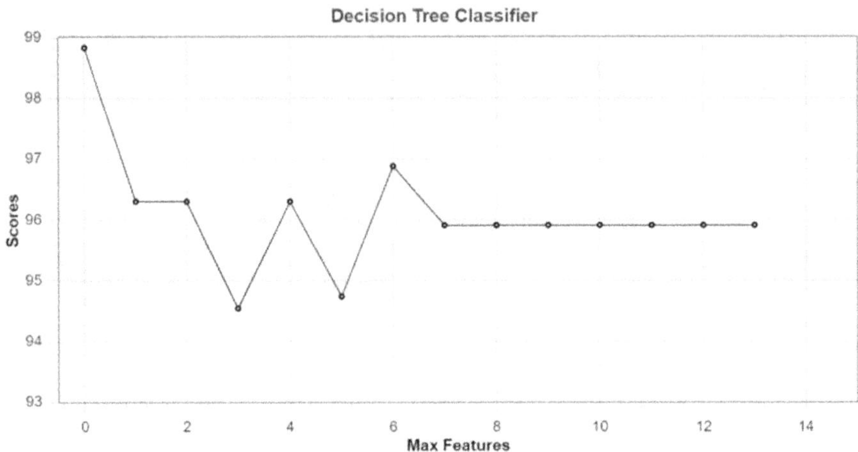

FIGURE 12.7 Precise ratings for the decision of presence of a cardiac condition.

In Figure 12.7, the graph shows the rating (degree of correction) for a prediction made on whether a patient has a heart condition or not by a model. In Figure 12.8, the graph shows that KNN has been applied to the former graph and it shows the closes K scores which are closest to being precise as per the result.

The forest when n is 1000, 500, 200, 100 or 10. In Figure 12.9, results for random neighbors from when n is 1 to n is 7 is shown, which are precise as per the result is taken into account.

In Figure 12.10, scores produced by the SVM algorithm which are precise, ranging from n = 1000, 500, 200, 100, or 10, are shown. Coronary artery disease (CAD) is caused by accumulation of fat in the wall of coronary artery that supplies blood to the heart. It is one of the major arteries that supply blood. Plaque is made up of cholesterol deposits. Arteries get narrow due to plaque buildup which results in a

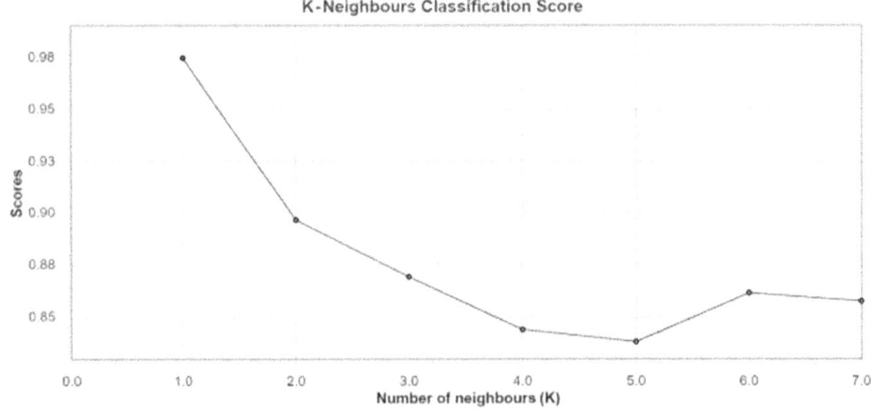

FIGURE 12.8 Displays K scores that are precise.

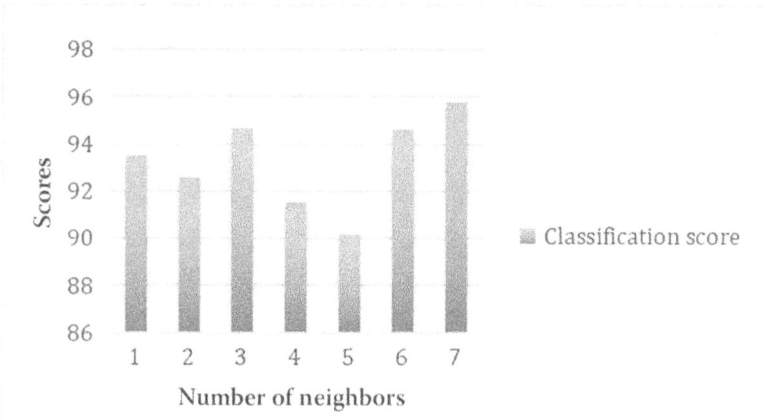

FIGURE 12.9 Results of random neighbors for $n = 1$ to $n = 7$.

decrease of blood flow and is critical to the patient's health. This process is called Atherosclerosis.

Symptoms: Chest pain and discomfort is the most common symptom of CAD.

Nuclear medicine specialists assigned labels to each occurrence of the information that was collected from a total of 625 individuals, including 127 patients who had infarctions, 241 patients who had ischemic conditions, and 257 patients who were deemed to be normal.

The single-photon emission computed tomography (SPECT) technique was used to retrieve the pictures, which show the condition of heart (images) during rest and during stress.

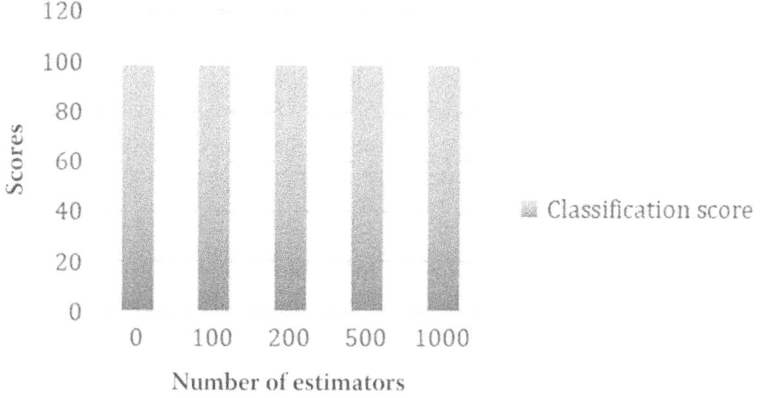

FIGURE 12.10 SVM—produced precise scores ranging from when n is 1000, 500, 200, 100, or 10.

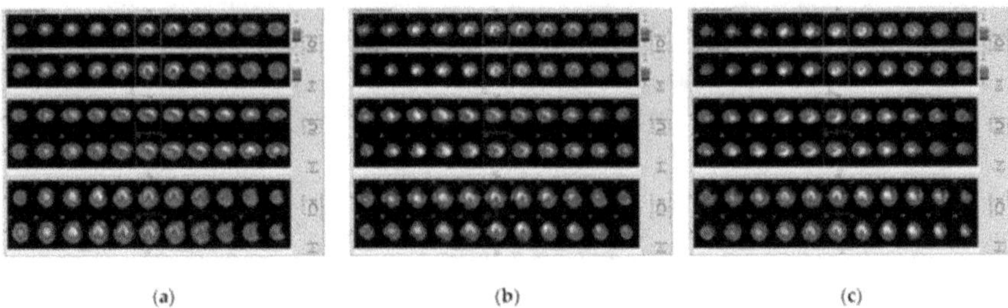

FIGURE 12.11 (a) Infarction, (b) ischemia, and (c) normal.

Additionally, the professionals finished the labeling using myocardial perfusion imaging (MPI) images from every patient. In this manner, a direct comparison between the model and human experts might be made.

The objective of this study is to make a model that can compete with the human eye and knowledge, using the diagnostic output of the experts as the source of truth.

In Figure 12.11, three heart conditions are shown. The first two are abnormal, i.e., having a cardiac disease, while the last one is heart under normal conditions. Figure 12.11(a) shows the images of heart in a condition called infarction, which is a serious heart ailment. Figure 12.11(b) shows the images of heart in a condition called Ischemia, which too is a serious cardiac ailment. Figure 12.11(c) shows the images of heart under normal conditions. These are images of healthy hearts which function normally.

These images are fed to the model while training and the model is trained on these data sets and images like these, which are images of hearts of real patients, so the model can develop an understanding of how to classify based on images. The above diagram (Figure 12.11) represents different cases regarding the tests the patients have gone through which consists of Infarction, Ischemia, and the patients which are normal.

Figure 12.11(a) Infarction. This figure depicts CAD myocardial infarction, which refers to a type of heart attack that occurs due to blockage in one or more coronary arteries which are the major suppliers of blood to the heart muscle. This generally occurs due to plaque buildup or fat accumulation in the valves of the major arteries. If the plaque ruptures it can form a clot which completely blocks the blood flow which can result in heart failure.

Figure 12.11(b) Ischemia: This figure depicts ischemia which is a medical term that refers to insufficient supply of blood to organ or tissue, which can lead to lack of oxygen and nutrients. This causes the organ or tissue to become damaged or to die. The major reason for occurrence of ischemia is due to blockage in blood vessels.

Figure 12.11(c) Normal: This figure depicts the normal case of functioning of heart. Here, the patient is completely normal and fit in relation to audio-related issues.

12.4 RESEARCH METHODOLOGY

Convolutional Neural Networks (CNN): Main Aspects

CNN is a term for a computer technique that simulates the operation of brain neurons. It comes under several artificial NN models that are in use for diverse data sets and different types of works. This approach allows the machine to learn directly from the data that is given to it.

Input, hidden, and output layers are all present in CNNs, and each layer is made up of edges connected to nodes. Since CNN is exceedingly precise and effective, it is typically employed for image recognition jobs. Based on their excellent results, CNN has been recognized as the most reliable in analysis of images related to medical study and diagnosis.

Now the distinct layers of CNN are described in detail below:

The Convolutional Layer (CL) is the layer at the top. The main building element is a convolutional layer made up of sieves (filters) that create activation maps through the convolution process. Activation maps are used to categorize unseen data and are composed of patterns that were retrieved from the input photos.

- After every CL, the pooling layer is added as the second layer. Pixel values are disregarded since they are labeled as noise. As a result, the time required for computation is reduced and CNN is provided with the appropriate pixel values based on the dataset.
- The dropout layer is included as the third layer to prevent over-fitting. It zeroes off random pixel values, which cuts down on computation time. It uses regularization method to prevent over-fitting by zeroing random pixel values.
- The flatten layer (FL) changes data into vectors. It is the fourth layer.
- All connected layers are then finally used together, with every node being attached to the layer above it in order to calculate the prediction using activation functions. Convolutional layers were constructed using rectified linear unit (ReLU), and output activation functions were created using softmax.

12.5 METHODOLOGICAL FRAMEWORK

This study's objective is to use an RGB-CNN model for analysis of images (nuclear medical images) to categorize different CAD pictures and create a self-contained computer-aided system using "Gradient-CAM."

Gradient-Weighted Class Activation Mapping (Grad-CAM) is a well-known CNN approach that draws attention to key areas of an image that matter most in the network's final classification judgment. Grad-CAM is used as a reliable, effective, and completely trained CNN model since it has demonstrated excellent abilities in terms of the interpretability of NN.

The flow (methodological) includes the following parts:

1. Loading of data set
2. Pre-processing of data

3. Design and evaluation of CNN model
4. Application of Grad-CAM

Below are the steps stated:

Step 1: Loading of Dataset

The nuclear specialist provided RGB (red, green, and blue) formatted SPECT MPI pictures. Each incident was given a score of 0, 1, or 2, depending on whether it was an infarction, an ischemia, or a typical occurrence. The resulting dataset was then kept in a computer's memory after that.

Step 2: Preparation of Data

- **Data Normalization:** Pixel values are converted and put into the range [0, 1].
- **Data Shuffle:** Data is shuffled here to make the fetching of pattern unbiased. Hence, data insertion is randomly done.
- **Data Split:** Data set is divided into three parts: Training, validation, and testing.
  - i. **Training:** The given dataset is used to train the model. The weights were changed in order to find the minimized error using the gradient backward propagation approach.
  - ii. **Validation:** The validation dataset rates CNN using pre-established data. As a consequence, the final model is established.
  - iii. **Testing:** The best model is created and evaluated using the testing data set on unknown data after training and validation are complete. Different parameters are used to gauge performance.

Step 3: Explicitness Using Grad-CAM

Given that CNNs are not explicable and transparent, we used Grad-CAM to predict CNN models through formation of heat maps to boost comprehensiveness. The heat maps generated by this model identify areas where the fully trained model's anticipated output has been positively impacted. We use the gradients of the last convolutional layer of the specified model to find out these key areas. This draws out the key details that influence the decision-making process.

Step 4: Inference Phase

The testing picture, which is often an unidentified example from the training data set, is supplied to the pre-trained model, which then generates the output that the model for that certain image will predict. The feature map weights generated by the model's final convolutional layer are then determined. Then the alpha values of the weights are found using the Global Average Pooling (GAP).

CNNs employ the pooling procedure (GAP) to reduce the spatial dimension of a feature map while maintaining the depth. GAP has been a well-liked methodology in contemporary CNN architectures because of its success in fetching global information in a compact and effective manner.

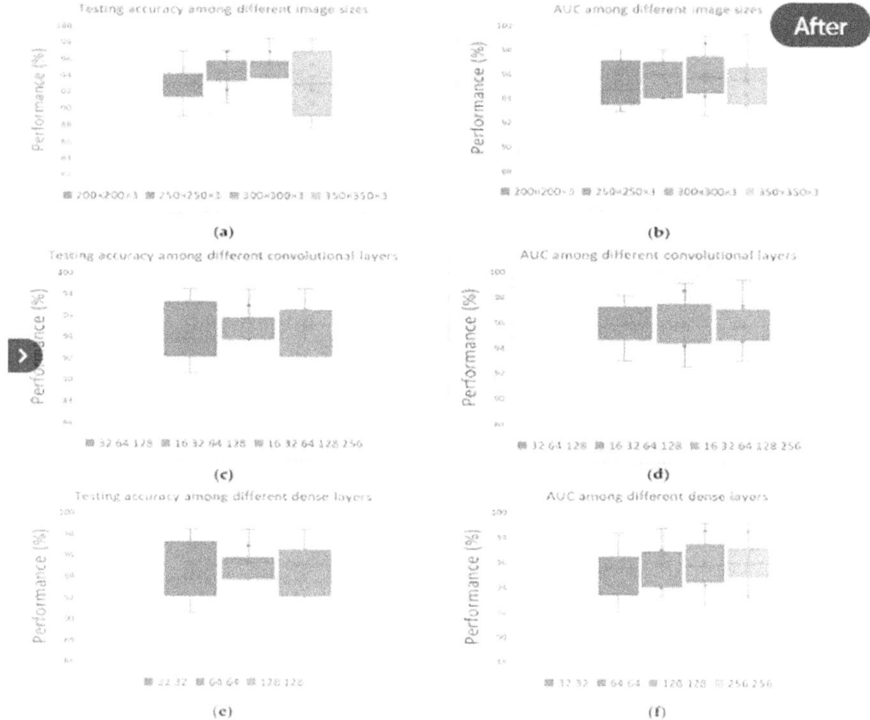

FIGURE 12.12 (a) Accuracy of testing for different image sizes; (b) AUC for various sizes of imaging; (c) testing accuracy for various CL; (d) AUC for various CL; (e) testing accuracy for various dense layers (DL); and (f) AUC for various DL.

A heat map is then produced. This heat map displays the crucial areas that correspond to the expected results. It is then shrunk to the testing image's size. The negative values are ignored.

In Figure 12.12, different graphs based on different layers and their accuracy of testing and area under the curve (AUC) graphs are shown.

12.6 RESULTS AND DISCUSSION

In Figure 12.13, results generated by Grad-CAM are shown in a grid form. The first column shows original images of infarction, ischemia, and normal conditions, which are similar to the images we saw in Figure 12.11. The second column shows the heat maps generated in all three conditions. The third column shows the overlay in all three conditions.

The CNN was declared as the best model for separation and classification of medical images after testing several parameters such as picture size, batch size, and CLs.

AUC, receiver operating characteristic curve (ROC) curve, sensitivity, and other well-known performance indicators were utilized to assess the tested CNN model.

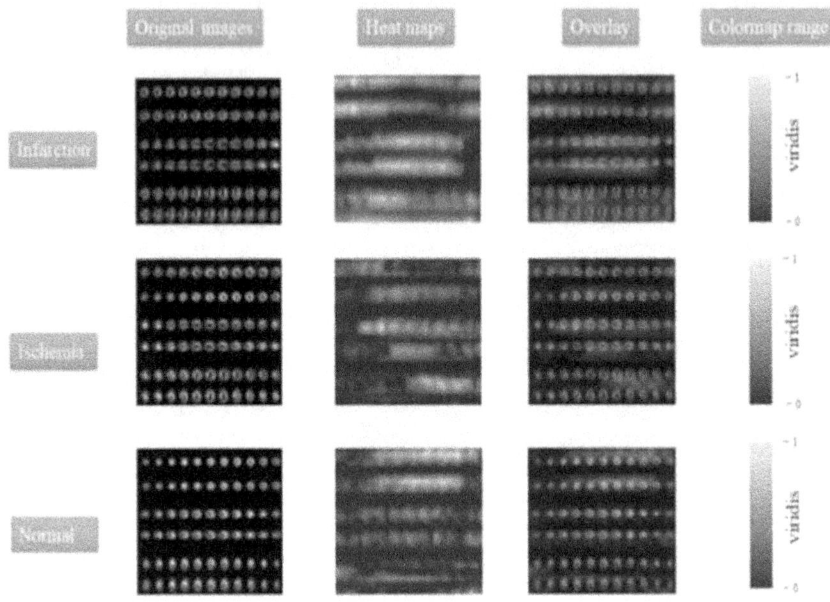

FIGURE 12.13 Results generated by GRAD-CAM.

ROC is a visual representation of AUC, which ranges from 0 to 1 and measures how well the model can differentiate between the supplied classes.

Reflected by the large number of data sets in the given above case studies, AI and ML have shown a huge possibility to impact and power diagnostic decision making in cardiology. Detecting the type of CAD with the help of ML is a major change in the field of medical sciences from obsolete statistical methods and techniques. Listed below are some challenges faced during the diagnosis using AI and ML algorithms:

- In today's modern area many hospitals and clinics still rely on stand-alone parameters which were used earlier for making important diagnostic decisions despite awareness and many encouraging research studies from experts.
- The diversity of cardiovascular imaging has made it tough for diagnosis.
- Risk stratification cannot be determined. Also, there is lack of proper standardization.
- Implementation of AI to CAD, however, is still in early stages and facing significant challenges which will take time to improve with more research in this arena in the future.
- The quality of imaging features must be high while building image biomarkers. Till now, trained models and algorithms have limited generalization due to the multiple factors which can possibly impact the future.
- The studies involving CT and PET imaging have marked the hard-comings faced while developing reliable radio-mic features while using different scanners and reconstruction settings as the particular needs for cardiac imaging have not yet been identified.

- The investigation found that the algorithms have to be reconstructed on the quality and comparability of radiomics features considering various technical settings.
- There is little evidence involving the robustness of radio-mic features in MRI. The radiomic feature's robustness depends extensively on sequences related to acquisition and reconstruction parameters. Due to absence of absolute signal intensities, the robustness decreases.
- Several studies have shown the influence of the acquisition sequence and resolution involved while producing images as well as image processing settings on the robustness of radio mic features.
- The sizes of samples in many cardiovascular imaging studies have led to the risk of over-fitting.
- The absence of interoperability of several systems used in medical systems poses a massive obstacle to data pooling.
- The quality and ability needed for understanding the principle of reasons behind predictive analysis (ML) generated grouping is important and necessary for achieving widespread use of this technology. However, with DL techniques, no proper insights or explanation on how the conclusion was reached.

12.7 CONCLUSION

This study used a predictive analysis (ML) approach to develop its proposal for "Cardiac Pattern recognition using predictive analysis (ML) Algorithms." Four algorithms were employed in this predictive analysis (ML) technique to train the data set and assess it containing the test results of various patients. These algorithms were also checked for preciseness by generating a grid (chart) using the MATLAB library. The three models with the greatest accuracy scores—DT, RF, and SVM —are roughly 98.83% precise, whereas KNN is approximately 97.4% precise. The Flask API was used to integrate the DT model into the web, and it correctly predicted outcomes when tested five times on the web. Using DL method, this research can be implemented into a real-time system where users can input their results as images. There are not only positives but also certain challenges like risk stratification and no further insights or explanation on how the conclusions were reached. This is still a developing field. A lot of research and discoveries are yet to be performed in this field to give us further insight and knowledge about how to apply predictive analysis (ML) and DL in the field of science.

REFERENCES

1. Princy, R. J. P., Parthasarathy, S., Hency Jose, P. S., Lakshminarayanan, A. R., & Jeganathan, S. (2020). "Prediction of Cardiac Disease using Supervised Machine Learning Algorithms," *2020 4th International Conference on Intelligent Computing and Control Systems (ICICCS)*, Madurai, India, pp. 570–575. doi:10.1109/ICICCS48265.2020.9121169
2. Tr, R., Lilhore, U. K., M., P., Simaiya, S., Kaur, A., & Hamdi, M. (2022). Predictive analysis of heart diseases with machine learning approaches. Malaysian Journal of Computer Science, 132–148. https://doi.org/10.22452/mjcs.sp2022no1.10

3. Al'Aref, S. J., Anchouche, K., Singh, G., Slomka, P. J., Kolli, K. K., Kumar, A., Pandey, M., Maliakal, G., van Rosendael, A. R., Beecy, A. N., Berman, D. S., Leipsic, J., Nieman, K., Andreini, D., Pontone, G., Schoepf, U. J., Shaw, L. J., Chang, H. J., Narula, J., Bax, J. J., & Min, J. K. (2019). Clinical applications of machine learning in cardiovascular disease and its relevance to cardiac imaging. European Heart Journal, 40(24), 1975–1986. https://doi.org/10.1093/eurheartj/ehy404
4. Sitar Taut, A. V., Zdrenghea, D., Pop, D., & Sitar-Taut, D.-A. (2009). Using machine learning algorithms in cardiovascular disease risk evaluation. Journal of Applied Computer Science & Mathematics. https://doaj.org/article/275abbd3182347f49998c192545454e6
5. Sarveshvar, M. R., Gogoi, A., Chaubey, A. K., Rohit, S., & Mahesh, T. R. (2021). "Performance of different Machine Learning Techniques for the Prediction of Heart Diseases," *2021 International Conference on Forensics, Analytics, Big Data, Security (FABS)*, Bengaluru, India, pp. 1–4. doi:10.1109/FABS52071.2021.9702566
6. Krittanawong, C., Virk, H. U. H., Bangalore, S., Wang, Z., Johnson, K. W., Pinotti, R., Zhang, H., Kaplin, S., Narasimhan, B., Kitai, T., Baber, U., Halperin, J. L., & Tang, W. H. W. (2020). Machine learning prediction in cardiovascular diseases: A meta-analysis. Scientific Reports, 10(1), 16057. https://doi.org/10.1038/s41598-020-72685-1
7. Mathur, P., Srivastava, S., Xu, X., & Mehta, J. L. (2020). Artificial intelligence, machine learning, and cardiovascular disease. Clinical Medicine Insights. Cardiology, 14, 1179546820927404. https://doi.org/10.1177/1179546820927404
8. Saboor, A., Usman, M., Ali, S., Samad, A., Abrar, M. F., & Ullah, N. (2022). A method for improving prediction of human heart disease using machine learning algorithms. Mobile Information Systems. https://www.hindawi.com/journals/misy/2022/1410169/
9. Suri, J. S., Bhagawati, M., Paul, S., Protogeron, A., Sfikakis, P. P., Kitas, G. D., Khanna, N. N., Ruzsa, Z., Sharma, A. M., Saxena, S., Faa, G., Paraskevas, K. I., Laird, J. R., Johri, A. M., Saba, L., & Kalra, M. (2022). Understanding the bias in machine learning systems for cardiovascular disease risk assessment: The first of its kind review. Computers in Biology and Medicine, 142, 105204. https://doi.org/10.1016/j.compbiomed.2021.105204
10. Mohan, S., Thirumalai, C., & Srivastava, G. (2019). Effective heart disease prediction using hybrid machine learning techniques. IEEE Access, 7, 81542–81554. 10.1109/ACCESS.2019.2923707
11. Nadakinamani, R. G., Reyana, A., Kautish, S., Vibith, A. S., Gupta, Y., Abdelwahab, S. F., & Mohamed, A. W. (2022). Clinical data analysis for prediction of cardiovascular disease using machine learning techniques. Computational Intelligence and Neuroscience, 2022, 2973324. https://doi.org/10.1155/2022/2973324
12. Shehzadi, S., Hassan, M. A., Rizwan, M., Kryvinska, N., & Vincent, K. (2022). Diagnosis of chronic ischemic heart disease using machine learning techniques. Computational Intelligence and Neuroscience, 2022, 3823350. https://doi.org/10.1155/2022/3823350.
13. Pires, I. M., Marques, G., Garcia, N. M., & Ponciano, V., (2020). Machine learning for the evaluation of the presence of heart disease, Procedia Computer Science, 177, 432–437. ISSN 1877-0509. https://doi.org/10.1016/j.procs.2020.10.058
14. Cheung, C. Y., Xu, D., Cheng, C. Y., Sabanayagam, C., Tham, Y. C., Yu, M., Rim, T. H., Chai, C. Y., Gopinath, B., Mitchell, P., Poulton, R., Moffitt, T. E., Caspi, A., Yam, J. C., Tham, C. C., Jonas, J. B., Wang, Y. X., Song, S. J., Burrell, L. M., Farouque, O., & Wong, T. Y. (2021). A deep-learning system for the assessment of cardiovascular disease risk via the measurement of retinal-vessel calibre. Nature Biomedical Engineering, 5(6), 498–508. https://doi.org/10.1038/s41551-020-00626-4
15. Khan, Y., Qamar, U., Yousaf, N., & Khan, A. (2019). Machine learning techniques for heart disease datasets: A survey. International Conference on Machine Learning and Computing. https://dl.acm.org/doi/abs/10.1145/3318299.3318343

16. Abdeldjouad, F. Z., Brahami, M., & Matta, N. (2020). "A Hybrid Approach for Heart Disease Diagnosis and Prediction Using Machine Learning Techniques," *The Impact of Digital Technologies on Public Health in Developed and Developing Countries: 18th International Conference, ICOST 2020,* Hammamet, Tunisia, June 24–26, Proceedings, 12157, 299–306. https://doi.org/10.1007/978-3-030-51517-1_26
17. Pal, M., Parija, S., Panda, G., Dhama, K., & Mohapatra, R. K. (2022). Risk prediction of cardiovascular disease using machine learning classifiers. Open Medicine (Warsaw, Poland), 17(1), 1100–1113. https://doi.org/10.1515/med-2022-0508
18. Sajid, M. R., Almehmadi, B. A., Sami, W., Alzahrani, M. K., Muhammad, N., Chesneau, C., Hanif, A., Khan, A. A., & Shahbaz, A. (2021). Development of nonlaboratory-based risk prediction models for cardiovascular diseases using conventional and machine learning approaches. International Journal of Environmental Research and Public Health, 18(23), 12586. https://doi.org/10.3390/ijerph182312586
19. Brunese, L., Martinelli, F., Mercaldo, F., & Santone, A. (2020). Deep learning for heart disease detection through cardiac sounds. Procedia Computer Science, 176, 2202–2211. ISSN 1877-0509. https://doi.org/10.1016/j.procs.2020.09.257
20. Venkatesh, V., Rai, P., Reddy, K. A., Praba, S., & Anushiadevi, R. (2022). "An Intelligent Framework for Heart Disease Prediction Deep Learning-Based Ensemble Method," *2022 International Conference on Computer, Power and Communications (ICCPC),* Chennai, India, pp. 274–280. doi:10.1109/ICCPC55978.2022.10072285.

13 Design of a Novel Medical Chatbot to Simulate User Interactions

Angelia Melani Adrian

13.1 INTRODUCTION

Chatbots have become a ubiquitous part of our daily lives, but their lineage may be located around the middle of the 20th century. The concept of chatbots, also known as conversational agents, can be found in the early days of artificial intelligence (AI) research in the 1950s. The very first chatbot, ELIZA, was invented by Joseph Weizenbaum in the year of 1966 at the Massachusetts Institute of Technology (MIT). ELIZA was designed to simulate conversation by using Computational Linguistics (NLP) techniques to answer user inputs. It used a set of predefined rules to generate responses, which made it more of a scripted program than a true AI chatbot. Despite its limitations, ELIZA was a groundbreaking achievement in the field of AI and set the stage for future chatbot development. Chatbots are intelligent software that function like a human when interacting with users. Their applications are diverse: commonly utilized in after-sales service, e-marketing, and instant communication with clients. There exist types of chatbot models: retrieval based and generative based, which vary based on their construction. Chatbots were developed to simulate human conversation and automate tasks that would otherwise require human intervention. They were designed to provide a more personalized and efficient user experience, particularly in the context of client or after-sales service and support.

One of the main advantages of chatbots is their capacity to offer round-the-clock assistance, without requiring handler or technician to be available at all times. This means that the arability of assistance to customers is at any time, regardless of their location or time zone. Additionally, chatbots can handle a high amount of inquiries simultaneously, reducing wait times and improving customer satisfaction. Chatbots can also help reduce operating costs for businesses, as they can automate routine tasks and reduce the need for human customer service agents. This not only saves money but also allows human agents to concentrate on more difficult and valuable activities. Chatbots have the ability to learn and improve over time. By analyzing user interactions and feedback, chatbots are able to recognize areas for improvement and change their answers appropriately.

Chatbots can be helpful in a variety of ways in medical services, particularly in providing quick and convenient access to information, improving patient outcomes,

DOI: 10.1201/9781032624891-13

and reducing the workload of healthcare professionals. Here are a few ways in which chatbots can be used in medical services:

- **Acquiring Patient Data:** Chatbots may be used to acquire patient data by inquiring about the patient's name, address, symptoms, current doctor, and insurance information. The chatbots then utilize EDI to save this information in the hospital's database to streamline patient admission, symptom monitoring, doctor-patient communication, and medical record keeping.
- **Health Monitoring:** Chatbots can be used to monitor a patient's health status by asking questions about symptoms and collecting data on vital indicator including pulse rate, blood pressure, and blood sugar levels. This data can be used to analyze to provide insights into the patient's health status and to alert healthcare professionals if there are any changes that require attention.
- **Medical Advice and Information:** Chatbots can provide patients with advice and information on a variety of medical topics, including symptoms, treatments, and medications. This will help patients make informed decisions about their healthcare and reduce the workload of healthcare professionals who may be able to focus on more complex cases.
- **Appointment Scheduling:** Chatbots can be used to schedule appointments, send reminders, and confirm attendance. This can help reduce the workload of receptionists and allow patients to schedule appointments at any time of day or night. Getting immediate help, and a doctor's contact and address were obtained very quickly.

Two different categories of chatbots are listed below.

- **Retrieval-Based Chatbots:** A retrieval-based chatbot relies on predefined patterns for input and response. It uses a heuristic approach to select the appropriate response. This technique is commonly used to create goal-oriented chatbots, and we can adjust their tone and natural conversational style to enhance customer service. Figure 13.1 shows a retrieval-based chatbot.

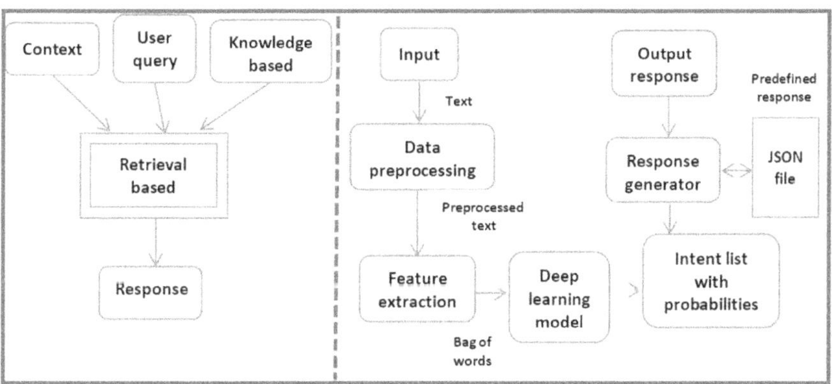

FIGURE 13.1 A retrieval-based chatbot.

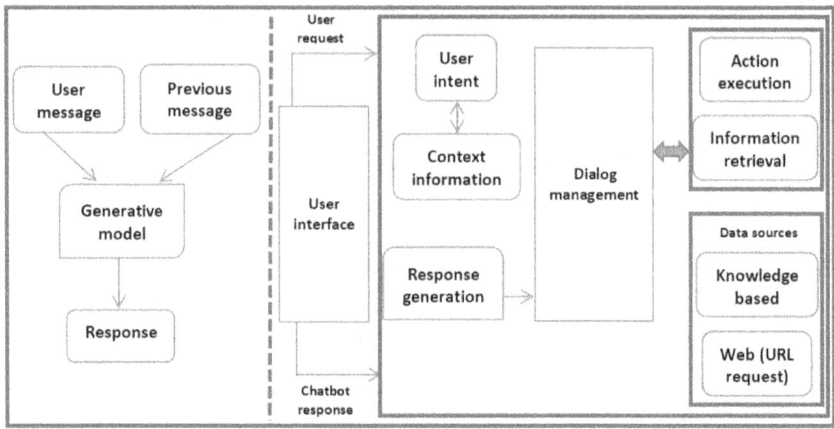

FIGURE 13.2 A generative-based chatbot.

- **Generative-Based Chatbots:** Generative models, unlike retrieval-based ones, do not depend on pre-determined responses. They are built upon Seq2Seq neural networks, which draw inspiration from machine translation. While machine translation involves converting source code from one language to another, generative models convert input into output. These models are rooted in Deep Neural Networks and demand a substantial amount of data. Figure 13.2 shows a generative-based chatbot.

A comparative analysis of these two types is shown in Table 13.1. The current study is in regard to the development of the chatbot "Medi-Chat" that would provide medical assistance to customers 24/7. It helps users to provide information regarding blood pressure, adverse drug reaction and notification about nearest hospitals and

TABLE 13.1
Comparison between Retrieval and Generative Chatbots

Generative Chatbot	Retrieval Chatbot
A generative-based chatbot uses Computational Linguistics (NLP) and Predictive Analytics algorithms to generate responses to user input.	A retrieval-based chatbot uses predefined responses or templates to respond to user input.
These chatbots are trained on large datasets of human conversations and can understand the context and intent behind user input.	The chatbot matches the user's input to a predefined set of keywords or phrases and then chooses a reply from a pre-existing list of answers.
These chatbots are slower in comparison to the retrieval but are capable of handling a wider range of queries.	These chatbots are typically faster and easier to develop than generative chatbots, but their responses are limited to the pre-defined options.

pharmacies. We have created an intent-based chatbot that provides the desired result to the user based on the information provided.

The response is contained in a JSON file from where it can revert back the results to the users. The chatbot is trained on deep learning models, where it can understand the intention of the user and provide solutions or advice. The user provides manual input and gets the result and this process continues till the conversation comes to an end. It has been designed such that it remains user friendly to everyone. Medi-Chat is a medical conversation bot that can solve your various medical emergencies like finding the nearest hospital list, returning all the allergies list of the owner, blood pressure, heart rate, calling the emergency number in case any emergency situation is detected, and many more. It is basically a chatting robot or chatbot that answers various questions on the basis of data provided to it.

Main objectives of the analysis are as follows:

- Applying deep learning to create a chatbot in this study with source code. The details, which include categories (intents), trends, and replies, will be used to train the chatbot.
- Designing and implementing a conversational flow by defining the dialogues that our chatbot will have with users. The conversational flow will depend on the purpose of the chatbot, the target audience, and the type of questions that users may ask.
- Using NLP techniques to understand user inputs by implementing linguistics techniques such as Tokenization, word category labeling, and named entity classification to extract meaning from user inputs. This will allow your chatbot to understand user queries more accurately.
- Using Keras to build a Predictive Analytics model that can generate responses to user queries. Then, we will test and refine the chatbot based on user feedback. Finally, we deploy the chatbot.

13.2 BACKGROUND STUDY AND RELATED WORKS

According to research, clinical offerings are important requirements for human life in spite of the fact that they broadly speaking have restrained property. Modern-day advances are used for increasing management magnitude and diminishing the interest fee. Pre-programmed message frameworks or chatbots, which are extensively recognized within the subject of online groups, may be applied to scientific blessings. Consequently, the target of these paintings is to carry out the clinical representative machine administration by using chatbot technology. It became accomplished dependent on the information of the side outcomes and remedy facts assembled from the application. [1].

According to the research, exclusive methodologies for the advancement of chatbots and various improvements in the making of chatbots were created in light of these endeavors. Natural Language Toolkit (NLTK) is a Python module ready to carry out Computational Linguistics. It's far utilized to receive speech input and produce understandable replies for humans [2]. The design and application of the Stanford CoreNLP toolkit, an extendable pipeline that provides essential natural language analysis, are discussed in the study "The Stanford CoreNLP Computational Linguistics Toolkit." This toolset is often used by both the exploration NLP group and moreover by open-source NLP innovation clientele in industry and government [3]. According to the study, an artificially intelligent computer software simulates user dialogues. A chatbot is a piece of software that permits textual conversation via natural language. Users find it difficult to understand that the chatbot isn't a real person, which highlights the critical necessity for a sizable knowledge base that includes the current set of guidelines a chatbot holds [4]. Based on a research study, customers can engage in conversations with a chatbot through a communication supervisor. To categorize the criteria, a standards classifier module is employed, which maps them into five pre-established classes. The standards classifier handles the criteria as vectors of phrase embedding. To enhance the training set, an active learning algorithm selects criteria for which the model has the least confidence in their category and requests labeling from a human oracle. Once the label is obtained, the algorithm propagates it to neighboring criteria, thereby increasing the number of samples in the training set [5]. MedWhat: Making Medical Diagnoses Faster: Checking out Med What if you're the type of person who has WebMD bookmarked. Imagine this chatbot as an articulate and intelligent version of WebMD, aiming to expedite and simplify medical diagnoses while ensuring transparency for patients and doctors alike. MedWhat utilizes a robust Predictive Analytics algorithm that offers users increasingly accurate responses based on the patterns it discerns through interactions with individuals [6]. According to the survey, the techniques for developing rules for chatbots have been superior. Techniques for creating chatbots have depended on handwritten guidelines and templates. With the rapid rise in technology, conventional approaches had been fast replaced by deep neural networks. All of the above, Deep Neural Networks is an effective generative-based total model to take care of the conversational response era troubles [7]. According to the study, these individuals used actual supervised statistics to solve a cause recognition problem in the Lithuanian language. Their major precept of consciousness is the improvement of the herbal language information (NLU) module, which is responsible for the comprehension of a person's questions. The NLU model is developed such that it should select phrase vectorization with Deep Neural Network (DNN) classifier. At some stage in their experiments, they have tentatively investigated fastText and bidirectional encoder representations from transformers (BERT) embeddings [8]. A chatbot application that offers conversational services for mental health care based on techniques for emotion recognition and chat assistant platforms. This application doesn't consider the user's psychiatric status through continuous user monitoring [9]. In this text-based healthcare setting, chatbots can be created to support patients and healthcare providers in therapeutic settings outside of on-demand consultations. It lacks in-person care and is a situation where THCBs are most likely to fail [10]. The primary care chatbot system described in this paper was developed to support healthcare staff by streamlining the patient intake procedure. More diseases should have been mentioned in this paper, and a thesaurus of synonyms for symptoms should also be created [11]. A chatbot is a software application that enables natural language interactions through text. Users often struggle to recognize that the chatbot is not a real person, highlighting the importance of a robust knowledge base that serves as the chatbot's rule set. In the near future, chatbots are poised to become an excellent means for businesses to engage with customers and promptly address their inquiries [12]. This chatbot utilizes a text-based interface, simulating a conversation with a human. It asks users about their health concerns and proceeds to inquire about their symptoms, providing suggestions and clarification to aid in the diagnosis of diseases. However, it does not offer specific information such as the duration or severity of symptoms [1]. Multiple programs aim to imitate human interaction by adopting a human-like appearance, but often the data used in a chatbot's conversations is derived from a database created by human experts. With the application of AI, we have the ability to develop various types of chatbots. In this particular project, we have developed a chatbot specifically designed to address college-related inquiries [13]. Other studies have focused on the design and development of medical assistance chatbots. For example, a study published in 2020 proposed a framework for designing a chatbot to support patients with chronic diseases. Another study in 2019 developed a chatbot to assist with medication management for older adults [14].

13.3 PROPOSED MODEL

The proposed model is shown in Figure 13.3. We have created a JSON file with all the intents in order to create an intent-based chatbot. The healthcare system is the foundation for the intention we have developed. Intents: Where we will store our natural language data is in the intent file lists. As it is mentioned earlier, we have our JSON file, which contains the "intents." There is no difference. The intent file can be modified however we please. We will use this intent file to train our chatbot so that it can comprehend the user's intentions and respond appropriately. There are numerous libraries available, including NLTK, which includes numerous tools for text cleaning

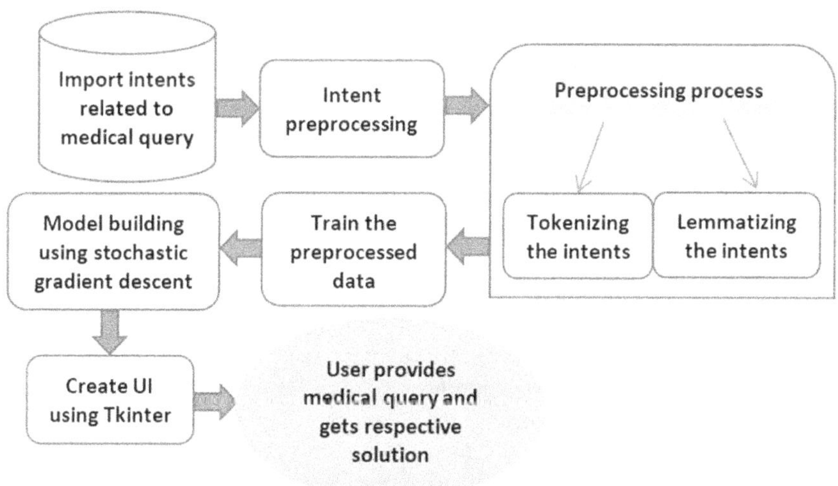

FIGURE 13.3 Proposed model for Medi-chat.

and preparation for deep learning algorithms, JSON, which loads JSON files directly into Python, pickle, and many others.

We first created a Mediset intent file, which contains all the patterns for how our intent-based chatbot will respond to user inquiries. After lemmatizing the word, we used NLTK modules to extract words, classes, and documents from the intent file. Now that we have these words, classes, and documents, we must create training the Mediset data. Following the creation of the training data, we built a 3-layer neural network model with the first layer containing 128 neurons, the second layer 64 neurons, and the third layer serving as the output layer. The neural network model was then improved using the stochastic gradient descent (SGD) optimizer. Then, we developed a few techniques that will take user inputs and produce a result based on prediction.

Relevant Steps to Create a Chatbot in Python

- Importing and loading the Mediset data file
- Preprocessing Mediset data
- Create model training and validation Mediset data
- Building the model
- Predicting the response
    - **Importing and Loading the Mediset Data File:** Firstly create a file with the name train_chatbot.py; establish the variables that will be used in our Python project; and import all the packages needed by the chatbot. It used the JSON package to inspect the JSON file into Python because the Mediset data file is in JSON format.
    - **Preprocessing Mediset Details:** Before constructing a Predictive Analytics or deep learning model, it is necessary to handle text data, specifically the medical query data. Several preprocessing steps need to be undertaken based on the specific requirements. The initial step involves tokenizing the text data, which involves breaking down the entire text into smaller units like words. Using the nltk.word_tokenize() function, we iterate through the patterns, append each word to the words list, and create a list of classes for our tags. Next, we perform lemmatization, which involves converting words into their lemma form and eliminating any repetitions from the list [15–17]. Finally, a pickle file is created to store the Python objects necessary for prediction.
    - **Create Model Training and Validation Mediset Details:** With the completion of the training data, we will now incorporate the input and output elements. The pattern will be utilized as our input, while the corresponding class that the pattern belongs to will serve as our output. However, since computers cannot comprehend text directly, we need to convert it into numerical representations.
    - **Build the Model:** Having completed the preparation of our training data, we will now build a deep neural network consisting of three layers. To achieve this, we will utilize the Keras sequential API. The model will be trained for 200 epochs, resulting in a perfect accuracy of 100%. To save the model, we will assign it the name "Medichat_model.h5."

- **Predict the Response (Graphical User Interface):** We need to build a new file called "chatapp.py" to anticipate the user's responses and predict the sentences. Once the trained model is loaded, a graphical user interface (GUI) will be utilized to generate the chatbot's responses. To retrieve a random response from the list of responses, we will implement functions that first identify the class to which the model belongs. We will import the necessary packages and load the pickle files created during the model training process, named "words.pkl" and "classes.pkl." To predict the class, the input should follow the same preprocessing steps as during training. Therefore, we will develop functions that preprocess the text before determining the class and subsequently fetch a random response from the list of intents. The next step involves creating a complete source code for the GUI, using the Tkinter library, which provides useful GUI libraries. The user's input message will be captured, and with the help of the implemented helper functions, the bot's response will be retrieved and displayed on the GUI.
- **Run the Chatbot:** Two main files—train_chatbot.py and chatapp.py—are required to run the chatbot. We first train the model by typing the following terminal command: train_chatbot.py in Python. If there are no errors found during training, the model was successfully created. We then execute the second file to launch the application. With the help of Python chat GUI, within a few seconds a GUI window will be displayed by the program. You can interface with the bot easily using the GUI.

13.4 RESULTS AND DISCUSSION

To handle the data file in JSON format, we utilized the JSON package to parse it into Python. The nltk.word_tokenize() method was employed to tokenize the sentence, and each word from the words list was appended after iterating through the patterns. Additionally, we created a list of classes to represent the tags. The model was constructed with 3 layers, consisting of 128 neurons in the first layer, 64 neurons in the second layer, and a number of neurons in the third output layer equal to the softmax output intent predictions. Figure 13.4 denotes the accuracy rate analysis in terms of number of epochs.

We made a new file called "chatapp.py" to forecast the user's responses to the sentences. Once again, we imported the necessary packages and loaded the pickle files named "words.pkl" and "classes.pkl" that were created during the model training phase. We utilized the same data for making predictions in the class as we did during training. Hence, we developed several text preparation methods to preprocess the input before predicting the class. To facilitate the creation of a GUI, we utilized the Tkinter package, which offers a variety of useful GUI libraries. Upon receiving the user's input message, we executed the chatbot by employing the helper methods we had previously written, enabling us to obtain the bot's response and display it on the GUI. A sample demonstration of a JSON file is shown in Figure 13.5.

Medichat has great data accuracy and a smooth workflow. The final outcome of Medi-chat is shown in Figure 13.6.

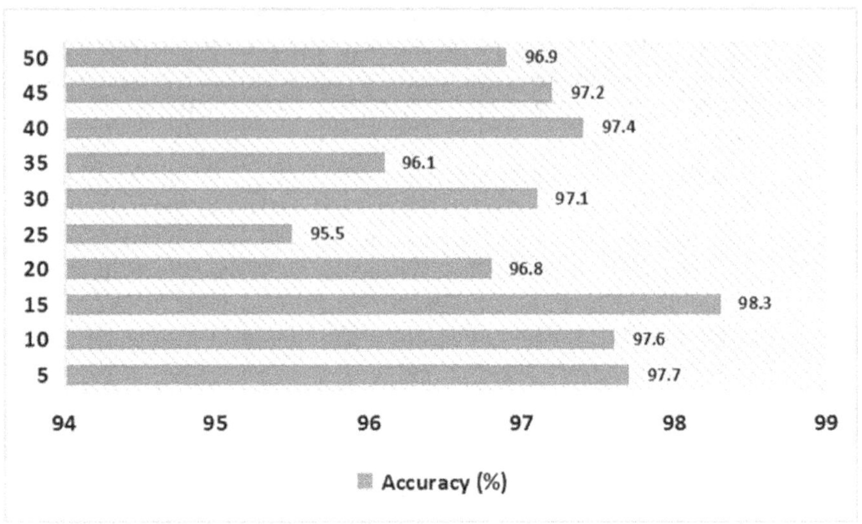

FIGURE 13.4 Accuracy analysis in context to epochs.

The proposed Medichat model is compared with other existing models and the analysis is highlighted here.

- **KBot:** It is a personalized chatbot with knowledge for managing asthma. KBot is a chatbot that primarily assists asthma sufferers by having meaningful conversations. Its limitations include that it lacked intelligence and was unable to provide responses that accurately reflected human emotions or attitudes. Its accuracy was around 67%.

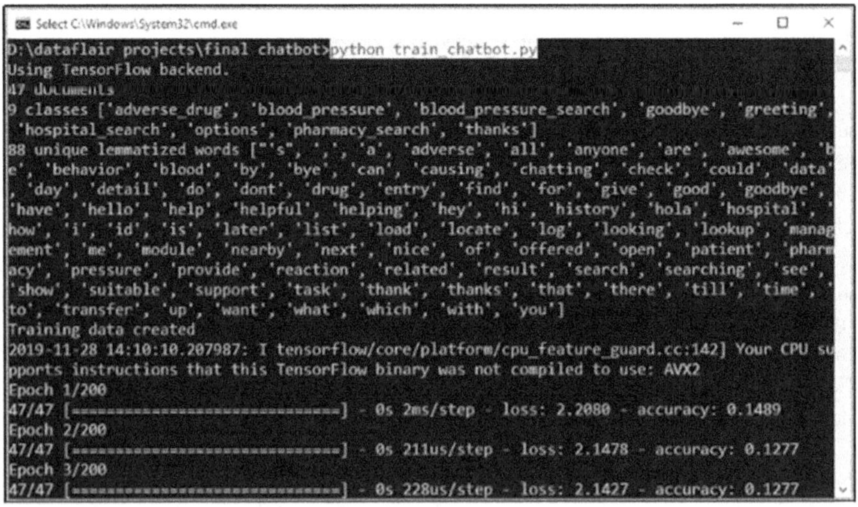

```
Select C:\Windows\System32\cmd.exe
D:\dataflair projects\final chatbot>python train_chatbot.py
Using TensorFlow backend.
47 documents
9 classes ['adverse_drug', 'blood_pressure', 'blood_pressure_search', 'goodbye', 'greeting',
 'hospital_search', 'options', 'pharmacy_search', 'thanks']
88 unique lemmatized words ["'s", ',', 'a', 'adverse', 'all', 'anyone', 'are', 'awesome', 'b
e', 'behavior', 'blood', 'by', 'bye', 'can', 'causing', 'chatting', 'check', 'could', 'data'
, 'day', 'detail', 'do', 'dont', 'drug', 'entry', 'find', 'for', 'give', 'good', 'goodbye',
'have', 'hello', 'help', 'helpful', 'helping', 'hey', 'hi', 'history', 'hola', 'hospital', '
how', 'i', 'id', 'is', 'later', 'list', 'load', 'locate', 'log', 'looking', 'lookup', 'manag
ement', 'me', 'module', 'nearby', 'next', 'nice', 'of', 'offered', 'open', 'patient', 'pharm
acy', 'pressure', 'provide', 'reaction', 'related', 'result', 'search', 'searching', 'see',
'show', 'suitable', 'support', 'task', 'thank', 'thanks', 'that', 'there', 'till', 'time', '
to', 'transfer', 'up', 'want', 'what', 'which', 'with', 'you']
Training data created
2019-11-28 14:10:10.207987: I tensorflow/core/platform/cpu_feature_guard.cc:142] Your CPU su
pports instructions that this TensorFlow binary was not compiled to use: AVX2
Epoch 1/200
47/47 [==============================] - 0s 2ms/step - loss: 2.2080 - accuracy: 0.1489
Epoch 2/200
47/47 [==============================] - 0s 211us/step - loss: 2.1478 - accuracy: 0.1277
Epoch 3/200
47/47 [==============================] - 0s 228us/step - loss: 2.1427 - accuracy: 0.1277
```

FIGURE 13.5 Sample JSON file.

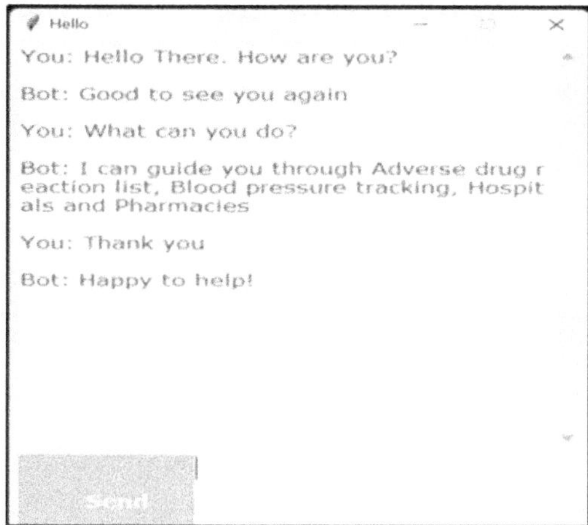

FIGURE 13.6 Final output of Medi-chat.

- **PathBot:** It is an intelligent chatbot to help visitors find locations. PathBot was created as a tool to help students and visitors find their way around the campus's facilities. Its limitations are rerouting and situations in which the user is lost are not efficiently handled. Also its accuracy was 75%.
- **Speech Recognition:** It is a Deep Neural Networks voice recognition software that is the capacity of a machine to grasp the meaning of spoken words and phrases and convert them into a machine-readable format. Its limitations include that it may be difficult to distinguish between two languages, as well as to identify accents. Its accuracy was 70%.
- **Covid-19:** It is a Deep Learning Application to deal with pandemic crisis. This study investigates how Deep Learning has combated the COVID-19 epidemic and offers recommendations for future COVID-19 research. Its constraints include generalization metrics, Learning from Limited Labeled Data, Interpretability, and Data Privacy. Its accuracy was 65%.

13.5 BENEFITS OF CHATBOTS IN HEALTHCARE

- **24/7 Availability:** Patients can get medical help whenever they need it because it is accessible every day of the week, round-the-clock.
- **Reduce Waiting Time:** With AI as technology, chatbots are able to respond in a much faster way and, in some cases, they are even better than human support.
- **Quick Access to Critical Information:** Healthcare chatbots may quickly and simply provide patients with information about surrounding medical institutions, their opening and closing times, and pharmacies and drugstores where they can pick up prescription refills [18].
- **Reduce Care Costs:** It can be challenging to find ways to save expenses without sacrificing quality of care and service and chatbots make it possible

- **Enhance Patient Satisfaction:** The capacity of patients and healthcare professionals to give and receive "humanized" care through chatbots is a major source of worry.

13.6 FUTURE SCOPE AND CHALLENGES OF CHATBOT IN HEALTHCARE

- **Patient triage and Diagnosis:** Chatbots can be used to collect patient information and symptoms to triage patients to the appropriate care level, provide basic diagnosis and treatment recommendations.
- **Patient Education and Engagement:** Chatbots can help educate patients about their conditions, provide self-care advice, and engage patients in ongoing management of their health.
- **Remote Monitoring:** Chatbots can be used to monitor patients remotely, collect data on their health status, and alert medical professionals if there are any concerning trends.
- **Mental Health Support:** Chatbots can provide support and guidance for individuals dealing with mental health issues, offering coping strategies, resources, and access to professional help.
- **Disease Management**: Chatbots can help patients manage chronic conditions, such as diabetes or hypertension, by providing reminders, offering advice on lifestyle changes, and tracking symptoms [19].

Relevant challenges and issues pertaining to medical chatbot use cases are as follows.

- **Data Privacy and Security:** Chatbots require access to sensitive patient information, which raises concerns about data privacy and security. Chatbots must be designed to comply with data privacy regulations and to protect patient information from unauthorized access.
- **Accuracy and Reliability:** Chatbots need to be accurate and reliable in providing medical information and advice. Any inaccuracies or errors in the chatbot's responses can have serious consequences for patients.
- **Lack of Emotional Intelligence:** Chatbots may lack emotional intelligence and empathy, which is critical in healthcare. Patients may feel more comfortable speaking with a human healthcare provider who can understand their emotional state and provide support.
- **Limited Diagnostic Capabilities:** Chatbots may not be able to provide accurate diagnoses for complex medical conditions, and patients may require in-person evaluations from healthcare providers.

13.7 CONCLUSION

In this Python data science project, we learned about chatbots and developed an accurate deep learning chatbot in Python. The dataset that comprises categories (intents), patterns, and replies is used to train the chatbot. In order to determine which category the user's message falls under, we employed a particular recurrent neural network (long short-term memory, LSTM), after which we randomly selected a response from a list of available options. Additionally, we tailored the data based on user wants and business goals and highly accurately taught the chatbot. Every organization, especially those in the healthcare industry, is eager to integrate chatbots into their workflow because they are utilized everywhere. Health-related issues may be resolved by this chatbot on its own, saving time and money by eliminating the trouble of visiting physicians and hospitals as well as other fees and expenditures. This chatbot does not replace doctors or does not provide treatment or medicines, but it's a single-step platform for all the other needs like keeping patient's history, allergy lists, nearest hospital number, 24/7 monitoring, etc., making the treatment process easy and simple. Instead of having to navigate the system themselves and make mistakes that increase costs, patients can let healthcare chatbots guide them through the system more effectively.

REFERENCES

1. Shivam, K, Saud, K, Sharma, M, Vashishth, S, Patil, S (June 2018) "Chatbot for college website" in Int J Comput Technol 5:74–77.
2. Susanna, Ms. Ch. L, Pratyusha, R (March 2020) "College enquiry chatbot" in Int Res J Eng Technol (IRJET) 7.
3. Hiremath, G, Hajare, A, Bhosale, P, Nanaware, R, Wagh, KS (2018) "Chatbot for education system" in Int J Adv Res Ideas Innov Technol 4(3):37–43.
4. Redström, J, Jaksetic, P, Ljungstrand, P (1999) The ChatterBox. In Gellersen, HW (ed.) Handheld and Ubiquitous Computing. HUC 1999. Lecture Notes in Computer Science (vol 1707). Springer, Berlin, Heidelberg. https://doi.org/10.1007/3-540-48157-5_46.
5. Punith, S, Chaitra, B, Kotagi, V, Chethana, RM (2020) "Chatbot for student admission enquiry" in J Adv Software Eng Testing 3:1–9.
6. Babu, E, Wilson, G (2021) "Chatbot for college enquiry" in Int J Creat Res Thoughts 9:1833–1837.
7. Adam, M, Wessel, M, Benlian, A (2020) "AI-based chatbots in customer service and their effects on user compliance" in Electron Markets 31:427–445. https://doi.org/10.1007/s12525-020-00414-7
8. Amershi, S, Weld, D, Vorvoreanu, M, Fourney, A, Nushi, B, Collisson, P, Teevan, J (2019) Guidelines for human–AI interaction. In: Proceedings of the CHI 2019 (paper no. 3). ACM, New York.
9. Araujo, T (2018) "Living up to the chatbot hype: The influence of anthropomorphic design cues and communicative agency framing on conversational agent and company perceptions" in Comput Hum Behav 85:183–189.
10. Ashktorab, Z, Jain, M, Liao, QV, Weisz, JD (2019) Resilient chatbots: Repair strategy preferences for conversational breakdowns. In: Proceedings of CHI 2019 (paper no. 254). ACM, New York.
11. Bobrow, DG, Kaplan, RM, Kay, M, Norman, DA, Thompson, H, Winograd, T (1977) "GUS, a frame-driven dialog system" in Artif Intell 8(2):155–173.
12. Breazeal, C (2003) Toward sociable robots. Robot Auton Syst 42(3–4):167–175.
13. Raj, S (2018) *Building Chatbots with Python Using Computational Linguistics and Predictive Analytics*. Apress, Pune, India.
14. Bavaresco, R, Silveira, D, Reis, E, Barbosa, J, Righi, R, Costa, C, Moreira, C (2020) "Conversational agents in business: A systematic literature review and future research directions" in Comput Sci Rev 36:100239. https://doi.org/10.1016/j.cosrev.2020.100239

15. Bickmore, T, Picard, RW (2005) "Establishing and maintaining long-term human–computer relationships" in ACM Trans Comput Hum Interact 12(2):293–327. https://doi.org/10.1145/1067860.1067867
16. Oh, CS, Bailenson, JN, Welch, GF (2018) "A systematic review of social presence: Definition, antecedents, and implications" in Front Robot AI 5:114.
17. Pérez, JQ, Daradoumis, T, Puig, JMM (2020) "Rediscovering the use of chatbots in education: A systematic literature review" in Comput Appl Eng Educ 28(6):1549–1565.
18. Porcheron, M, Fischer, JE, Reeves, S, Sharples, S (2018) Voice interfaces in everyday life. In: Proceedings of CHI 2018 (paper no. 640). ACM, New York.
19. Roller, S, Dinan, E, Goyal, N, Ju, D, Williamson, M, Liu, Y, Boureau, YL (2020) Recipes for building an open-domain chatbot. arXiv preprint. arXiv:2004.13637

14 Significance of Vehicular Ad Hoc Networks (VANETs) in Smart Healthcare

Research Challenges and Case Studies

Aradhana Behura

14.1 INTRODUCTION

Effective and timely communication of critical patient data is vital for enhancing healthcare outcomes, especially in emergency situations. This paper introduces an innovative Emergency Routing Protocol (ERP) designed specifically for vehicular ad hoc networks (VANETs) in healthcare applications. The primary objective of this protocol is to facilitate the rapid and reliable transmission of essential patient status information from ambulances to hospitals using vehicular communication technology [1, 2]. By leveraging the capabilities of VANETs, this protocol aims to expedite pre-medical treatment, ultimately increasing the chances of patient survival during critical medical emergencies [3].

The paper introduces an "Emergency Routing Protocol (ERP)" designed for VANETs in healthcare, emphasizing the critical role of efficient data communication in emergency medical situations [4]. The following aspects are worth noting in the brief review:

Significance: The paper recognizes the significance of timely communication of patient data during emergencies, a crucial aspect in healthcare settings where every second counts.

Innovation: The ERP represents an innovative solution that leverages VANET technology, demonstrating the potential for vehicular networks to enhance healthcare outcomes.

The review of related work highlights the unique contribution of the ERP in the context of VANETs and healthcare, setting the stage for its architecture. The architecture of the proposed ERP is a pivotal element of the paper, as it serves as the

DOI: 10.1201/9781032624891-14

foundation for efficient data communication in healthcare emergencies [5, 6]. The following architectural components and their significance are discussed:

- **Ambulance Nodes:** These are the primary data sources in the architecture. Ambulances are equipped with sensors and devices that collect vital patient information. The architecture facilitates the seamless integration of this data into the VANET.
- **Hospital Nodes:** Hospital nodes act as the ultimate recipients of patient data. They play a critical role in receiving, processing, and acting upon the transmitted patient status information. The architecture should ensure a robust connection between ambulances and hospitals [7].
- **Vehicle Nodes (Intermediate Nodes):** These nodes represent the vehicular network's backbone. They facilitate the transmission of patient data from ambulances to hospitals by relaying information efficiently. The routing algorithm governing these nodes is of paramount importance, as it determines the effectiveness of data delivery [8].
- **Data Flow and Communication Pathways:** The architecture should establish clear and efficient communication pathways. It must define how data is collected, prioritized, and transmitted from ambulances to hospitals. Quality of Service (QoS) considerations should be integrated to ensure the most critical data is given priority [9].
- **Security and Privacy:** The architecture should incorporate robust security measures to protect patient data during transmission. Encryption, authentication, and access control mechanisms are essential components in this context [10].
- **Validation:** The architecture's effectiveness must be validated through implementation and simulation. This step ensures that the proposed protocol and architecture perform as expected in various real-world scenarios.
- **Use Cases:** Real-world use cases should be considered to demonstrate the practical application of the architecture. These use cases help illustrate how ERP can enhance emergency medical responses.

14.1.1 Overview of Data Communication in Healthcare Emergencies

Data communication plays a pivotal role in healthcare emergencies due to its significant impact on patient care, outcomes, and overall healthcare system efficiency [1–4, 11–14]. Here's a brief overview of the significance of data communication in healthcare emergencies:

- **Timely Decision-Making:** Rapid and accurate communication of patient data is crucial for healthcare providers to make informed decisions quickly. In emergencies, delays in data transmission can result in critical consequences [15–19].
- **Coordination of Care:** Effective data communication facilitates the coordination of care among healthcare professionals, ambulance personnel, and

hospital staff. It ensures that everyone involved in a patient's care has access to up-to-date information.

- **Remote Consultations:** In some emergencies, specialists or consultants may not be on-site. Telemedicine and remote consultations rely on data communication to connect experts with on-site healthcare providers to guide diagnosis and treatment.
- **Medical History Access:** Access to a patient's medical history, medications, allergies, and prior diagnoses through electronic health records (EHRs) can prevent adverse drug interactions and help healthcare providers tailor treatments to the patient's specific needs.
- **Resource Allocation:** Hospitals and healthcare facilities need real-time data on incoming patients' conditions to allocate resources efficiently. This includes prioritizing surgeries, ICU beds, and medical supplies.
- **Patient Tracking:** In mass casualty incidents or disasters, data communication systems enable the tracking and identification of patients, ensuring that no one is lost in the chaos and that families are informed of their loved ones' status [20–29].
- **Emergency Alerts:** Healthcare emergencies often necessitate rapid communication with the public or specific patient populations. Alerts about disease outbreaks, vaccination campaigns, or safety measures are disseminated through various communication channels [30–36].
- **Research and Data Analysis:** Data collected during healthcare emergencies are invaluable for research and epidemiological analysis. Studying patterns and trends in emergency data can inform public health strategies and preparedness.
- **Public Health Surveillance:** Efficient data communication is essential for monitoring and responding to public health threats, such as infectious disease outbreaks or bioterrorism events.
- **Patient Empowerment:** In some cases, patients themselves use wearable devices or apps that transmit health data to healthcare providers. This can aid in early detection of health issues and timely interventions [37–39].

In summary, data communication in healthcare emergencies is a lifeline that ensures healthcare providers have access to critical information, enabling them to make rapid, well-informed decisions, deliver appropriate treatments, and save lives. It also supports the broader healthcare system by enhancing resource allocation, research, and public health surveillance efforts.

14.1.2 Introduction to VANET Technology and Its Potential in Healthcare Applications

VANETs represent a cutting-edge technology that leverages the connectivity of vehicles to create dynamic and self-organizing wireless communication networks. These networks are primarily designed to enhance road safety, traffic efficiency, and driver assistance. However, their potential extends beyond transportation, with applications emerging in various domains, including healthcare. VANETs rely on onboard vehicle communication systems equipped with sensors and wireless communication modules. These systems enable vehicles to exchange information with each other, infrastructure, and even pedestrians. The real-time data exchange within VANETs is facilitated by dedicated short-range communication (DSRC) or cellular networks, allowing vehicles to form ad hoc networks on the move.

In the context of healthcare applications, VANET technology holds immense promise:

- **Emergency Medical Response:** VANETs can play a pivotal role in transmitting critical patient data from ambulances to hospitals in real-time. This rapid data exchange allows healthcare professionals to prepare for incoming patients, potentially improving pre-hospital and in-hospital care during emergencies.
- **Remote Consultations:** By connecting ambulances to medical experts at distant hospitals, VANETs enable real-time telemedicine consultations. Specialists can assess patients' conditions remotely, provide guidance to paramedics, and recommend necessary treatments, all while the ambulance is en route to the hospital.
- **Patient Monitoring:** In non-emergency scenarios, VANET-enabled wearable devices and sensors within vehicles can continuously monitor patients' vital signs and health metrics. This data can be shared securely with healthcare providers, offering a more comprehensive understanding of a patient's health status.
- **Public Health Surveillance:** VANETs can contribute to public health efforts by gathering data on environmental factors, traffic patterns, and air quality, which can be used to detect disease outbreaks or assess the impact of environmental factors on public health.

The "Emergency Routing Protocol for VANET in Healthcare" introduces an architecture that addresses the critical need for efficient data communication in emergency medical situations. By leveraging VANET technology, this architecture has the potential to significantly improve patient outcomes in healthcare emergencies. However, successful implementation and validation are key to realizing these benefits, and future research directions should consider scalability, adaptability, and real-world deployment challenges.

14.1.3 Statement of the Research Problem and Objectives

The potential benefits of integrating VANET technology into healthcare applications are clear, but significant challenges must be addressed to harness this potential effectively. Therefore, the research problem and objectives can be defined as follows:

- **Research Problem:** In healthcare emergencies, timely and efficient data communication from ambulances to hospitals is critical for improving patient outcomes. Current data communication methods may have limitations, and there is a need to explore how VANET technology can be optimally utilized to address these limitations and enhance emergency medical responses.

Objectives:

- **Develop an Emergency Routing Protocol (ERP):** Design and implement an innovative ERP tailored for VANETs to facilitate the rapid and reliable transmission of critical patient data from ambulances to hospitals during emergencies.
- **Evaluate ERP Performance:** Conduct extensive simulations and real-world tests to evaluate the performance of the ERP in various emergency scenarios. Assess factors such as data transmission speed, reliability, and network resilience.
- **Ensure Data Security:** Implement robust security measures within the VANET-based healthcare system to protect patient data during transmission. This includes encryption, authentication, and access control mechanisms.
- **Explore Telemedicine Applications:** Investigate the feasibility of using VANETs for real-time telemedicine consultations between ambulances and remote medical experts. Assess the impact on patient care and outcomes.
- **Address Scalability and Integration:** Explore how the VANET-based healthcare system can scale to accommodate a larger number of ambulances, hospitals, and healthcare providers. Investigate interoperability with existing healthcare information systems.

In summary, this research aims to harness the potential of VANET technology to improve healthcare outcomes during emergencies by developing a dedicated routing protocol and addressing key challenges related to data security, telemedicine applications, and system scalability. The ultimate goal is to enhance the efficiency and effectiveness of emergency medical responses through the integration of VANET technology.

14.2 SYSTEM ARCHITECTURE

The ERP is designed to facilitate the rapid and reliable transmission of critical patient data from ambulances to hospitals via VANETs. Here's a brief description of the key components of the ERP:

- **Ambulance Nodes**: Data Sources and Transmission Points

  Data Sources: Ambulance nodes represent the mobile healthcare units equipped with various sensors, medical devices, and communication equipment. These devices collect real-time patient data, including vital signs, medical history, and current symptoms.

  Transmission Points: Ambulance nodes serve as the initial source of patient data. The ERP allows these nodes to transmit the collected patient information securely to hospital nodes via the VANET. This transmission occurs in real-time as the ambulance travels to the medical facility.

- **Hospital Nodes:** Data Recipients and Medical Service Providers
  Data Recipients: Hospital nodes represent the healthcare facilities that are the ultimate recipients of the patient data transmitted by ambulances. These nodes are equipped with data reception and processing capabilities, including the ability to decode and interpret the transmitted data.

  Medical Service Providers: Hospital nodes include healthcare professionals who use the received patient data to prepare for the arrival of the ambulance and provide pre-medical treatment instructions. This can involve emergency room staff, physicians, nurses, and specialists.
- **Vehicle Nodes (Intermediate Nodes):** Facilitators of Data Transmission
  These nodes consist of vehicles in the vicinity of the ambulance's route. They serve as intermediaries in the data transmission process, relaying the patient data from ambulances to hospitals. Intermediate nodes play a crucial role in ensuring the efficient and reliable transmission of patient data. They form a dynamic communication network that extends the range of data transmission, overcoming obstacles or dead zones that may exist on the ambulance's route. The ERP's routing algorithm guides these intermediate nodes to forward data efficiently.
- **Data Flow and Communication Pathways**
  Patient data flows from the ambulance nodes to the intermediate nodes and, ultimately, to the hospital nodes. The ERP defines the data flow pathways and protocols for data transmission, ensuring that data packets reach their destination securely and promptly.
- **Communication Pathways**
  The VANET technology enables vehicle-to-vehicle (V2V) and vehicle-to-infrastructure (V2I) communication. In the context of the ERP, V2V communication allows ambulances to communicate with nearby vehicles (intermediate nodes), while V2I communication facilitates data exchange between ambulances and hospital nodes via infrastructure support.

  In summary, the ERP's components include ambulances as data sources and transmission points, hospitals as data recipients and medical service providers, and intermediate nodes (vehicles) that act as facilitators of data transmission. The data flow within the ERP follows defined communication pathways, leveraging VANET technology to ensure the timely and efficient transmission of critical patient data in emergency healthcare scenarios.

14.3 PROTOCOL DESIGN

14.3.1 Routing Algorithm for Efficient and Timely Data Forwarding

To ensure efficient and timely data forwarding in the proposed ERP for VANETs in healthcare, a robust routing algorithm is essential. The routing algorithm should prioritize the delivery of critical patient data while considering the dynamic and mobile nature of VANETs. Here's a brief description:

A suitable routing algorithm for the ERP could be a combination of Geographic Routing and Priority-Based Routing. In this approach, geographic routing leverages location information to forward data packets to the nearest intermediate nodes or hospital nodes. This minimizes transmission delays. Priority-Based Routing assigns different priority levels to data packets, ensuring that emergency data packets are given the highest priority for immediate forwarding.

- **Quality of Service Considerations and Prioritization of Emergency Data**
  Maintaining QoS is vital in healthcare applications, especially during emergencies. The ERP should ensure that critical patient data receives the highest level of service. Here's a brief description.
- **QoS Parameters**
  The ERP defines QoS parameters such as latency, reliability, and bandwidth allocation. Emergency data packets are assigned the highest priority, guaranteeing minimal latency and maximum reliability for their transmission.
- **Emergency Data Prioritization**
  The ERP employs a traffic classification mechanism to identify emergency data packets. These packets are tagged with a specific priority level to ensure they are processed and forwarded with minimal delay, even in congested network conditions.

14.3.2 Handling Network Disruptions and Ensuring Data Reliability

VANETs are susceptible to network disruptions due to the mobility of vehicles. Ensuring data reliability and handling network disruptions are critical aspects of the ERP. Here's a brief description:

- **Network Disruption Handling**
  The ERP incorporates mechanisms for handling network disruptions, such as intermittent connectivity or node departures. This includes route re-establishment protocols that dynamically adapt to changing network topologies.
  - **Data Reliability:** To enhance data reliability, the ERP employs techniques like data packet replication and acknowledgment mechanisms. Data packets are replicated and sent via multiple routes to ensure that at least one copy reaches its destination, reducing the likelihood of data loss.
  - **Buffering and Caching:** The ERP uses buffer management strategies to temporarily store data packets in case of network disruptions. Intermediate nodes can cache emergency data packets and forward them once connectivity is re-established.

In summary, the routing algorithm in the ERP combines Geographic Routing and Priority-Based Routing to ensure efficient data forwarding. QoS considerations prioritize emergency data, guaranteeing minimal latency and maximum reliability. To handle network disruptions, the ERP includes route re-establishment protocols, data replication, acknowledgment mechanisms, and buffering/caching strategies to ensure data reliability and timely delivery, even in challenging VANET environments.

14.4 USE CASES

14.4.1 Real-World Scenarios Illustrating the Protocol's Effectiveness in Emergency Healthcare Situations and Use of Smart Transportation System

Illustrating the effectiveness of the ERP for VANETs in emergency healthcare situations and its integration with a smart transportation system can be done through real-world scenarios. These scenarios showcase how the ERP improves emergency medical responses and healthcare outcomes.

- **Scenario 1: Cardiac Arrest Response**
  Context: A patient experiences a sudden cardiac arrest in a residential area, far from the nearest hospital. An ambulance equipped with the ERP and integrated with the smart transportation system is dispatched to the scene.
  Illustration: The patient's vital signs are continuously monitored by medical devices within the ambulance. The ERP identifies the emergency nature of the situation and assigns a high priority to the patient's data. The ambulance communicates with the smart transportation system to request a clear and efficient route to the nearest hospital, considering traffic conditions and road closures. The ERP utilizes VANET communication to transmit the patient's critical data to the hospital in real-time. Hospital nodes receive the data, and the emergency room staff is immediately alerted. Upon arrival, the medical team is prepared with the necessary equipment and information, improving the chances of successful resuscitation.
- **Scenario 2: Trauma Care in a Traffic Jam**
  Context: An accident occurs on a busy highway, causing a traffic jam. Several vehicles are involved, and multiple injured individuals need immediate medical attention.
  Illustration: The ERP in nearby vehicles detects the accident and prioritizes the transmission of emergency data to the nearest hospital. Hospital nodes receive data from multiple sources and assess the severity of injuries. Emergency services are dispatched to the accident site with the precise location provided by the smart transportation system. Intermediate vehicle nodes help relay critical patient data from the accident site to the hospital, bypassing traffic congestion. The hospital prepares for incoming patients, ensuring that resources and staff are allocated appropriately. Patients receive timely medical care, and the ERP continues to transmit updates on their conditions during transport to the hospital [40–43].
- **Scenario 3: Remote Diagnosis During Evacuation**
  Context: A natural disaster, such as a flood, forces residents to evacuate their homes. Medical personnel operate mobile healthcare units equipped with the ERP and smart transportation integration to provide healthcare services during the evacuation.
  Illustration: Mobile healthcare units move through the affected area, offering medical assistance to evacuees. Data collected from patients, such

as their medical history and current health status, is transmitted in real-time via VANET to hospital nodes. Hospital nodes analyze the incoming data and provide remote medical consultations to the healthcare personnel on-site. Telemedicine capabilities allow specialists to assist in diagnosing and treating patients, even in remote areas [44–47].

The smart transportation system assists in redirecting mobile healthcare units to areas with the highest demand for medical services. Timely interventions and access to medical expertise contribute to better outcomes for evacuees, even in challenging disaster scenarios.

These real-world scenarios highlight the ERP's effectiveness in improving emergency healthcare responses by leveraging VANET technology and integrating with a smart transportation system. The protocol ensures that critical patient data is rapidly transmitted, enabling healthcare providers to make informed decisions and provide timely care, ultimately saving lives and enhancing healthcare outcomes during emergencies.

14.5 REAL-WORLD EXAMPLES AND CASE STUDIES

While the integration of VANETs and ERPs in healthcare is a relatively emerging field, there are real-world examples and case studies that provide insights into the potential applications and benefits of such technology. Here are a few examples:

1. **The European VENUS-C Project:**
   Context: The Vehicular Communication for Emergency and Safety Applications in Europe (VENUS-C) project aimed to enhance emergency responses using VANETs in European cities.
   Case Study: In the city of Bordeaux, France, the VENUS-C project implemented VANET technology to improve emergency medical responses. Ambulances were equipped with VANET devices, enabling them to transmit patient data, GPS coordinates, and traffic information to nearby hospitals. This data allowed hospitals to prepare for incoming patients efficiently.
   Outcome: The project demonstrated significant reductions in response times and better utilization of hospital resources during emergencies. It highlighted the potential for VANETs to enhance healthcare in urban settings.
2. **Mobile Telemedicine Units in Disaster Response:**
   Context: In disaster-prone areas like Japan, mobile telemedicine units equipped with VANET technology have been used during natural disasters.
   Case Study: Following the Great East Japan Earthquake and Tsunami in 2011, mobile telemedicine units were dispatched to provide medical care in affected areas. These units used VANETs to communicate with hospitals and remote specialists, allowing for real-time consultations and data exchange.

Outcome: VANET-enabled mobile telemedicine units improved the quality of care in disaster-stricken areas by facilitating timely access to medical expertise and resources, even when traditional communication infrastructure was disrupted.

3. **Trauma Care in Smart Cities:**

   Context: Several smart cities around the world have been exploring the integration of VANETs and ERPs into their emergency response systems.

   Case Study: In a smart city with an integrated VANET-based emergency response system, accidents and medical emergencies trigger immediate responses. Ambulances, equipped with VANET technology, transmit patient data and traffic conditions to hospitals, which, in turn, coordinate with emergency rooms and specialists for incoming cases.

   Outcome: Such systems have demonstrated improved emergency medical responses, reduced response times, and optimized resource allocation in urban environments, ultimately enhancing patient outcomes.

These real-world examples and case studies demonstrate the potential of VANET technology and ERPs in healthcare, particularly in the context of emergency responses. While these applications are still evolving, they showcase the tangible benefits of integrating VANETs into healthcare systems, including faster access to medical care, improved resource allocation, and enhanced coordination between emergency services and healthcare providers.

14.6 SECURITY AND PRIVACY

Measures to ensure the security and privacy of patient data during transmission and Encryption and authentication mechanisms

Ensuring the security and privacy of patient data during transmission is paramount in healthcare, especially when using technologies like VANETs for data exchange. Here are measures and brief explanations of encryption and authentication mechanisms to achieve this.

14.6.1 Security and Privacy Measures

- **Data Encryption:** Encrypt patient data during transmission to protect it from unauthorized access. Encryption algorithms like Advanced Encryption Standard (AES) or Transport Layer Security (TLS) can be employed to secure data packets.
- **Secure Communication Channels:** Ensure that VANET communications occur over secure channels, such as Virtual Private Networks (VPNs) or dedicated encrypted communication protocols, to prevent eavesdropping and data interception.
- **Authentication:** Implement strong authentication mechanisms to verify the identity of both sender and receiver nodes in VANETs. Use techniques like Public Key Infrastructure (PKI) for node authentication.

- **Access Control:** Define strict access control policies to restrict who can send and receive patient data within the VANET. Only authorized nodes, such as ambulances and hospitals, should have access.
- **Data Anonymization:** Anonymize patient data whenever possible by removing or obfuscating personally identifiable information (PII) before transmission. This helps protect patient privacy in case of data breaches.
- **Data Integrity Checks:** Implement data integrity checks like hash functions or checksums to detect tampering or corruption of data during transmission. This ensures that data received is exactly as transmitted.

14.6.2 Encryption Mechanisms

- **Symmetric Encryption:** In symmetric encryption, the same key is used for both encryption and decryption. It's efficient for securing data within a VANET but requires a secure method for distributing keys to authorized nodes.
- **Asymmetric Encryption:** Asymmetric encryption uses a pair of keys (public and private) for encryption and decryption. It's commonly used for secure key exchange and authentication in VANETs. Public keys can be freely distributed, while private keys are kept confidential.

14.6.3 Authentication Mechanisms

- **Digital Signatures:** Nodes can use digital signatures to sign data packets, providing proof of their authenticity. Recipient nodes can then verify the signature using the sender's public key.
- **Certificate-Based Authentication:** PKI is often used for VANET authentication. Each node has a digital certificate issued by a trusted Certificate Authority (CA). Nodes can verify each other's certificates to establish trust.
- **Shared Secrets:** Nodes can use shared secrets, like pre-shared keys (PSKs), for mutual authentication. Both the sender and receiver need to know the secret to establish a secure connection.
- **Biometric Authentication:** In some cases, biometric authentication methods, such as fingerprint or iris scans, can be used to uniquely identify authorized personnel accessing patient data.

In summary, encryption and authentication mechanisms are crucial for securing patient data during transmission in VANET-based healthcare systems. These measures help prevent unauthorized access, tampering, and data breaches, ensuring patient privacy and data integrity throughout the communication process. The long long-term license issuing and maintenance are the responsibility of CAS. According to [48], at predetermined times, automobiles contact CAs for quick pseudonyms. Self-issuance techniques of pseudonyms [49] have been developed to allow automobiles to create pseudonyms independently to reduce the cost of data communication with CAs. To shorten a pseudonym's lifespan and impede tracking, an innovative pseRSUym altering strategy [50] was given in 2012.

Researcher discussed MbRE cloud-based protocol [51] using Jetson Nano and Google Colab. Vehicular information is separated and sequenced into multiple information branches—motion information (M), i.e., velocity and position, frequency (F) inherited from the information timestamps, and pseudo-identities (I). The CNN algorithm is used to train vehicular datasets with encoding rules. Eight categories for anonymous authentication systems can be made based on secure, cutting-edge techniques. A private key generator (PKG) is the third trusted authority for assigning and generating private keys in the IBS scheme. This group is reliant on identity-based cryptosystems. The automobile's asymmetric key is generated using the required data (such as its contact number and email address). As a result, the need for certificate allocation is eliminated. For data authentication, none of these techniques make use of certificates. Each member receives a symmetric key from the KGC, which also serves as a trusted third-party member. In [52], a privacy-preserving identity-based verification strategy for VANETs was implemented. A pool of transitory pseudonyms is loaded further into the TPD (trusted party) of the automobile by local transportation authorities. When an automobile wants to transmit the data, a shared digital secret key will be generated from each participant in data transmission. Next, the trustworthy dealer (TD) calculates and distributes the confidential data shares to the agencies using the corruption-resistant threshold verification system. Similarly, the RTA employs a defense technique based on threshold authentication to identify group members and locate fraudulent vehicles. This system can guarantee traceability, integrity, confidentiality, and non-repudiation. It does not offer a mathematical justification or graph illustrating the vehicular network performance. Furthermore, no assessment is made to demonstrate how successful and efficient the system is compared to other schemes. To ensure privacy preservation, an id-based offline or online signature technique has been planned [53]. Similarly, V2I authentication uses an id-based offline or online signature system. The cross-RSU (road side unit) node V2V authentication and cross-region validation are also included in this method. In this protocol, an automobile whose pseudonym key is absent from the verifier's storage is authenticated. The car that has traveled from another location is authenticated in base station (BS). However, because the offline process necessitates a lot of storage space, the IBOOS scheme is unsuited for VANETs. Additionally, because the PKG is aware of every automobile's private key, these methods must address the key escrow issue. This approach requires separate automobile authentication, and RSUs add to its complexity. It has been suggested in [53] to employ elliptic curve cryptography (ECC)–based data authentication without using bilinear pairing, which uses a hash function to deliver source and data authentication techniques. In this case, the private key is generated using pseudo-identity. Using a message-signature pair, the TA can reveal the genuine identity of the vehicle at issue in a dispute. Under the random oracle paradigm, this approach is unaffected by an adaptively chosen message attack. When the density rises, the message loss ratio is not considered. Researchers in [54] have presented an accumulative-based pseudonym exchange system to improve location-based privacy in vehicular social networks. Here, pseudonym-changing areas are created to alter pseudonyms while using group signatures. As a result, the tracing attacker has more reason to be suspicious of a particular pseudonym, which enhances location privacy. To allocate and administer group identity (GID), related keys, and uniquely private and asymmetric keys in the area, RSUs choose a group leader (GL). When an automobile joins a group, it trades pseudonyms with the other group members. The automobile must activate pseudonyms before the registration authority exchange (RA). When a vehicle departs the group, the GL deletes the entry from the list of members. The RA updates the blocklist with a malicious vehicle's identification and transmits the new list throughout the network. However, due to the intricate procedures involved, this system has large computing and communication overhead. In [55], a composite privacy-preserving authentication technique was put forth. The management and revocation of certificates are not required for this scheme. The trapdoor mechanism aids in the detection, tracking, and elimination of harmful vehicles from a network.

Instead of using vehicle-based segmentation in this, regions are grouped. First, the identity verification and enrollment (IdVE) module provides the certificate for the vehicle. In the message broadcast step, the sender selects a pseudonym corresponding to the beacon's broadcast time. The beacon is then transmitted after the notification has been signed with the area's symmetric key. Additionally, the LEA can determine the automobile's identity that sent the malicious signal. The replay, Sybil, and modification attacks resist this method. However, it takes a long time and requires a lot of complexity to locate and eliminate malicious nodes from the vehicular network.

A certificateless aggregate signature approach similar to has been put out in, where all of the signatures are combined, and the data verification procedure is carried out using the combined signature. Next, the suggested CLAS (certificate-less signature) approach in [56] does not use bilinear pairing. Corser et al. proposed a certificate-less system [57], which focused on K-means concept. A message signature scheme's claim that it is secure against forgery attacks under the KDT concept has also been demonstrated as false. Additionally, RSU performs batch verification to quicken and boost effectiveness. In contrast to other CLAS systems, this scheme has a high level of intricacy.

Using signature aggregation, a privacy-preserving approach has been put out [58] that provides data validation and lessens the burden on processing and data transmission hardware. Several attributes are computed beforehand to lower the cost of generating a signature when an automobile enters the data communication range of the new RSU. This system is secure and unforgeable against the adaptive asymmetric-key replacement attack, selected identity assault, and selected message attack. However, the complicated pseudonym generation, aggregation, and verification considerably raise computing and communication costs.

Emara et al. proposed the MixGroup pseudonym exchanging protocol [59], and an improved Signature-based certification system utilizing identity-based group signatures (IBGS) was presented. For adequate signature verification, it makes use of a batch scheduling method. Vehicles, group managers, and RSUs are issued private keys by the trusted escrow authority (TEA). The vehicle must follow a group or cluster join protocol to request a membership-authenticated certificate from GM. The vehicle uses the secret key and certificate to create a group signature when it wishes to deliver a message. The message receiver can confirm the information's validity by checking the signature with batch data verification. This system offers traceability, member revocation, source, and message authentication. However, it does not provide delays, computation costs, or communication overhead. To impact uniquely private and asymmetric key privacy-preserving mechanism has been developed [60]. The sender sends group signature-based cipher text C1 to the RSU node. When the validation is completed, RSU sends the C1 to an LBS provider L1. L1 uses the verification algorithm to extract the group signature from the C1 and verify it. Additionally, KGC can deactivate harmful vehicles utilizing the ML and RL member lists. Additionally, this plan can guarantee non-repudiation, message secrecy, and integrity.

The bilinear pairing technique based on authentication and data delivery access control mechanism has been put forth in [61]. A safe system based on blind signatures and hierarchical pseudonyms has been presented in [62]. When a signer uses a blind signature, the message owner and signer are different parties, and the signer is not required to be aware of the message's contents. Three stages—requirement definition, comprehensive protocol design, and security analysis—are used to define it. However, this protocol does not mention how an RSU node validates data signatures obtained from automobiles. Researcher [63] suggests a distributed aggregate privacy-preserving authentication mechanism. It employs a one-time aggregate signature approach based on numerous trustworthy authorities. TA provides the certificate and public key to an RSU. Similarly, TA delivers a vehicle with its authentication key Ki and internal pseudo-identity (IPID). The TA also has members list (ML) in its database, where each vehicle's IPID, ID, and Ki are kept. After receiving the member secrets and allotted time, the vehicle stores these data. The message and its signature are sent throughout the network. The receiver checks message signature pairings using bilinear pairing to ensure non-repudiation and accuracy. The TA can use the details about the vehicle in the ML to achieve traceability. This system is resistant to DoS, Sybil, and side-channel attacks. A vehicle must, however, go through a new identification process each time it switches networks. The batch authentication and anonymous mutual system have been suggested in [64]. The privacy and security of V2V data transmission are ensured by anonymous mutual authentication. An anonymous batch authentication is performed, confirming the vehicle's identity and assisting in verifying messages sent by an RSU. The main advantage of this plan is that it evenly distributes the authentication load among cars, easing the stress on RSUs and TA. Once registered to TA, each vehicle must produce a short-term anonymous certificate and digital signature. The network's performance is improved by using car and RSU authentication. However, this technique did not explain the data loss ratio and message transmission overhead. The secure and intelligent traffic control techniques based on cloud-fog computing have been described in [65]. When there is a high vehicle density, the first technique is inefficient but offers security from DoS attacks. The second technique authenticates automobiles effectively even in high vehicle densities and is fog-compatible. This system can reduce communication and computing overhead through secure protocol development and traffic light verification. A conditional bilinear mapping-based authentication technique that protects privacy has been suggested in [66].

In addition, we deliberate the tradeoff between privacy and security in VANETs, highlighting the need for a compromise when designing a security scheme [67, 68].

Researchers proposed the SECMACE protocol [69] for efficient credential management. Researchers edpicted CPPA certificate-less protocol [1], which achieves traceability and anonymity but suffers from signature forgery, high message communication cost, security vulnerability, and computational complexity. Chen, Y., Chen, J. (2021) proposed the CPP-CLAS protocol [70], a certificate-less privacy-preserving aggregate compressed signature technique that ensures unforgeability with reduced communication and computational cost. It secures data transmission between V2V, V2I, and I2I. Researchers [71] described the PPAAS protocol, which supports encryption and helps to detect malicious nodes in the trace phase. This protocol has five steps: system initialization, registration, message delivery, fog-based data processing, and trace. Researchers depicted eCLAS-based (enhanced certificate-less signature) protocol [72], which achieves message authentication, anonymity, unlinkability, traceability, integrity, and resistance against replay attacks, impersonation attacks, modification attacks, message spoofing, and man-in-the-middle attack. This secure protocol has seven stages: pseudonym identity generation, automobile key generation, partial private key extract, the message with signature, data aggregation, signature aggregation, and verification. The elliptic curve supports Tate pairing and bilinear pairing. Yang, Minghao, et al. describe a pairing-free robust and secure key-protected certificates protocol using an elliptic curve algorithm [73].

Samra, B., and Fouzi, S. et al. proposed the CLA-TRS protocol [73, 74], which supports the Diffie-Hellman algorithm to achieve traceability, unforgeability, and anonymity. It is a certificate-less ring signature based on bilinear pairing aggregate signatures over the elliptic curve (EC) algorithm for VANET. This model has three entities: OBU, RSU, and TRC. Each automobile is equipped with OBU. The TRC is a KGC, a semi-trusted system responsible for the single-point failure and generating partial private, secure keys for OBUs and registered RSU nodes. All relevant sensitive data is stored in the TPD of associated OBUs of each RSU. The TRC checks the conditional traceability of automobiles. The OBU is a wireless device that helps data transmission with another automobile with an RSU node through the DSRC protocol. The aggregate ring signature generator RSU collects all signatures regarding traffic data and then aggregates them with automobile signatures. The vehicle will check RSU's aggregate signature rather than the individual one. Vijayakumar, Pandi, et al. described [75] an anonymous authentication 6G and bilinear pairing-based secure key exchange method. This protocol provides high throughput, availability, and reliability, outperforming other algorithms regarding message delay, batch verification, and communication cost. This model has six stages: system initialization, vehicle registration, RSU's registration, mutual authentication, anonymous key exchange, and batch authentication. Xiong, Wanjun, et al. depicted the CPPA-D protocol [76], and the TPD is vulnerable to channel attack; thus, cyclic groups are constructed in the elliptic curve. Batch verification is useful for multiple data authentication, and it is challenging to forge a vehicle secure key and master session key, so double insurance is beneficial to achieve confidentiality and integrity. Gupta, Maanak, et al. proposed an attribute-based AB-ITS protocol [77] based on secure V2I and V2V data communication using cloudlets. Guo, Rui, et al. described ring signcryption-based certificate-less privacy-preserving protocol using ECC [78] as advantageous in terms of low data transmission latency, less packet loss, and secure communication.

Wang, Yujue, et al. depicted the RCoM protocol [79] based on the Diffie-Hellman concept for security and the cloud server for storage. The objective of root authority is to observe the road surroundings through the cloud server to respond to some emergencies. The cloud server is preserved by many cloud service providers, which has essential storage and computing resources; it delivers road condition data to end users. Wang, P., Liu, Y., et al. proposed the SEMA protocol based on a group and pseudonyms algorithm. The pseudonyms (K1-K3) and group-based algorithms (K4-K5) have some challenges described in K1-K5. The SEMA protocol [80] combines RSA, bilinear pairing, q-SDH, and ElGamal protocol.

K1: Updating and preloading pseudonyms in the server are infeasible for automobiles in reality.
K2: The CRL that provisions the pseudonyms regarding revoked automobiles should be modified by all authentic automobiles, and it is a challenging task.
K3: Each pseudonym of the vehicle is cast off to put a signature in multiple data in a particular interval; the intruders trace the vehicle trajectory of the owners in this time interval.
K4: Verifying and generating the vehicular group signatures carries overhead to the RSUs or automobiles.
K5: To revoke an automobile, all genuine automobiles must update the group secure key and parameters simultaneously.

Researchers proposed the CLSS-CPPA protocol [81], which supports batch processing to speed up multiple digital signature verification. Liang, Y., Liu, Y. et al. proposed a CLAS protocol [82], unable to handle forgery attacks and overhearing issues. Cao, Yibo, et al. proposed the FSA-LGS protocol [83], which prevents forging signatures by taking help from bonsai tree architecture. It produces secret keys for each epoch. This lattice concept-inspired group signature can handle quantum attacks using bonsai tree signature methods. The computation overhead depends upon the signature size, but bonsai architecture takes low storage efficiently. Alaya, B., and Sellami, L. et al. proposed a secure hybrid cluster-based vital management protocol [84] that avoids congestion and jamming, which aims to balance resource load.

The protocol considers many parameters, such as the number of automobiles, RSUs, traffic type, GLs, simulation area, data size, transmission range, and vehicle speed. This protocol has various stages: network initialization, key generation, key distribution, secure communication, node adding, and node removing. It provides better performance regarding faster data delivery rate, improved lifetime, and less inter-cluster distance overhead. The scheme proposed by Nath, H. J., Choudhury, H. et al. uses a secure, lightweight cryptographic algorithm [85] to reach its purposes with low latency. Furthermore, automobiles can demand pseudonyms after the validity period. Our upcoming research is used to develop the updation regarding the group key stage, where multiple RSU nodes can update and manage through group communication. This procedure will enhance the performance in terms of communication cost and computation time of this protocol with a large number of vehicular sensor deployments as they traverse from the communication range of one RSU node to another. Vijayakumar, Pandi, et al. proposed a mutual batch authentication protocol [86] which consists of seven stages such as system initialization, vehicle registration, RSU's registration, mutual anonymous authentication, anonymous key exchange, batch authentication, and integrity preservation and outperforms better in terms of message delay, communication cost, and batch verification.

Blockchain technology can be used in the future to achieve better location privacy. In combination with VANET with 6G, high throughput, high availability, and high reliability are supported in this area. However, the data transmitted in the system must be secured. If the CRL message size increases, it creates data storage and computation overhead. The MHT is used to check RSU nodes, and MMPT is used to authenticate vehicles. The ECC is used for data verification and integrity. A quotient filter [87] based sensor node validation used to verify the automobile's legitimacy is enhanced. The goal is to handle unauthorized and illegal sensors attempting to connect the network and share relevant information. Fog computing is used to reduce latency and provides improved throughput. Luo, Ming, and Yanzibo Zhou et al. proposed that CPPA, KOSTIS protocol [88], which follows encryption but cannot handle ring selection attacks. Chen, Xiaohu, et al. described the SOERS protocol [89], which focused on a multi-signature scheme rather than a chameleon signature. This scheme requires two operations, one hash, and two multiplication operations to create a sign for all OBU. Li, Guanjie, et al. depicted the SecCDV protocol [90] based on the Cybertwin-Driven scheme. The cyber twin system has the features of more reliability, lower latency, and higher scalability, so it is useful for delay-sensitive-based applications associated with the digital twin concept, which is positioned in the central cloud. Ren, Yanli, et al. discussed [91] how lexicographical-based Merkle tree and batch verification is helpful to reduce computational cost and achieve message integrity, anonymity, authentication, unlinkability, authority distribution, and resistance from the attacks (impersonation–modification–a middleman–replay attack). Othman, Wajdy, et al. depicted a lightweight AI-inspired cryptosystem [92]. This protocol consists of four steps: system setup, V2I key renewal, mutual authentication, V2V secure data communication, and revocation extractor. The fuzzy extractor is used for key generation, but if many CRLs are available, this protocol takes time in the checking process. Wang, Yu et al. described error location proper-grained protocol [93] for vehicular cloud and outperforms in terms of security, communication overhead, privacy-preserving, and computation delay. The design goal consists of message authentication, privacy-preserving, error signature prediction, key update periodically, traceability, non-repudiation, unlinkability, and resistance to various attacks such as reply–forgery attacks.

Researchers depicted [94] invalid signature detection techniques and signature verification using batch processing. The researcher will concentrate on post-quantum or no pairing secure batch authentication and identification scheme in the upcoming situation. Wang, Peng, et al. proposed an HDMA scheme [95], a pseudonyms-based group signature. In this protocol, 5G helps to achieve ultra-latency and signaling. The CRL (certificate revocation list) creates storage overhead so TPD can be used, but it is known to be susceptible to side wireless channel attacks. Trajectory confidentiality is not reached. As a pseudonym is cast off to put signature multiple data transmitted in a particular time period, an intruder can disclose the automobile's trajectory in a specific period by considering the signatures created by the unchanged pseudonym.

Khalid, Adia, et al. proposed [96] a blockchain-based security model which handles selfish behavior and the storage capacity of the vehicles. The vehicles can receive incentives after the event validation successfully. Researchers exploited the PPVF protocol [97], which supports a reputation-based pallier encryption procedure. The pallier homomorphic encryption has three phases: key generation, decryption, and encryption. This protocol focused on the design goal, such as feedback confidentiality, integrity, authentication, traceability, and resistance to various attacks. Wei, Lu et al. designed a key agreement based on the secure tree protocol [98]. The authenticated key agreement (AKA) is used to provide session keys among the automobiles or V2I, I2V, and I2I communication. The protocol has eight steps: system setup or establishing the connection, vehicle registration, RSU node registration, authenticated data of automobiles, authentication information of RSU, authenticated feedback for RSU and vehicles, and key updating message. Bhattacharya, Pronaya, et al. proposed the 6Blocks protocol [96], and it resists the C-V2X attack.

14.7 ROLE OF MACHINE LEARNING AND CLOUD COMPUTING IN SMART TRANSPORTATION HEALTHCARE

Machine learning (ML) and cloud computing play pivotal roles in the integration of smart transportation into smart healthcare systems. Here's how they contribute to the efficiency and effectiveness of these interconnected systems.

- **Data Analytics and Predictive Modeling**
  ML algorithms can analyze vast amounts of data generated by smart transportation and healthcare systems. They can identify patterns, trends, and anomalies in patient health data, transportation routes, and traffic conditions. Predictive models can help anticipate healthcare needs and optimize transportation routes.
- **Real-time Decision Support**
  ML algorithms can provide real-time decision support for emergency medical responses. They can analyze patient data, traffic information, and hospital availability to recommend the best course of action for ambulance routes, ensuring timely care.
- **Resource Allocation**
  ML algorithms can optimize resource allocation in healthcare, such as matching available ambulances with patient locations and severity levels. This ensures efficient utilization of medical resources.
- **Personalized Healthcare**
  ML can personalize healthcare services by analyzing patient data to tailor treatment plans, medication dosages, and rehabilitation programs. It takes into account an individual's health history, genetics, and lifestyle.
- **Telemedicine and Remote Monitoring**
  Cloud platforms enable remote access to healthcare data, facilitating telemedicine consultations and remote patient monitoring. Cloud-hosted EHRs ensure healthcare providers have up-to-date information.

- **Data Storage and Scalability**
  Cloud services offer scalable and cost-effective data storage solutions for the massive volumes of data generated by smart healthcare and transportation systems. This ensures data availability and accessibility.
- **Security and Compliance**
  Cloud providers invest heavily in security measures and compliance certifications, making it easier for healthcare organizations to meet regulatory requirements and protect patient data.
- **Real-time Data Sharing**
  Cloud-based platforms facilitate real-time data sharing among healthcare providers, transportation agencies, and emergency services. This ensures that all stakeholders have access to critical information when needed.
- **Remote Diagnostics and Treatment**
  ML models can assist in diagnosing medical conditions remotely, while cloud-based applications enable physicians to access and share diagnostic tools and images in real time, even from remote locations.
- **Integration and Interoperability**
  ML models and cloud-based middleware can bridge the gap between different healthcare and transportation systems, ensuring interoperability and smooth data exchange.

In the context of smart transportation and smart healthcare, ML and cloud computing collectively empower data-driven decision-making, enhance patient care, optimize transportation routes, and improve overall system efficiency. They enable healthcare providers to respond rapidly to emergencies, provide personalized care, and harness the potential of interconnected systems to benefit patients and society as a whole.

14.7.1 Discussion

Emphasis on the importance of timely patient data communication in emergency healthcare.

The importance of timely patient data communication in emergency healthcare cannot be understated, and integrating smart transportation systems into this process can significantly enhance the efficiency and effectiveness of emergency medical services (EMS). Here's an emphasis on the importance of both timely patient data communication and the role of smart transportation systems in emergency healthcare:

1. **Rapid Response and Care Delivery**
   - Timely patient data communication allows emergency responders to arrive at the scene with essential patient information, enabling them to provide immediate and appropriate care.
   - Smart transportation systems help EMS teams reach the location faster by optimizing routes, reducing response times, and minimizing traffic delays.

2. **Enhanced Pre-Hospital Care**
    - Access to patient data enables EMS personnel to make informed decisions about pre-hospital care, such as administering specific medications or treatments based on the patient's medical history.
    - Smart transportation systems can guide responders to the nearest healthcare facility equipped to handle the patient's condition, further improving the chances of a positive outcome.
3. **Seamless Data Sharing**
    - Timely communication of patient data between EMS, hospitals, and specialists ensures a seamless transition of care. This prevents delays and ensures that the receiving healthcare team is well-prepared.
    - Smart transportation systems can transmit patient data securely in real time to healthcare facilities, reducing paperwork and the risk of data errors.
4. **Resource Allocation**
    - Efficient communication of patient data allows hospitals to prepare for incoming patients, ensuring that the necessary medical personnel, equipment, and resources are available.
    - Smart transportation systems can provide hospitals with estimated arrival times, enabling them to allocate resources effectively and prioritize incoming cases.
5. **Telemedicine Integration**
    - In cases where on-site specialists are not available, telemedicine can be employed. Timely patient data communication supports remote consultations with specialists, who can guide EMS teams and on-site healthcare providers.
    - Smart transportation systems can facilitate connectivity for telemedicine consultations by ensuring that ambulances are equipped with the necessary communication tools and stable internet connections.
6. **Data Security and Privacy**
    - Timely patient data communication must prioritize security and privacy. Smart transportation systems should incorporate encryption and data access controls to protect sensitive patient information during transit (58–59).
    - Compliance with healthcare data regulations (e.g., HIPAA [Health Insurance Portability and Accountability Act] in the United States) is essential to maintain the confidentiality of patient records.
7. **Continuous Monitoring**
    - Smart transportation systems can enable real-time monitoring of patient vitals during transit, allowing medical teams at the receiving facility to prepare for immediate interventions upon arrival.
8. **Disaster Response**
    - In disaster scenarios, where multiple patients require transport to various healthcare facilities, smart transportation systems can help coordinate the movement of ambulances and allocate resources efficiently.

In conclusion, the timely communication of patient data in emergency healthcare is a critical factor in improving patient outcomes. When combined with smart transportation systems, which optimize response times and facilitate seamless data sharing, the overall quality of emergency medical services can be greatly enhanced. This integration not only saves lives but also ensures that patients receive the right care at the right time, even in challenging circumstances.

14.7.2 Challenges and Limitations of the Proposed Protocol

- **VANET Coverage:** VANETs may have limited coverage in rural or less populated areas, potentially impacting data transmission in such regions.
- **Network Congestion:** High traffic volumes or network congestion can lead to delays in data transmission, affecting the timeliness of emergency responses.
- **Security Concerns:** While encryption and authentication mechanisms are in place, VANETs are susceptible to security threats, such as cyber-attacks, which could compromise patient data.
- **Scalability:** Scaling the protocol to accommodate a larger number of ambulances, hospitals, and vehicles may pose challenges in terms of network management and data routing.
- **Interoperability:** Ensuring interoperability with existing healthcare information systems and different VANET technologies used in various regions may require standardized protocols and interfaces.
- **Data Privacy:** Despite encryption, data privacy remains a concern. Striking a balance between data security and the need for timely medical responses is a challenge.
- **Network Disruptions:** VANETs can experience intermittent connectivity due to the mobility of vehicles, making it essential to handle network disruptions effectively.

14.8 POTENTIAL FUTURE ENHANCEMENTS AND RESEARCH DIRECTIONS

- **Edge Computing Integration:** Exploring the integration of edge computing in VANETs to process data closer to the source, reducing latency and enhancing real-time decision-making.
- **AI and Predictive Analytics:** Leveraging artificial intelligence and predictive analytics to anticipate healthcare needs, optimize ambulance routes, and improve resource allocation.
- **Blockchain for Data Security:** Investigating the use of blockchain technology to enhance data security and traceability, ensuring the integrity and privacy of patient data.
- **5G Connectivity:** Exploring the integration of 5G networks for faster and more reliable VANET communication, especially in urban areas.
- **Robust Routing Algorithms:** Developing more robust and adaptive routing algorithms that can handle dynamic network conditions and prioritize critical data.

- **Human-Machine Interaction:** Researching human-machine interaction in emergency healthcare scenarios, including the role of human decision-makers alongside automated systems.
- **Patient-Centric Care:** Focusing on patient-centric care by further personalizing treatment plans and improving patient engagement through smart healthcare applications.
- **Public Health Monitoring:** Extending the protocol's capabilities to monitor public health trends, detect disease outbreaks, and facilitate early interventions.
- **Regulatory Frameworks:** Developing regulatory frameworks and standards specific to VANET-based healthcare to address privacy, security, and interoperability concerns.
- **Cross-Border Collaboration:** Exploring cross-border collaboration and data sharing to enhance healthcare responses in regions with shared transportation routes.
- **User Training and Adoption:** Investigating strategies for user training and adoption to ensure that healthcare professionals and emergency responders can effectively utilize the protocol's capabilities.
- **Environmental Monitoring**: Expanding the protocol's scope to include real-time environmental monitoring, which can help assess air quality, weather conditions, and other environmental factors affecting healthcare.

As VANET technology continues to evolve and smart healthcare systems become more integrated with transportation networks, ongoing research and development efforts will be crucial to address current limitations and unlock the full potential of these interconnected systems for improving emergency healthcare responses and patient outcomes [99].

14.9 CONCLUSION

The importance of timely patient data communication in emergency healthcare cannot be overstated. In critical situations, such as medical emergencies, accidents, or natural disasters, the ability to quickly and accurately share patient data can have a significant impact on patient outcomes. To ensure the importance of timely patient data communication in emergency healthcare, healthcare systems must invest in robust health information exchange systems, data security measures, interoperability standards, and training for healthcare professionals. Additionally, patients can play a role by maintaining up-to-date medical records and authorizing the sharing of their health information when needed in emergencies. Ultimately, the efficient exchange of patient data is a critical component of modern emergency healthcare delivery, with the potential to save lives and improve overall patient outcomes [100, 101].

REFERENCES

1. Kaur, G., & Kakkar, D. (2022). Hybrid optimization enabled trust-based secure routing with deep learning-based attack detection in VANET. Ad Hoc Networks, 136, 102961.

2. Ali, A., Iqbal, M. M., Jabbar, S., Asghar, M. N., Raza, U., & Al-Turjman, F. (2022). VABLOCK: A blockchain-based secure communication in a V2V network using ICN network support technology. Microprocessors and Microsystems, 93, 104569.
3. Xia, H., Zhang, S. S., Li, Y., Pan, Z. K., Peng, X., & Cheng, X. Z. (2019). An attack-resistant trust inference model for securing routing in vehicular ad hoc networks. IEEE Transactions on Vehicular Technology, 68(7), 7108–7120.
4. Feng, H., Chen, D., & Lv, Z. (2022). Blockchain in digital twins-based vehicle management in VANETs. IEEE Transactions on Intelligent Transportation Systems, 23(10), 19613–19623.
5. Bhabani, B., & Mahapatro, J. (2023). TRP: A TOPSIS-based RSU-enabled priority scheduling scheme to disseminate alert messages of WBAN sensors in hybrid VANETs. Peer-to-Peer Networking and Applications, 16(4), 1868–1886.
6. Bhoi, S. K., & Khilar, P. M. (2016). VehiHealth: An emergency routing protocol for vehicular ad hoc network to support healthcare system. Journal of Medical Systems, 40, 65. https://doi.org/10.1007/s10916-015-0420-2
7. Singh, P., Raw, R. S., Khan, S. A., Mohammed, M. A., Aly, A. A., & Le, D.-N. (2022). W-GeoR: Weighted geographical routing for VANET's health monitoring applications in urban traffic networks. IEEE Access, 10, 38850–38869. doi: 10.1109/ACCESS.2021.3092426
8. Sundaravadivel, P., Kougianos, E., Mohanty, S. P., & Ganapathiraju, M. K. (2018, Jan). Everything you wanted to know about smart health care: Evaluating the different technologies and components of the internet of things for better health. IEEE Consumer Electronics Magazine, 7(1), 18–28. doi: 10.1109/MCE.2017.2755378
9. Behura, A., Srinivas, M., & Kabat, M. R. (2022). Giraffe kicking optimization algorithm provides efficient routing mechanism in the field of vehicular ad hoc networks. Journal of Ambient Intelligence and Humanized Computing, 13(8), 3989–4008.
10. Behura, A., Singh, A., & Nayak, S. (2024). Integration of cloud, IoT, and AI for smart services. in Fostering Cross-Industry Sustainability with Intelligent Technologies (pp. 162–182). IGI Global.
11. Saravana Kumar, N. M., Pagadala, P. K., Vijayakumar, V., & Kavinya, A. (2022). Multi objective glow swarm based situation and quality aware routing in VANET. Wireless Personal Communications, 125(1), 879–895.
12. Zhang, T., Xu, C., Zhang, B., Shen, J., Kuang, X., & Grieco, L. A. (2022). Toward attack-resistant route mutation for VANETs: An online and adaptive multiagent reinforcement learning approach. IEEE Transactions on Intelligent Transportation Systems, 23(12), 23254–23267.
13. Chougule, A., Kohli, V., Chamola, V., & Yu, F. R. (2023) Multibranch reconstruction error (MbRE) intrusion detection architecture for intelligent edge-based policing in vehicular Ad-Hoc networks. In IEEE Transactions on Intelligent Transportation Systems, vol. 24, no. 11, pp. 13068–13077. doi: 10.1109/TITS.2022.3201548.
14. Azhdari, M. S., Barati, A., & Barati, H. (2022). A cluster-based routing method with authentication capability in Vehicular Ad hoc Networks (VANETs). Journal of Parallel and Distributed Computing, 169, 1–23.
15. Cárdenas, L. L., León, J. P. A., & Mezher, A. M. (2022). GraTree: A gradient boosting decision tree based multimetric routing protocol for vehicular ad hoc networks. Ad Hoc Networks, 137, 102995.
16. Nahar, A., & Das, D. (2023). MetaLearn: Optimizing routing heuristics with a hybrid meta-learning approach in vehicular ad-hoc networks. Ad Hoc Networks, 138, 102996.
17. Darabkh, K. A., Alkhader, B. Z., Ala'F, K., Jubair, F., & Abdel-Majeed, M. (2022). ICDRP-f-SDVN: An innovative cluster-based dual-phase routing protocol using fog computing and software-defined vehicular network. Vehicular Communications, 34, 100453.

18. Sun, G., Zhang, Y., Yu, H., Du, X., & Guizani, M. (2019). Intersection fog-based distributed routing for V2V communication in urban vehicular ad hoc networks. IEEE Transactions on Intelligent Transportation Systems, 21(6), 2409–2426.
19. Zhang, J., Cui, J., Zhong, H., Chen, Z., & Liu, L. (2019). PA-CRT: Chinese Remainder theorem-based conditional privacy-preserving authentication scheme in vehicular ad-hoc networks. IEEE Transactions on Dependable and Secure Computing, 18(2), 722–735.
20. Yadav, V. K., Verma, S., & Venkatesan, S. (2020). Efficient and secure location-based services scheme in VANET. IEEE Transactions on Vehicular Technology, 69(11), 13567–13578.
21. Fan, N., & Wu, C. Q. (2019). On trust models for communication security in vehicular ad-hoc networks. Ad Hoc Networks, 90, 101740.
22. Shrestha, R., Bajracharya, R., Shrestha, A. P., & Nam, S. Y. (2020). A new type of blockchain for secure message exchange in VANET. Digital Communications and Networks, 6(2), 177–186.
23. Hosmani, S., & Mathapati, B. (2023). R2SCDT: Robust and reliable secure clustering and data transmission in vehicular ad hoc network using weight evaluation. Journal of Ambient Intelligence and Humanized Computing, 14(3), 2029–2046.
24. Haghighi, M. S., & Aziminejad, Z. (2019). Highly anonymous mobility-tolerant location-based onion routing for VANETs. IEEE Internet of Things Journal, 7(4), 2582–2590.
25. Wang, X., Hu, J., Lin, H., Garg, S., Kaddoum, G., Piran, M. J., & Hossain, M. S. (2021). QoS and privacy-aware routing for 5G-enabled industrial internet of things: A federated reinforcement learning approach. IEEE Transactions on Industrial Informatics, 18(6), 4189–4197.
26. Li, W., & Song, H. (2015). ART: An attack-resistant trust management scheme for securing vehicular ad hoc networks. IEEE Transactions on Intelligent Transportation Systems, 17(4), 960–969.
27. Guo, J., Li, X., Liu, Z., Ma, J., Yang, C., Zhang, J., & Wu, D. (2020). TROVE: A context-awareness trust model for VANETs using reinforcement learning. IEEE Internet of Things Journal, 7(7), 6647–6662.
28. Naresh, V. S., Allavarpu, V. D., & Reddi, S. (2022). Blockchain iota sharding-based scalable secure group communication in large vanets. IEEE Internet of Things Journal, 10(6), 5205–5213.
29. Abbasi, F., Zarei, M., & Rahmani, A. M. (2022). FWDP: A fuzzy logic-based vehicle weighting model for data prioritization in vehicular ad hoc networks. Vehicular Communications, 33, 100413.
30. Zhang, C., Li, W., Luo, Y., & Hu, Y. (2020). AIT: An AI-enabled trust management system for vehicular networks using blockchain technology. IEEE Internet of Things Journal, 8(5), 3157–3169.
31. Mehra, A., Mandal, M., Narang, P., & Chamola, V. (2020). ReViewNet: A fast and resource-optimized network enabling safe autonomous driving in hazy weather conditions. IEEE Transactions on Intelligent Transportation Systems, 22(7), 4256–4266.
32. Behura, A. (2023). Role of cryptography, blockchain, and digital forensics in vehicular networks. Sustainable Science and Intelligent Technologies for Societal Development, 358–379.
33. Divya, N. S., Bobba, V., & Vatambeti, R. (2022). An adaptive cluster based vehicular routing protocol for secure communication. Wireless Personal Communications, 1–20.
34. Zhao, L., Bi, Z., Lin, M., Hawbani, A., Shi, J., & Guan, Y. (2021). An intelligent fuzzy-based routing scheme for software-defined vehicular networks. Computer Networks, 187, 107837.
35. Guo, C., Li, D., Chen, X., & Zhang, G. (2022). An adaptive V2R communication strategy based on data delivery delay estimation in VANETs. Vehicular Communications, 34, 100444.

36. Bao, X., Li, H., Zhao, G., Chang, L., Zhou, J., & Li, Y. (2020). Efficient clustering V2V routing based on PSO in VANETs. Measurement, 152, 107306.
37. Kolandaisamy, R., Noor, R. M., Kolandaisamy, I., Ahmedy, I., Kiah, M. L. M., Tamil, M. E. M., & Nandy, T. (2021). A stream position performance analysis model based on DDoS attack detection for cluster-based routing in VANET. Journal of Ambient Intelligence and Humanized Computing, 12(6), 6599–6612.
38. Tang, Y., Cheng, N., Wu, W., Wang, M., Dai, Y., & Shen, X. (2019). Delay-minimization routing for heterogeneous VANETs with machine learning based mobility prediction. IEEE Transactions on Vehicular Technology, 68(4), 3967–3979.
39. Abhishek, N. V., Aman, M. N., Lim, T. J., & Sikdar, B. (2021). DRiVe: Detecting malicious roadside units in the internet of vehicles with low latency data integrity. IEEE Internet of Things Journal, 9(5), 3270–3281.
40. Behura, A., & Kabat, M. R. (2020). Energy-efficient optimization-based routing technique for wireless sensor network using machine learning. In Progress in Computing, Analytics and Networking: Proceedings of ICCAN 2019 (pp. 555–565). Springer.
41. Behura, A. (2022). Optimized data transmission scheme based on proper channel coordination used in vehicular ad hoc networks. International Journal of Information Technology, 14(2), 1107–1116.
42. Behura, A., & Kabat, M. R. (2022). Optimization-based energy-efficient routing scheme for wireless body area network. In Cognitive Big Data Intelligence with a Metaheuristic Approach (pp. 279–303). Academic Press.
43. Behura, A. (2021). A deep learning application for prediction of COVID-19. Impact of AI and Data Science in Response to Coronavirus Pandemic, 127–148.
44. Behura, A., & Panda, S. K. (2022). Role of machine learning in big data peregrination. in Handbook of Research for Big Data (pp. 235–276). Apple Academic Press.
45. Behura, A. (2022). Intelligent automotive sector with IoT (internet of things) and its consequential impact in vehicular ad hoc networks. Internet of Things and Its Applications, 5, 427–449.
46. Behura, A., Kabat, M. R., & Mohanty, S. N. (2022). The fusion of IOT and wireless body area network. Internet of Things and Its Applications, 1, 195–220.
47. Behura, A., & Nandan Mohanty, S. (2022). Application of the internet of things (iot) in biomedical engineering: Present scenario and challenges. Internet of Things and Its Applications, 1, 151–169.
48. Boualouache, A., Senouci, S. M., & Moussaoui, S. (2017). A survey on pseudonym changing strategies for vehicular ad-hoc networks. IEEE Communications Surveys Tutorials, 20(1), 770–790.
49. Zeng, K. (2006). Pseudonymous PKI for ubiquitous computing. in European Public Key Infrastructure Workshop (pp. 207–222). Springer.
50. Lu, R., Lin, X., Luan, T. H., Liang, X., & Shen, X. (2011). Pseudonym changing at social spots: An effective strategy for location privacy in VANETs. IEEE Transactions on Vehicular Technology, 61(1), 86–96.
51. Goyal, R., Mittal, N., Gupta, L., & Surana, A. (2023). Routing protocols in wireless body area networks: Architecture, challenges, and classification. Wireless Communications and Mobile Computing, 1.
52. Tsai, J. L. (2015). A new efficient certificateless short signature scheme using bilinear pairings. IEEE Systems Journal, 11(4), 2395–2402.
53. Choudhury, H. (2021). HashXor: A lightweight scheme for identity privacy of IoT devices in 5G mobile network. Computer Networks, 186, 107753.
54. Sedjelmaci, H., & Senouci, S. M. (2015). An accurate and efficient collaborative intrusion detection framework to secure vehicular networks. Computers Electrical Engineering, 43, 33–47.

55. Sikora, P., Malina, L., Kiac, M, Martinasek, Z., Riha, K., Prinosil, J., Jirik, L., & Srivastava, G. (2021) Artificial intelligence-based surveillance system for railway crossing traffic. IEEE Sensors Journal, 21, 15515–15526
56. Corser, G., Fu, H., Shu, T., D'Errico, P., Ma, W., Leng, S., & Zhu, Y. (2014). Privacy-by-decoy: Protecting location privacy against collusion and deanonymization in vehicular location based services. In 2014 IEEE Intelligent Vehicles Symposium Proceedings (pp. 1030–1036). IEEE.
57. Yu, R., Kang, J., Huang, X., Xie, S., Zhang, Y., & Gjessing, S. (2015). MixGroup: Accumulative pseudonym exchanging for location privacy enhancement in vehicular social networks. IEEE Transactions on Dependable and Secure Computing, 13(1), 93–105.
58. Movahedi, Z., Hosseini, Z., Bayan, F., & Pujolle, G. (2015). Trust-distortion resistant trust management frameworks on mobile ad hoc networks: A survey. IEEE Communications Surveys Tutorials, 18(2), 1287–1309.
59. Emara, K., Woerndl, W., & Schlichter, J. (2015). On evaluation of location privacy preserving schemes for VANET safety applications. Computer Communications, 63, 11–23.
60. Bansal, U., Kar, J., Ali, I., & Naik, K. (2022). ID-CEPPA: Identity-based computationally efficient privacy-preserving authentication scheme for vehicle-to-vehicle communications. Journal of Systems Architecture, 123, 102387.
61. Park, M. H., Gwon, G. P., Seo, S. W., & Jeong, H. Y. (2011). RSU-based distributed key management (RDKM) for secure vehicular multicast communications. IEEE Journal on Selected Areas in Communications, 29(3), 644–658.
62. Sun, Y., Feng, Z., Hu, Q., & Su, J. (2012). An efficient distributed key management scheme for group-signature based anonymous authentication in VANET. Security and Communication Networks, 5(1), 79–86.
63. Malina, L., Castella-Roca, J., Vives-Guasch, A., & Hajny, J. (2012, October). Short-term linkable group signatures with categorized batch verification. In International Symposium on Foundations and Practice of Security (pp. 244–260). Springer.
64. Peng, T., Liu, Q., Meng, D., & Wang, G. (2017). Collaborative trajectory privacy preserving scheme in location-based services. Information Sciences, 387, 165–179.
65. Hussain, R., Lee, J., & Zeadally, S. (2020). Trust in VANET: A survey of current solutions and future research opportunities. IEEE Transactions on Intelligent Transportation Systems, 22(5), 2553–2571.
66. Ali, I., Hassan, A., & Li, F. (2019). Authentication and privacy schemes for vehicular ad hoc networks (VANETs): A survey. Vehicular Communications, 16, 45–61.
67. Khodaei, M., Jin, H., & Papadimitratos, P. (2018). SECMACE: Scalable and robust identity and credential management infrastructure in vehicular communication systems. IEEE Transactions on Intelligent Transportation Systems, 19(5), 1430–1444.
68. Zhou, X., Luo, M., Vijayakumar, P., Peng, C., & He, D. (2022). Efficient certificateless conditional privacy-preserving authentication for VANETs. IEEE Transactions on Vehicular Technology, 71(7), 7863–7875.
69. Chen, Y., & Chen, J. (2021). CPP-CLAS: Efficient and conditional privacy-preserving certificateless aggregate signature scheme for VANETs. IEEE Internet of Things Journal, 9(12), 10354–10365.
70. Yang, Y., Zhang, L., Zhao, Y., Choo, K. K. R., & Zhang, Y. (2022). Privacy-preserving aggregation-authentication scheme for safety warning system in fog-cloud based VANET. IEEE Transactions on Information Forensics and Security, 17, 317–331.
71. Han, Y., Song, W., Zhou, Z., Wang, H., & Yuan, B. (2021). eCLAS: An efficient pairing-free certificateless aggregate signature for secure VANET communication. IEEE Systems Journal, 16(1), 1637–1648.

72. Yang, M., Chen, J., Chen, Y., Ma, R., & Kumar, S. (2021). Strong key-insulated secure and energy-aware certificateless authentication scheme for VANETs. Computers and Electrical Engineering, 95, 107417.
73. Samra, B., & Fouzi, S. (2022). New efficient certificateless scheme-based conditional privacy preservation authentication for applications in VANET. Vehicular Communications, 34, 100414.
74. Vijayakumar, P., Azees, M., Kannan, A., & Deborah, L. J. (2016). Dual authentication and key management techniques for secure data transmission in vehicular ad hoc networks. IEEE Transactions on Intelligent Transportation Systems, 17, 1015–1028.
75. Xiong, W., Wang, R., Wang, Y., Zhou, F., & Luo, X. (2021). CPPA-D: Efficient conditional privacy-preserving authentication scheme with double-insurance in VANETs. IEEE Transactions on Vehicular Technology, 70(4), 3456–3468.
76. Gupta, M., Benson, J., Patwa, F., & Sandhu, R. (2020). Secure V2V and V2I communication in intelligent transportation using cloudlets. IEEE Transactions on Services Computing, 15(4), 1912–1925.
77. Guo, R., Xu, L., Li, X., Zhang, Y., & Li, X. (2022). An efficient certificateless ring signcryption scheme with conditional privacy-preserving in VANETs. Journal of Systems Architecture, 129, 102633.
78. Wang, Y., Ding, Y., Wu, Q., Wei, Y., Qin, B., & Wang, H. (2018). Privacy-preserving cloud-based road condition monitoring with source authentication in VANETs. IEEE Transactions on Information Forensics and Security, 14(7), 1779–1790.
79. Wang, P., & Liu, Y. (2021). SEMA: Secure and efficient message authentication protocol for VANETs. IEEE Systems Journal, 15(1), 846–855.
80. Ali, I., Chen, Y., Ullah, N., Kumar, R., & He, W. (2021). An efficient and provably secure ECC-based conditional privacy-preserving authentication for vehicle-to-vehicle communication in VANETs. IEEE Transactions on Vehicular Technology, 70(2), 1278–1291.
81. Liang, Y., & Liu, Y. (2022). Analysis and improvement of an efficient certificateless aggregate signature with conditional privacy preservation in VANETs. IEEE Systems Journal, 17(1), 664–672.
82. Cao, Y., Xu, S., Chen, X., He, Y., & Jiang, S. (2022). A forward-secure and efficient authentication protocol through lattice-based group signature in VANETs scenarios. Computer Networks, 214, 109149
83. Alaya, B., & Sellami, L. (2021). Clustering method and symmetric/asymmetric cryptography scheme adapted to securing urban VANET networks. Journal of Information Security and Applications, 58, 102779.
84. Nath, H. J., & Choudhury, H. (2022). A privacy-preserving mutual authentication scheme for group communication in VANET. Computer Communications, 192, 357–372.
85. Vijayakumar, P., Azees, M., Kozlov, S. A., & Rodrigues, J. J. (2021). An anonymous batch authentication and key exchange protocols for 6G enabled VANETs. IEEE Transactions on Intelligent Transportation Systems, 23(2), 1630–1638.
86. Goudarzi, S., Soleymani, S. A., Anisi, M. H., Azgomi, M. A., Movahedi, Z., Kama, N., & Khan, M. K. (2022). A privacy-preserving authentication scheme based on elliptic curve cryptography and using quotient filter in fog-enabled VANET. Ad Hoc Networks, 128, 102782.
87. Luo, M., & Zhou, Y. (2022). An efficient conditional privacy-preserving authentication protocol based on generalized ring signcryption for VANETs. IEEE Transactions on Vehicular Technology, 71(9), 10001–10015.
88. Chen, X., Yang, A., Tong, Y., Weng, J., Weng, J., & Li, T. (2022). A multisignature-based secure and OBU-friendly emergency reporting scheme in VANET. IEEE Internet of Things Journal, 9(22), 23130–23141.

89. Li, G., Lai, C., Lu, R., & Zheng, D. (2021). SecCDV: A security reference architecture for cybertwin-driven 6G V2X. IEEE Transactions on Vehicular Technology, 71(5), 4535–4550.
90. Ren, Y., Li, X., Sun, S. F., Yuan, X., & Zhang, X. (2021). Privacy-preserving batch verification signature scheme based on blockchain for vehicular ad-hoc networks. Journal of Information Security and Applications, 58, 102698.
91. Othman, W., Fuyou, M., Xue, K., & Hawbani, A. (2021). Physically secure lightweight and privacy-preserving message authentication protocol for VANET in smart city. IEEE Transactions on Vehicular Technology, 70(12), 12902–12917.
92. Wang, Y., Zhang, W., Wang, X., Khan, M. K., & Fan, P. (2021). Efficient privacy-preserving authentication scheme with fine-grained error location for cloud-based VANET. IEEE Transactions on Vehicular Technology, 70(10), 10436–10449.
93. Liu, Z., Yuan, M., Ding, Y., & Wang, B. (2021). Efficient small-batch verification and identification scheme with invalid signatures in VANETs. IEEE Transactions on Vehicular Technology, 70(12), 12836–12846.
94. Wang, P., Chen, C. M., Kumari, S., Shojafar, M., Tafazolli, R., & Liu, Y. N. (2020). HDMA: Hybrid D2D message authentication scheme for 5G-enabled VANETs. IEEE Transactions on Intelligent Transportation Systems, 22(8), 5071–5080.
95. Khalid, A., Iftikhar, M. S., Almogren, A., Khalid, R., Afzal, M. K., & Javaid, N. (2021). A blockchain based incentive provisioning scheme for traffic event validation and information storage in VANETs. Information Processing Management, 58(2), 102464.
96. Cheng, H., Shojafar, M., Alazab, M., Tafazolli, R., & Liu, Y. (2021). PPVF: Privacy-preserving protocol for vehicle feedback in cloud-assisted VANET. IEEE Transactions on Intelligent Transportation Systems, 23(7), 9391–9403.
97. Wei, L., Cui, J., Zhong, H., Xu, Y., & Liu, L. (2021). Proven secure tree-based authenticated key agreement for securing V2V and V2I communications in VANETs. IEEE Transactions on Mobile Computing, 21(9), 3280–3297.
98. Bhattacharya, P., Shukla, A., Tanwar, S., Kumar, N., & Sharma, R. (2022). 6Blocks: 6G-enabled trust management scheme for decentralized autonomous vehicles. Computer Communications, 191, 53–68.
99. Behura, A., Sahu, S., & Kabat, M. R. (2021). Advancement of machine learning and cloud computing in the field of Smart Health Care. Machine Learning Approach for Cloud Data Analytics in IoT, 58, 273–306.
100. Islam, S. H., Obaidat, M. S., Vijayakumar, P., Abdulhay, E., Li, F., & Reddy, M. K. C. (2018). A robust and efficient password-based conditional privacy preserving authentication and group-key agreement protocol for VANETs. Future Generation Computer Systems, 84, 216–227.
101. Corser, G. P., Fu, H., & Banihani, A. (2016). Evaluating location privacy in vehicular communications and applications. IEEE Transactions on Intelligent Transportation Systems, 17(9), 2658–2667.

Index

For Product Safety Concerns and Information please contact our EU
representative GPSR@taylorandfrancis.com
Taylor & Francis Verlag GmbH, Kaufingerstraße 24, 80331 München, Germany

www.ingramcontent.com/pod-product-compliance
Lightning Source LLC
LaVergne TN
LVHW010557110826
845149LV00003B/688

* 9 7 8 1 0 3 2 6 2 4 8 8 4 *